Progress in Alzheimer's Disease and Similar Conditions

American Psychopathological Association

Progress in Alzheimer's Disease and Similar Conditions

Edited by

Leonard L. Heston, M.D.

American Psychopathological Association

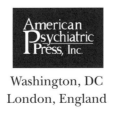

Washington, DC
London, England

Copyright © 1997 American Psychiatric Press, Inc.
‣ALL RIGHTS RESERVED
Manufactured in the United States of America on acid-free paper
00 99 98 97   4 3 2 1

American Psychiatric Press, Inc.
1400 K Street, N.W., Washington, DC 20005

Library of Congress Cataloging-in-Publication Data
Progress in Alzheimer's disease and similar conditions / edited by
    Leonard L. Heston.
        p.   cm. — (American Psychopathological Association series)
    Includes bibliographical references and index.
    ISBN 0-88048-760-7 (cloth : alk. paper)
    1. Alzheimer's disease.   2. Senile dementia.   I. Heston, Leonard
L.   II. Series.
    [DNLM: 1. Alzheimer's Disease.   2. Dementia.   WT 155 P9645 1997]
RC523.P765   1997
616.8'31—dc20
DNLM/DLC
for Library of Congress   96-26156
                                                                      CIP

British Library Cataloguing in Publication Data
A CIP record is available from the British Library.

Contents

Contributors

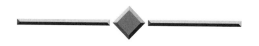

Abby Ambinder, Ed.D.
Family Counselor, Aging and Dementia Research Center, New York University Medical Center, New York, New York

John C. S. Breitner, M.D., M.P.H.
Associate Professor and Head, Division of Geriatric Psychiatry, Duke University Medical Center, Durham, North Carolina

Barbara Cordell, Ph.D.
Vice President for Research, Scios-Nova Inc., Mountain View, California

Steven H. Ferris, Ph.D.
Professor, Department of Psychiatry, Executive Director, Aging and Dementia Research Center, New York University School of Medicine, New York, New York

Marshal F. Folstein, M.D.
Professor and Head, Department of Psychiatry, Tufts University, Boston, Massachusetts

Susan E. Folstein, M.D.
Professor of Psychiatry, Tufts University, Boston, Massachusetts

Denise Heinrichs
Iowa Alzheimer Disease Association, Davenport, Iowa

Leonard L. Heston, M.D.
Professor of Psychiatry, University of Washington, Seattle, Washington

Jeffrey Higaki, Ph.D.
Scios-Nova Inc., Mountain View, California

Linda S. Higgins, Ph.D.
Scios-Nova Inc., Mountain View, California

Carolyn C. Hoch, Ph.D.
Assistant Professor of Psychiatry, University of Pittsburgh School of Medicine, Pittsburgh, Pennsylvania

Joan Mackell, Ph.D.
Family Counselor, Aging and Dementia Research Center, New York University Medical Center, New York, New York

Paul R. McHugh, M.D.
Professor and Head, Department of Psychiatry, Johns Hopkins University, Baltimore, Maryland

Suzanne S. Mirra, M.D.
Professor of Pathology (Neuropathology), Department of Pathology and Laboratory Medicine, Emory University School of Medicine, Atlanta, Georgia; Director, Emory Alzheimer's Disease Center, Atlanta VA Medical Center, Atlanta, Georgia

Mary S. Mittelman, Dr.P.H.
Associate Research Professor, Director of Caregiver Research, Aging and Dementia Research Center, New York University School of Medicine, New York, New York

Paula M. Moran, Ph.D.
Marion Merrell Dow Research Institute, Strasbourg Cedex, France

James A. Mortimer, Ph.D.
Geriatric Research, Education, and Clinical Center, VA Medical Center, Minneapolis, Minnesota; Professor, Departments of Neurology and Epidemiology, University of Minnesota, Minneapolis, Minnesota

Paul C. Moser, Ph.D.
Marion Merrell Dow Research Institute, Strasbourg Cedex, France

Benoit H. Mulsant, M.D.
Assistant Professor, Department of Psychiatry, University of Pittsburgh School of Medicine, Pittsburgh, Pennsylvania

Richard H. Myers, Ph.D.
Professor of Neurology, Boston University School of Medicine,
Boston, Massachusetts

Robert D. Nebes, Ph.D.
Professor of Psychiatry, University of Pittsburgh School of Medicine, Pittsburgh, Pennsylvania

Paul A. Newhouse, M.D.
Associate Professor of Psychiatry, Clinical Neuroscience Research Unit, University of Vermont College of Medicine, Burlington, Vermont

Harry T. Orr, Ph.D.
Professor of Laboratory Medicine and Pathology, Professor of Biochemistry, Institute of Human Genetics, University of Minnesota, Minneapolis, Minnesota

Elaine R. Peskind, M.D.
Psychiatry Service, Seattle/American Lake VA Medical Center, Seattle, Washington; Assistant Professor of Psychiatry and Behavioral Sciences, University of Washington, Seattle, Washington

Bruce G. Pollock, M.D., Ph.D.
Associate Professor of Psychiatry and Pharmacology, Department of Psychiatry, University of Pittsburgh School of Medicine, Pittsburgh, Pennsylvania

Stanley B. Prusiner, M.D.
Professor of Neurology, Professor of Biochemistry and Biophysics, University of California, San Francisco, California

Peter V. Rabins, M.D., M.P.H.
Professor of Psychiatry, Johns Hopkins Medical Center, Baltimore, Maryland

Stanley I. Rapoport, M.D.
Chief, Laboratory of Neurosciences, National Institute on Aging, National Institutes of Health, Bethesda, Maryland

Ray Raschko, M.S.W.
Director, Elder Services, Spokane Community Mental Health Center, Spokane, Washington

Murray A. Raskind, M.D.
Psychiatry Service, Seattle/American Lake VA Medical Center, Seattle, Washington; Professor of Psychiatry and Behavioral Sciences, University of Washington, Seattle, Washington

Charles F. Reynolds III, M.D.
Professor of Psychiatry and Neurology, University of Pittsburgh School of Medicine, Pittsburgh, Pennsylvania

Emma Shulman, M.S.
Senior Family Counselor, Aging and Dementia Research Center, New York University Medical Center, New York, New York

Judith A. Sinsheimer, L.I.C.S.W.
Social Service Department, Massachusetts General Hospital, Boston, Massachusetts

Gertrude Steinberg, M.A.
Senior Family Counselor, Aging and Dementia Research Center, New York University Medical Center, New York, New York

Catherine A. Taylor, L.C.S.W.
Department of Neurology, Boston University School of Medicine, Boston, Massachusetts

Ziyang Zhong, Ph.D.
Scios-Nova Inc., Mountain View, California

Huda Y. Zoghbi, M.D.
Professor of Pediatrics, Professor of Molecular and Human Genetics, Baylor College of Medicine, Houston, Texas

Introduction

This book aims to broadly update professionals concerned with brain diseases. Staying current has become, at best, extremely difficult. By now, however, some diseases have become well enough known to provide models that teach through understandable examples. That process is this book's teaching rationale.

Rapid and spectacular advances in research on human genetics, which carry with them implications for clinical practice and research that are hard to overstate, provide one backdrop for this volume. Two chapters in this volume describe startling, unique disease mechanisms—prions and triplet repeats—that would have been unimaginable given the medical profession's understanding of genetics at the beginning of the 1980s. Several brain diseases are associated with these entities; researchers surely will discover more. Moreover, prions provide important insights into how environment can lead to disease.

Other chapters focus on Alzheimer's disease, probably the best known among the more common brain diseases. In these chapters, the authors present important findings in epidemiology, pathology, pharmacology, and pathophysiology. Alzheimer's disease illustrates major molecular genetic schemes, including candidate gene and linkage strategies. Genetic studies of Alzheimer's disease have defined DNA mutations directly associated with disease and isolated discrete regions of DNA that harbor other mutations. These studies also offer a major insight: widespread heterogeneity is likely to be the rule in psychopathology, with critical implications for research, prognosis, and treatment.

Alzheimer's disease also provides major clinical challenges. Several chapters in this volume describe the pain this dread disease brings to patients and their relatives. In these chapters, the authors describe in detail current efforts to alleviate the disease's effects; these efforts represent a treasury of clinical experience.

Leonard L. Heston, M.D.

These chapters were originally presented as part of the annual meeting of the American Psychopathological Association in New York City on March 2–4, 1995.

Chapter 1
Zubin Award Lecture

Emotional Disorders Associated With Dementing Illnesses

Paul R. McHugh, M.D.

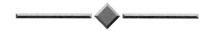

I n this chapter, I review a motif running through the research enterprises of my colleagues in the Department of Psychiatry at Cornell University School of Medicine and Johns Hopkins School of Medicine since the late 1960s. I spotlight the leaders of these efforts, describe the results, and characterize some of the obstacles this work surmounted.

My impulse for studying the emotional disorders of dementing illnesses emerged from experiences that Marshal Folstein and I shared at the New York Hospital, Westchester Division, in the late 1960s and early 1970s. Dr. Folstein and I were caring for a large number of patients with brain disorders of several kinds (Parkinson's disease, Huntington's disease, Alzheimer's disease). We often discussed how these patients displayed depressive states that differed little from those expressed by manic-depressive patients on other wards. We noted that some patients with brain disorders responded to medication, and some occasionally had manic attacks; their depression often was associated with delusional beliefs. We began to look more closely at these patients and shared our interest with our colleagues.

From the beginning (and continuing to the present), many skeptics found our preoccupation with these matters peculiar. These observers commented that patients with brain disorders naturally would be depressed because their primary illnesses were life-threatening, incapacitating, and progressive; depression would be an obvious response to such conditions. Many of our colleagues in neurological and psychiatric research suggested that Dr. Folstein and I were studying the emotional states of the doomed—an exercise that might interest Mother Theresa or Jack Kevorkian but hardly one that would offer new information or provide data of interest to their disciplines. Indeed, this perspective appeared in comments from editors, in "pink sheets" from study sections reviewing our grant applications, and even in remarks from physicians requesting our assistance in caring for depressed patients with dementing illnesses; these practitioners often assumed that we would help their patients adapt to their fate.

The studies that I review in this chapter consistently indicate, however, that many emotional disorders in patients with dementing illnesses represent fundamental symptoms of the disease itself, which require identification and can respond to treatment, rather than meaningful responses of despair. My colleagues and I were lucky: our interest arose at a time when psychopharmacological advances provided tools for treatment of emotional responses. Growing interest in psychiatric phenomenology drew attention to these issues, and developing enthusiasm for neuropsychiatry drew the attention of colleagues on both sides of the Atlantic; they were interested in our findings as they described the results of their own efforts.

Depressive Disorders Associated With Stroke

My colleague Robert Robinson began to amplify the theme of emotional disorders associated with dementing illnesses by attending more closely to the phenomena of depressions associated with stroke (Starkstein and Robinson 1993). In particular, he documented that depressive disorder with stroke had many characteristics similar to major depression: he found that many stroke patients were downhearted, had difficulty concentrating, and were self-blaming and hopeless about the future. He also demonstrated that the course of a depressive episode ran 8 to 9 months, after which the patient often experienced spontaneous recovery if left untreated. Such patients were at risk for further episodes in the future, however.

Working with John Lipsey (Lipsey et al. 1984), Dr. Robinson conducted a careful, double-blind, controlled study of the treatment of poststroke depression; they demonstrated that nortriptyline was more effective than placebo in terminating depression and facilitating recovery, as evidenced by standard scales. In conducting this work, Dr. Robinson also documented that this depressive disorder was not equally associated with all strokes; it was far more common in patients who had a left anterior cerebral lesion (Robinson et al. 1984; Starkstein et al. 1988). The combination of stereotypical symptoms and course, association with lesions in a particular area of the brain, and accessible treatment with antidepressants confirmed the hypothesis that poststroke depression is not simply a reaction to distressing life circumstances but a condition in itself. Dr. Robinson has conducted more intriguing research (Robinson and Starkstein 1990) in humans and animals documenting a neurochemical substrate for this condition; that research is beyond the scope of this chapter, however.

Huntington's Disease

Marshal Folstein and I also were interested in emotional disorders in patients with Huntington's disease. We had documented the depressive disorder previously identified by Huntington that was associated with hopelessness and guilt, as well as delusions of sinfulness, blameworthiness, or poverty among these patients (McHugh and Folstein 1975).

Susan Folstein pursued these suggestions further and conducted the most definitive study of all aspects of Huntington's disease, including emotional features (S. E. Folstein 1989; S. E. Folstein et al. 1979). She investigated the distribution of psychiatric disorders among Maryland residents who were at risk for Huntington's disease and found that affective disorders were not randomly distributed among patients with Huntington's disease: they were more common in certain families, in people with an older age at onset, and in whites rather than in blacks. She demonstrated that depression is a fundamental feature of Huntington's disease, not simply a response to a devastating illness.

Susan Folstein also reported that about 10% of patients with Huntington's disease have hypomania, a condition that is hard to associate with simple demoralization. Patients with Huntington's disease, like stroke patients, have delusions and hallucinations that follow their depressive and manic feelings. Furthermore, Susan Folstein called attention to the fact that the depressive disorder often precedes other symptoms of Huntington's disease, such as motor or cognitive symptoms; physicians even observe depression in patients who are unaware of their risk for Huntington's disease.

These findings indicate that depression is not simply a reaction to Huntington's disease but one of the symptoms of the condition. Susan Folstein demonstrated that affective disorders associated with Huntington's disease usually occur in episodes lasting less than 1 year; she found 21 patients untreated for depression in her Maryland survey.

These results, which appear in her now classic monograph on Huntington's disease (S. E. Folstein 1989), confirmed the importance of searching for symptoms of depression or mania and actively treating them—with great benefit to patients with Huntington's disease and their families. They also reinforced our enthusiasm for studying and treating the emotional disorders of patients with neurological disease (M. F. Folstein et al. 1985).

Affective Disorders Associated With HIV Infection

My colleagues and I faced problems in attempting to persuade other researchers that affective disorders associated with stroke or Huntington's disease were part of the nature of these conditions; making the same argument about affective symptoms in patients with HIV infection was more difficult. Glenn Treisman led us in this enterprise when he took responsibility for managing the psychiatric symptoms of patients with HIV infection at the infectious disease group at Johns Hopkins University. These patients had champions who regarded their psychological distress as natural and quite understandable given the mortal and relentless nature of their condition, as well as the stigma associated with HIV and AIDS. Yet physicians restricting themselves to that explanation would overlook psychiatric disorders in the same way that many practitioners neglected treatable depression in stroke patients.

Dr. Treisman focused on the phenomenology of psychiatric disorders associated with HIV infection. In particular, the delusional and neurovegetative features that afflicted many patients and the intermittency of depression when it occurred echoed the pattern in stroke and Huntington's disease (Treisman et al. 1994). Mania also played an important role in drawing attention to the affective component of HIV infection (Treisman et al. 1993).

Working with Costas Lyketsos, Dr. Treisman studied psychiatric disorders in patients admitted to the HIV clinic and demonstrated that mania increased in frequency among HIV patients compared with a general population. Patients who had no history of mania tended to develop this symptom late in the course of the HIV infection when they developed AIDS; patients with a preinfection history of mania, however, might have an attack of mania at any time in the course of their infection. Treisman and Lyketsos concluded that mania was a symptom of advanced HIV disease (Lyketsos et al. 1993). They also found that 20% of these patients had a major depressive disorder; 85% of those depressed patients responded successfully to antidepressant medication.

Thus, patients with HIV infection had treatable emotional disorders, and treatment made the illness more bearable. These findings do not invalidate the myriad of other needs of these patients; rather, they emphasize the importance of differential diagnoses of depressive disorders in AIDS patients.

Emotional Disorders Associated With Alzheimer's Disease

My colleagues and I also have focused our attention on depressive disorders associated with Alzheimer's disease, which presents a set of symptoms that complicates patient care. In one of our first studies, Christopher Ross—recognizing that Alzheimer's disease depletes neurons in the subcortical nuclei—demonstrated that depressed Alzheimer's patients had a significantly increased loss of neurons from the mid-locus coeruleus (Zweig et al. 1989). This work, subsequently confirmed by other investigators, indicates that a strategic loss of neurons bearing norepinephrine could provide a substrate for depressive symptoms in Alzheimer's disease.

Costas Lyketsos and his colleagues conducted a more systematic study of affective conditions in patients with Alzheimer's disease. Their work (which has not yet been published) involved a survey of the prevalence of mood disorders in Alzheimer's disease within a consecutive case series of 237 patients referred with probable Alzheimer's disease to a specialty clinic where comprehensive psychiatric and neuropsychiatric assessments were conducted. These investigators found major depressive syndromes in 27% of their patients. Depression was slightly more common in female patients and in patients with a family history of mood disorder; depression was not correlated with the severity of dementia or other demographics

(Pearlson et al. 1990). Manic syndromes occurred in only 2.2% of their patients—no more frequently than in the general population. Yet the researchers found a risk factor for mania in Alzheimer's disease among patients with a history of bipolar disorder, suggesting that the manic condition rather than the depression represented the reappearance of an old vulnerability (Lyketsos et al. 1995). Depressive disorders responded to pharmacological treatment, greatly relieving Alzheimer's patients of their depressive symptoms.

Assistance to Families of Patients With Alzheimer's Disease

Similar to any group of physicians, my colleagues and I have always been aware that many aspects of dementing conditions are discouraging and demoralizing to patients and their families. Peter Rabins has led our group in studying the burdens these families bear when a loved one has Alzheimer's disease. Rabins et al. (1982) documented the particular kinds of symptoms and behavioral problems that families cite as particularly burdensome. These hardships included not only simpler cognitive symptoms such as memory disturbance but also catastrophic reactions, suspiciousness, and wandering behavior that confuse and exhaust caregivers.

Dr. Rabins realized that physicians could help family members recognize these problems and care for their loved ones by transmitting information to them in an easily accessible form. For this reason, he collaborated with Nancy Mace on *The 36-Hour Day* (Mace and Rabins 1991). Readers often refer to this book as the "bible" of family guidance books for the care of Alzheimer's patients, as well as patients with other dementing illnesses.

These contributions demonstrate the importance of responding to the emotional conditions of patients that derive from the implications of dementing illnesses, as well as those that represent a feature of the disease itself. Testimonials from families who have been helped by these efforts demonstrate the value of such contributions.

Conclusion

My colleagues and I began with an interest in emotional conditions associated with dementing illnesses. Although some of our peers thought our work would simply state the obvious, we believed that such issues were an appropriate focus of attention. Indeed, our work has become an exciting arena of study; moreover, as this work proceeds, it provides opportunities to strengthen our knowledge of these conditions and our capacities for patient care. This work also offers model approaches to the study of likely cerebral substrates of idiopathic affective disorders. This enterprise continues to study the characteristics of the Huntington's gene, further localization of stroke lesions with affective symptoms, and even aspects of the *APOE* genotype that may differ among patients who have depression with Alzheimer's disease. A field of study that began as a glimmer of an idea for Marshal Folstein and me in the late 1960s has proven to be a lively domain of clinical research.

References

Folstein MF, Robinson RG, Folstein SE, et al: Depression and neurological disorders: new treatment opportunities for elderly depressed patients. J Affect Disord (suppl 1):S11–14, 1985

Folstein SE: Huntington's Disease: A Disorder of Families. Baltimore, MD, Johns Hopkins University Press, 1989

Folstein SE, Folstein MF, McHugh PR: Psychiatric syndromes in Huntington's disease. Adv Neurol 23:281–289, 1979

Lipsey JR, Robinson RG, Pearlson GD, et al: Nortriptyline treatment of post-stroke depression: a double-blind study. Lancet 1(8372):297–300, 1984

Lyketsos CG, Hanson AL, Fishman M, et al: Manic syndrome early and late in the course of HIV. Am J Psychiatry 150:326–327, 1993

Lyketsos CG, Korazzini K, Steele C: Mania in Alzheimer's disease. J Neuropsychiatry Clin Neurosci 7:350–352, 1995

Mace NL, Rabins PV: The 36-Hour Day—A Family Guide to Caring for Persons with Alzheimer's Disease, Related Dementing Illnesses, and Memory Loss in Later Life, Revised Edition. Baltimore, MD, Johns Hopkins University Press, 1991

McHugh PR, Folstein MF: Psychiatric syndromes of Huntington's chorea, in Psychiatric Aspects of Neurologic Disease. Edited by Benson DF, Blumer D. New York, Grune & Stratton, 1975, pp 267–286

Pearlson GD, Ross CR, Lohr WD, et al: Association between family history of affective disorder and the depressive syndrome of Alzheimer's disease. Am J Psychiatry 147:452–456, 1990

Rabins PV, Mace NL, Lucas MJ: The impact of dementia on the family. JAMA 248:333–335, 1982

Robinson RG, Starkstein SE: Current research in affective disorders following stroke. J Neuropsychiatry Clin Neurosci 2:1–14, 1990

Robinson RG, Kubos KL, Starr LB: Mood disorders in stroke patients: importance of location of lesion. Brain 107:81–93, 1984

Starkstein SE, Robinson RG: Depression in Neurologic Disease. Baltimore, MD, Johns Hopkins University Press, 1993

Starkstein SE, Robinson RG, Price TR: Comparison of patients with and without post-stroke major depression matched for size and location of lesion. Arch Gen Psychiatry 45:247–252, 1988

Treisman GJ, Lyketsos CG, Fishman M, et al: Psychiatric care for patients with HIV infection. Psychosomatics 34:432–439, 1993

Treisman G, Fishman M, Lyketsos CG, et al: Evaluation and treatment of psychiatric disorders associated with HIV infection, in HIV, AIDS and the Brain. Edited by Price RW, Perry SW. New York, Raven, 1994

Zweig RM, Ross CA, Hedreen JC, et al: Neuropathology of aminergic nuclei in Alzheimer's disease. Prog Clin Biol Res 317:353–365, 1989

Chapter 2

Is Alzheimer's Disease a Lifelong Illness?

Risk Factors for Pathological and Clinical Disease

James A. Mortimer, Ph.D.

———◆———

D
espite 15 years of epidemiological investigation, researchers
have identified relatively few
definitive risk factors for Alzheimer's disease. Such risk factors include
the presence of Down's syndrome and family history of dementia, which
likely reflect genotype at birth. Other risk factors for which investigators
have found substantial support include head injury and low levels of education. In most societies, education is completed by early adulthood; the
association between low education and Alzheimer's disease may reflect
the influence of genes and early life experiences in shaping brain development and its correlate, intelligence (Andreasen et al. 1993).

In this chapter, I argue that in most cases Alzheimer's disease is
a lifelong illness and that the risk of disease pathology and its clinical
expression is largely—though not exclusively—determined before adulthood. Progress in identifying the disease's causes and developing preventive strategies will depend on the profession's ability to distinguish and

This work was supported in part by grants from the National Institute on Aging
(R01-AG09238 and R01-AG08539) and by the U.S. Department of Veterans Affairs.

9

understand three sets of risk factors: those related to the etiology of pathogenic process, those related to the clinical expression of this process, and preclinical indicators of the disease.

Risk Factors for the Alzheimer's Pathogenic Process

As noted earlier, investigators have identified a small number of risk factors for Alzheimer's disease. In particular, family history of dementia, Down's syndrome, and head injury are implicated in the pathogenic process of the disease.

Family History of Dementia

Family history of dementia, particularly dementia of the Alzheimer's type, has been the most consistent risk factor for pathologically confirmed Alzheimer's disease. Heston et al. (1981), for example, found that individuals with autopsy-confirmed Alzheimer's disease were more likely than control subjects without apparent Alzheimer's disease to have first-degree relatives with dementia. Although this association could result from genetic inheritance or shared familial environment, Khoury et al. (1988) argued that genetic causation was a more likely explanation. (Chapter 12 of this volume reviews in detail the role of genes in the etiology of Alzheimer's disease.)

Down's Syndrome

Down's syndrome offers two important clues concerning the pathogenesis of Alzheimer's disease. First, nearly all individuals with Down's syndrome eventually develop the characteristic neuropathological lesions associated with Alzheimer's disease (Mortimer 1994). Many researchers believe that the early accumulation of Alzheimer's lesions in the brains of individuals with Down's syndrome is related to the increased gene dosage for amyloid precursor protein (Hardy and Duff 1993), the gene for which is located on chromosome 21. A second connection between Down's syndrome and Alzheimer's disease—the aggregation of these two conditions in families—was first reported by Heston (1977) and subsequently confirmed in a pooled analysis of case-control studies by van Duijn et al. (1991).

Schupf et al. (1994) measured the frequency of Alzheimer's disease in the parents of children with Down's syndrome. They found that only mothers who gave birth to a child with Down's syndrome before age 35 were at increased risk for Alzheimer's disease, whereas those who gave birth to a child with Down's syndrome after age 35 (when this event is more common) appeared not to be at increased risk. One explanation for this finding is that the genetic link between Down's syndrome and Alzheimer's disease might be a predisposition to chromosome 21 nondisjunction: nondisjunction during meiosis might lead to Down's syndrome, whereas nondisjunction during mitosis would result in mosaics and lead to Alzheimer's disease (Potter 1991).

Thus, mothers with a genetic predisposition to chromosome 21 nondisjunction would be more likely to give birth to children with Down's syndrome and have more trisomic cells in organs, including the brain. This explanation is consistent with two reports of individuals who were mosaic in lymphocytes for trisomy 21 (Rowe et al. 1989; Schapiro et al. 1989); although these patients did not develop a typical Down's phenotype, they nevertheless presented with Alzheimer's disease early in life. Although researchers know that trisomy for chromosome 21 is unlikely to be common in either brain cells or leukocytes of patients with Alzheimer's disease (St. George-Hyslop et al. 1987), the possibility remains that late-onset Alzheimer's disease might result from a relatively small percentage of trisomic cells in the brain that could go undetected.

Head Injury

A third risk factor leading to Alzheimer's pathology is head injury. Researchers had suspected an association between this risk factor and Alzheimer's disease since the initial case-control studies (Mortimer et al. 1983, 1991). Roberts and collaborators studied the brains of individuals who died after severe head injuries; they established that β-amyloid (Roberts et al. 1991) and hyperphosphorylated tau (Newman et al. 1994) accumulated rapidly following injury in approximately 30% of these cases.

A subsequent study by Mayeux et al. (1995) demonstrated that only individuals carrying one or more ε4 alleles for apolipoprotein E were at increased risk for Alzheimer's disease as a result of head injuries. The frequency of this allele in Western populations is consistent with the finding by Roberts et al. (1991) that only 30% of head injury cases show substantial β-amyloid deposition following trauma. A plausible explanation for the association between head injury and β-amyloid deposition is that overproduction of β-amyloid precursor protein occurs as a result of heat shock protein gene activation after head trauma (Harrison et al. 1993). If this hypothesis is true, other risk factors that activate heat shock protein genes—such as risk factors associated with episodes of hypoxia—also might be associated with Alzheimer's disease.

Risk Factors for Clinical Presentation of Dementia Among Individuals With Pathological Lesions

Since the clinicopathological studies of Blessed et al. (1968), researchers have appreciated that at least some Alzheimer's lesions may be present in the brains of individuals with normal mentation immediately before death. This observation gave rise to the threshold hypothesis of dementia (Roth 1986), which suggested that dementia became evident only after a sufficient quantity of lesions were present. A refinement of this model (Mortimer 1988) introduced the concept of brain reserve to explain the fact that individuals with higher levels of education appeared to be at lower risk for dementia. In this paradigm, the critical element in dementia presentation is not the quantity of lesions but the number of remaining functional neurons that reflects the premorbid brain reserve of neurons, as well as the loss experienced secondary to the disease process.

Katzman et al. (1988) conducted a clinicopathological study of 137 elderly residents of a nursing home, 78% of whom had dementia. They identified 10 individuals whose functional and cognitive performance was in the upper quintile but who were classified neuropathologically as having Alzheimer's disease. Comparison of the brains of these individuals with those of others with pathological and clinical evidence of Alzheimer's disease showed that the residents without dementia had higher brain weights and greater numbers of neurons in the cerebral cortex. This finding suggests that either a larger endowment of neurons at birth or reduced loss of neurons over the life course might offer protection from the clinical manifestations of Alzheimer's disease in old age.

Risk Factors Associated With Reduced Brain Reserve

Researchers have identified several exposures that may be associated with reduced brain reserve (reflected by brain size, numbers of neurons and/or synapses) and hasten the disclosure that a patient has the neuropathology of

Alzheimer's disease. These risk factors include head injury, alcohol abuse, stroke(s), and low levels of education.

Corkin et al. (1989) reported that penetrating head injuries in young adulthood exacerbated cognitive decline 30 years later. Because of the relatively young age of the cohort at their last evaluation, however, none of these subjects had dementia. Alcohol abuse is a risk factor not only for alcoholic dementia but also for Alzheimer's disease (Fratiglioni et al. 1993). Individuals who do not meet pathological criteria for either Alzheimer's disease or vascular dementia may present with intellectual impairment as a result of combined Alzheimer's and vascular lesions (Tomlinson et al. 1970). Low levels of education may predispose clinical presentation through several mechanisms, including brain development related to fetal or early-life exposures associated with the socioeconomic status of the family of origin (Mortimer and Graves 1993).

If brain reserve modifies the clinical presentation of Alzheimer's disease, persons born with larger heads and therefore larger brains might be expected to show less cognitive impairment than those with smaller heads. Graves et al. (1994) examined this hypothesis using data from the Kame Project, a population-based study of elderly Japanese Americans living in King County, Washington. The investigators measured head circumference (as an indicator of brain size) in 1,458 individuals and used the Cognitive Abilities Screening Instrument (CASI) to assess cognitive impairment; scores on this scale, which range between 0 and 100, correlate strongly with those of the more familiar Mini-Mental State Exam (Folstein et al. 1975). Smaller head circumference strongly predicted a CASI score of less than 50, which reflects severe impairment characteristic of dementia (odds ratio [adjusted for age, gender, and education] = 0.27; 95% confidence interval: 0.12–0.58). This finding is consistent with a model for cognitive functioning in which greater initial brain reserve (indexed by head size) provides a buffer against pathological processes that cause dementia.

One explanation for the strong association between smaller head circumference and greater cognitive impairment is that persons with smaller heads who have the pathology of Alzheimer's disease might begin exhibiting symptoms at an earlier age and therefore progress more by the time they are screened. A study of 28 female patients with Alzheimer's disease for whom computed tomography (CT) scans were available, from which premorbid brain size could be estimated (Schofield et al. 1995), supported this interpretation. The principal finding of this study was that individuals who began with larger brains exhibited dementia onset significantly later in life than those with smaller brains. The predicted shift in age at onset was 10 years, given the range of premorbid brain sizes examined.

Protective Factors for Alzheimer's Disease

As noted above, certain risk factors increase the loss of brain reserve and predispose individuals to clinical presentation of dementia. Investigators also have identified three exposures that may provide protection against clinical presentation of dementia: anti-inflammatory drugs, exogenous estrogen, and nicotine. These exposures seem to slow down or compensate for the loss of functioning neurons that can occur in Alzheimer's disease.

Anti-inflammatory drugs.   Researchers have found ample evidence that Alzheimer's disease entails immune-mediated autodestructive processes (Aisen and Davis 1994; McGeer and Rogers 1992). In a 6-month, double-blind clinical trial, Rogers et al. (1993) showed that indomethacin—a common nonsteroidal anti-inflammatory drug (NSAID)—retarded disease progression in Alzheimer's patients, compared with placebo. In a retrospective natural history study of Alzheimer's disease, Rich et al. (1995) also found significant differences in progression rates among 32 patients taking NSAIDs or aspirin on a daily basis, compared with 177 patient control subjects. Two case-control studies found significant inverse associations between Alzheimer's disease and steroidal (Breitner et al. 1994) and nonsteroidal medications (Canadian Study of Health and Aging 1994); one case-control study, using pharmacy records from a health maintenance organization, found no association, however (Kukull et al. 1994).

Exogenous estrogen.   A study of death records from a retirement community in California (Paganini-Hill and Henderson 1994) raised the possibility that estrogen replacement therapy (ERT) might retard the onset of Alzheimer's disease. This study demonstrated that among 2,529 female cohort members who died between 1981 and 1992, the risk of Alzheimer's disease and related dementias was reduced in estrogen users relative to non-estrogen users. This study did not control, however, for education—a major confounding factor that affects the use of estrogen and the clinical outcome. A small case-control study by the same investigators demonstrated an inverse association between ERT and Alzheimer's disease risk (Henderson et al. 1994); this association was not evident in another population based case-control study (Brenner et al. 1994).

Two other studies examined the association between ERT and the risk of cognitive impairment. Barrett-Connor and Kritz-Silverstein (1993) reported no association between ERT and performance on a variety of cognitive tests when age and education were controlled. The second study (Rice et al. 1994) found a strong association between estrogen usage and performance on a cognitive screening test ($P < .0001$); this association disappeared entirely, however ($P = .99$), when the predictive equation incorporated education and income. Although estrogen remains a plausible candidate for reducing the risk of Alzheimer's disease, epidemiological studies have not provided convincing evidence that it is protective.

Nicotine.   Several studies have reported inverse associations between the risk of Alzheimer's disease and smoking (e.g., Graves and Mortimer 1994). This association might result from selective survival of individuals who do not smoke and are at higher risk for Alzheimer's disease (e.g., through having one or more apolipoprotein ε4 alleles). A study by van Duijn et al. (1995) provided the first strong evidence in favor of a real protective effect of smoking rather than selection bias. In that study, smoking appeared to provide a strong protective effect against early-onset Alzheimer's disease in individuals who were at very high risk because they carried the apolipoprotein ε4 allele and had a positive family history of dementia. This finding was consistent with upregulation of nicotinic receptors in persons who smoke (Schwartz and Kellar 1983), which partially compensates for their loss as a result of Alzheimer's disease (Perry et al. 1987).

Risk Factors as Indicators of the Disease Process

Finally, some risk factors may reflect prodromal symptoms of the disease. These factors include depression (Jorm et al. 1991), physical and social inactivity (Broe et al. 1990; Kondo and Yamashita 1990), and cognitive performance many years before the onset of dementia.

Two studies showed that physicians may be able to distinguish, 20 years before onset of dementia, individuals who will develop Alzheimer's disease from those who will not. LaRue and Jarvik (1987) found that persons who were judged to have dementia at a mean age of 85 could be distinguished from their age peers without dementia on a variety of neuropsychological tests taken 20 years earlier. A study by Kawas et al. (1994) found that persons who developed pathologically confirmed Alzheimer's disease could be distinguished 20 years before death using the Benton

Visual Retention Test. These studies suggest that the pathological process of Alzheimer's disease may progress "behind the scenes" for decades before it reaches a severity sufficient to generate clinical symptoms. Investigators have advanced similar arguments for Parkinson's disease, in which the dopaminergic deficit in the striatum must reach 75% or more before clinical symptoms become evident (Mortimer and Webster 1982).

The most recent examination of this issue involved a prospective longitudinal study of 678 elderly Catholic nuns. Using linguistic measures derived from essays written by sisters at the time they took their final vows (around age 22), Snowdon et al. (1996) found that—when education and age at assessment were controlled—sisters with poor linguistic ability were up to 31 times more likely to be cognitively and functionally impaired in old age. Furthermore, these investigators reported that one measure, the density of ideas or propositions in the essays, was strongly predictive of pathologically confirmed Alzheimer's disease. The mean age at assessment in this study was 80 years, suggesting that detection of incipient dementia may be possible as many as 60 years before clinical onset.

Conclusion

Understanding the causes of Alzheimer's disease clearly is important to developing effective preventive strategies. In this chapter, I assert that at least three sets of risk factors are associated with Alzheimer's disease: those related to the pathological disease process, which are likely to be largely genetic; those affecting clinical expression of the underlying pathology, including brain size, toxic exposures, and compounds that may retard or compensate for damage done by the pathological process; and preclinical indicators of the disease. The ability to distinguish early in adult life individuals who will develop Alzheimer's disease from those who will not strongly suggests that Alzheimer's disease may be a lifelong or nearly lifelong illness.

References

Aisen PS, Davis KL: Inflammatory mechanisms in Alzheimer's disease: implications for therapy. Am J Psychiatry 151:1105–1113, 1994

Andreasen NC, Flaum M, Swayze VW, et al: Intelligence and brain structure in normal individuals. Am J Psychiatry 150:130–134, 1993

Barrett-Connor E, Kritz-Silverstein D: Estrogen replacement therapy and cognitive function in older women. JAMA 269:2637–2641, 1993

Blessed G, Tomlinson BE, Roth, M: The association between quantitative measures of dementia and of senile change in the cerebral grey matter of elderly subjects. Br J Psychiatry 114:797–811, 1968

Breitner JCS, Gau BA, Welsh KA, et al: Inverse association of anti-inflammatory treatments and Alzheimer's disease: initial results of a co-twin control study. Neurology 44:227–232, 1994

Brenner DE, Kukull WA, Stergachis A, et al: Postmenopausal estrogen replacement therapy and the risk of Alzheimer's disease: a population-based case-control study. Am J Epidemiol 140:262–267, 1994

Broe GA, Henderson AS, Creasey H, et al: A case-control study of Alzheimer's disease in Australia. Neurology 40:1698–1707, 1990

Canadian Study of Health and Aging: The Canadian Study of Health and Aging: risk factors for Alzheimer's disease in Canada. Neurology 44:2073–2080, 1994

Corkin S, Rosen TJ, Sullivan EV, et al: Penetrating head injury in young adulthood exacerbates cognitive decline in later years. J Neurosci 9:3876–3883, 1989

Folstein MF, Folstein SE, McHugh PR: Mini-Mental State: a practical method for grading the cognitive state of patients for the clinician. J Psychiatr Res 2: 189–198, 1975

Fratiglioni L, Ahlbom A, Viitanen M, et al: Risk factors for late-onset Alzheimer's disease: a population-based, case-control study. Ann Neurol 33:258–266, 1993

Graves AB, Mortimer JA: Does smoking reduce the risks of Parkinson's and Alzheimer's diseases? Journal of Smoking-Related Disorders 5(suppl 1): 79–90, 1994

Graves AB, Mortimer JA, Kramer J, et al: Head size as a risk factor for cognitive impairment in elderly Japanese-Americans: the Kame Project (abstract). Neurobiol Aging 15(suppl 1):S74, 1994

Hardy J, Duff K: Heterogeneity in Alzheimer's disease. Ann Med 25:437–440, 1993

Harrison PJ, Procter AW, Exworthy T, et al: Heat shock protein (hsx70) mRNA expression in human brain: effects of neurodegenerative disease and agonal state. Neuropathol Appl Neurobiol 19:10–21, 1993

Henderson VW, Paganini-Hill A, Emanuel CK, et al: Estrogen replacement therapy in older women: comparisons between Alzheimer's disease cases and nondemented control subjects. Arch Neurol 51:896–900, 1994

Heston LL: Alzheimer's disease, trisomy 21, and myeloproliferative disorders: associations suggesting a genetic diathesis. Science 196:322–323, 1977

Heston LL, Mastri AR, Anderson VE, et al: Dementia of the Alzheimer type: clinical genetics, natural history, and associated conditions. Arch Gen Psychiatry 38:1085–1090, 1981

Jorm AF, van Duijn CM, Chandra V, et al: Psychiatric history and related exposures as risk factors for Alzheimer's disease: a collaborative re-analysis of case-control studies. Int J Epidemiol 20(suppl 2):S43–S47, 1991

Katzman R, Terry R, DeTheresa R, et al: Clinical, pathological, and neurochemical changes in dementia: a subgroup with preserved mental status and numerous neocortical plaques. Ann Neurol 23:138–144, 1988

Kawas C, Corrada-Bravo M, Metter J, et al: Neuropsychological differences 20 years before death in subjects with and without Alzheimer's pathology (abstract). Presented at the 46th annual meeting of the American Academy of Neurology, Washington, DC, May 1–7, 1994. Neurology 44(suppl 2):A141, 1994

Khoury MJ, Beaty TH, Liang KY: Can familial aggregation of disease be explained by familial aggregation of environmental risk factors? Am J Epidemiol 127:674–683, 1988

Kondo K, Yamashita I: A case-control study of Alzheimer's disease in Japan: association with inactive psychosocial behaviors, in Psychogeriatrics, Biomedical and Social Advances. Edited by Hasegawa K, Homma A. Amsterdam, The Netherlands, Excerpta Medica, 1990, pp 49–53

Kukull WA, Larson EB, Stergachis A, et al: Non-steroidal anti-inflammatory drug use and risk of Alzheimer's disease (abstract). Presented at the 46th annual meeting of the American Academy of Neurology, Washington, DC, May 1–7, 1994. Neurology 44(suppl 2):A237, 1994

LaRue A, Jarvik LF: Cognitive function and prediction of dementia in old age. Int J Aging Hum Dev 25:79–89, 1987

Mayeux R, Ottman R, Maestre G, et al: Synergistic effects of traumatic head injury and apolipoprotein-ε4 in patients with Alzheimer's disease. Neurology 45:555–557, 1995

McGeer PL, Rogers J: Anti-inflammatory agents as a therapeutic approach to Alzheimer's disease. Neurology 42:447–449, 1992

Mortimer JA: Do psychosocial risk factors contribute to Alzheimer's disease? in Etiology of Dementia of the Alzheimer's Type. Edited by Henderson AS, Henderson JH. Chichester, England, John Wiley and Sons, 1988, pp 39–52

Mortimer JA: What are the risk factors for dementia? in Dementia and Normal Aging. Edited by Huppert FA, Brayne C, O'Connor D. Cambridge, England, Cambridge University Press, 1994, pp 208–229

Mortimer, JA, Graves, AB: Education and other socioeconomic determinants of dementia and Alzheimer's disease. Neurology 43(suppl 4):S39–S44, 1993

Mortimer JA, Webster DD: Comparison of extrapyramidal motor function in normal aging and Parkinson's disease, in The Aging Motor System. Edited by Mortimer JA, Pirozzolo FJ, Maletta GJ. New York, Praeger, 1982, pp 217–241

Mortimer JA, French LR, Hutton JT, et al: Reported head trauma in an epidemiologic study of Alzheimer's disease (abstract). Neurology 33(suppl 2):85, 1983

Mortimer JA, van Duijn CM, Chandra V, et al: Head trauma as a risk factor for Alzheimer's disease: a collaborative re-analysis of case-control studies. Int J Epidemiol 20(suppl 2):S28–S35, 1991

Newman SJ, Gentleman SM, Graham DI, et al: Tissue distribution and cellular localisation of hyperphosphorylated tau in human head injury and aged matched controls (abstract). Neurobiol Aging 15(suppl 1):S22, 1994

Paganini-Hill A, Henderson VW: Estrogen deficiency and risk of Alzheimer's disease in women. Am J Epidemiol 140:256–261, 1994

Perry EK, Perry RH, Smith CJ, et al: Nicotinic receptor abnormalities in Alzheimer's and Parkinson's diseases. J Neurol Neurosurg Psychiatry 50:806–809, 1987

Potter H: Review and hypothesis: Alzheimer disease and Down syndrome—chromosome 21 nondisjunction may underlie both disorders. Am J Hum Genet 48:1192–1200, 1991

Rice MM, Graves AB, Larson EB, et al: Estrogen replacement therapy and cognitive performance in postmenopausal Japanese-American women: the Kame Project (letter). Neurobiol Aging 15(suppl 1):S44, 1994

Rich JB, Rasmusson DX, Folstein MF, et al: Nonsteroidal anti-inflammatory drugs in Alzheimer's disease. Neurology 45:51–55, 1995

Roberts GW, Gentleman SM, Lynch A, et al: Beta A4 amyloid protein distribution in brain after head trauma. Lancet 338:1422–1423, 1991

Rogers J, Kirby LC, Hempleman SR, et al: Clinical trial of indomethacin in Alzheimer's disease. Neurology 43:1609–1611, 1993

Roth M: The association of clinical and neuropsychological findings and its bearings on the classification and aetiology of Alzheimer's disease. Br Med Bull 42:42–50, 1986

Rowe IF, Ridler MAC, Gibberd FB: Presenile dementia associated with mosaic trisomy 21 in a patient with a Down syndrome child (letter). Lancet 2:229, 1989

Schapiro MB, Kumar A, White B, et al: Alzheimer's disease (AD) in mosaic/translocation Down's syndrome (Ds) without mental retardation (abstract). Neurology 39(suppl 1):169, 1989

Schofield P, Mosesson RE, Stern Y, et al: The age at onset of Alzheimer's disease and an intracranial area measurement. Arch Neurol 52:95–98, 1995

Schupf N, Kapell D, Lee JH, et al: Increased risk of Alzheimer's disease in mothers of adults with Down's syndrome. Lancet 344:353–356, 1994

Schwartz RD, Kellar KJ: Nicotinic cholinergic receptor binding sites in the brain: regulation in vivo. Science 220:214–216, 1983

Snowdon DA, Kemper SJ, Mortimer JA, et al: Linguistic ability in early life and cognitive function and Alzheimer's disease in late life: findings from the Nun Study. JAMA 275:528–532, 1996

St. George-Hyslop PH, Tanzi RE, Polinsky RJ, et al: Absence of duplication of chromosome 21 genes in familial and sporadic Alzheimer's disease. Science 238:664–666, 1987

Tomlinson BE, Blessed G, Roth M: Observations on the brains of demented old people. J Neurol Sci 11:205–242, 1970

van Duijn CM, Clayton D, Chandra V, et al: Familial aggregation of Alzheimer's disease and related disorders: a collaborative re-analysis of case-control studies. Int J Epidemiol 20(suppl 2):S13–S20, 1991

van Duijn CM, Havekes LM, van Broeckhoven C, et al: Apolipoprotein E genotype and association between smoking and early-onset Alzheimer's disease.
BMJ 310(6980):627–631, 1995

Chapter 3

Alzheimer's Disease and Other Dementias
Neuropathological Considerations

Suzanne S. Mirra, M.D.

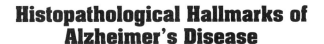

Histopathological Hallmarks of Alzheimer's Disease

Recognition of senile plaques and neurofibrillary tangles as the two major histopathological features of Alzheimer's disease has not changed over the years. Medicine's understanding of these changes and their implications for the pathogenesis of Alzheimer's disease, however, has evolved considerably. Physicians now know, for example, that the neurofibrillary tangle—a silver-positive cytoplasmic fibrillary structure (Figure 3–1, **c**)— is composed primarily of paired helical filaments whose major constituent is an abnormally phosphorylated form of the microtubule-associated protein tau.

Senile plaques may vary in appearance. Neuritic plaques (Figure 3–1, **a**) exhibit distended neuronal processes or neurites, which at a fine structural level are filled with dense bodies, lysosomes, and paired helical filaments. Fibrillar amyloid may be present between the neurites or in well-formed

This work was supported by grants from the National Institutes of Health (AG06790 and AG10130) and a Veterans Affairs Merit Award.

amyloid cores. Diffuse plaques (Figure 3–1, **b**), however, are rather amorphous and lack abnormal neurites and fibrillar amyloid. Senile plaques of both types share antigenic determinants with the β or A-4 amyloid protein isolated from Alzheimer's disease plaques and blood vessels. Other important changes that are virtually universal in Alzheimer's disease include amyloid deposition in blood vessels, or amyloid angiopathy (Figure 3–1, **d**), and abnormal processes known as "neuropil threads" within the hippocampus, entorhinal cortex, and other regions.

Making the Diagnosis of Alzheimer's Disease

Although researchers have established working criteria for the clinical diagnosis of Alzheimer's disease (McKhann et al. 1984) and have begun

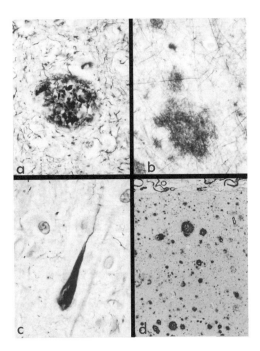

Figure 3–1.   Histopathologic features of Alzheimer's disease: a) Neuritic plaque (Bielschowsky silver stain); b) Diffuse plaque (Bielschowsky silver stain); c) Neurofibrillary tangle (Sevier-Munger silver stain); d) Numerous Aβ-positive plaques and blood vessels in the neocortex (Aβ immunohistochemistry).

to develop promising diagnostic assays, definitive diagnosis still rests on neuropathological confirmation (Mirra et al. 1993). Confirmation of the clinical diagnosis is critical (Gearing et al. 1995). Allocation of public health resources, patient selection for therapeutic trials, and other clinical studies rely on access to reliable information. Beyond the diagnosis itself, numerous clinical and basic scientific studies depend on accurate overall and/or regional assessment of key neuropathological features in Alzheimer's disease and control tissues. Conversely, information obtained at autopsy is less valuable when clinical data are inaccurate or inadequate (Whitehouse 1993).

Clinical diagnostic accuracy has improved over the past few years, particularly when diagnosticians use formal clinical criteria. Mendez et al. (1992), for example, conducted a retrospective autopsy study of 650 patients whose conditions were diagnosed as Alzheimer's disease using variable clinical criteria; they confirmed Alzheimer's disease, with or without other neuropathological conditions, in 78% of the cases. Gearing et al. (1995) confirmed Alzheimer's disease in 87% of 106 subjects with a diagnosis of probable or possible Alzheimer's disease.

Standardization of Neuropathological Evaluation of Alzheimer's Disease

Despite universal, long-standing recognition of histopathological changes in Alzheimer's disease, neuropathologists do not agree broadly on precise pathological criteria for the diagnosis of Alzheimer's disease. Based on a survey of neuropathologists, H. M. Wisniewski et al. (1989, p. 608) concluded that there is a need for "development of a consensus with regard to the diagnosis of Alzheimer's disease." Tierney et al. (1988) observed that the lack of standard neuropathological criteria for the diagnosis of Alzheimer's disease limits investigators' ability to compare research protocols.

In 1985 a panel of neuropathologists developed minimal microscopic criteria for establishing the diagnosis of Alzheimer's disease (Khachaturian 1985); diagnosis was based on an age-related minimum number of senile plaques per microscopic field of neocortex encompassing 1 mm^2 at a recommended microscopic magnification. These guidelines have been widely applied and continue to be useful for most Alzheimer's disease cases. Yet this (arguably arbitrary) numerical criterion for plaque frequency does not consider potentially large variations in stain, technique, and interpretation (Mirra et al. 1994). The neuropathological protocol developed by the Consortium to Establish a Registry for Alzheimer's Disease (CERAD) instead took a semiquantitative approach to the assessment of plaque frequency; using an algorithm incorporating the age-related neuritic plaque score with the presence or absence of dementia, the CERAD protocol determines levels of certainty of Alzheimer's disease diagnosis and promotes commonality of language (Mirra et al. 1991).

Concerns about intercenter variations in methodology and interpretation prompted my colleagues and me to compare neuropathological data among laboratories (Mirra et al. 1994). We asked 24 neuropathologists from 18 medical centers in the United States and Canada to stain sections derived from the frontal cortex of 8 patients with Alzheimer's disease and 2 control subjects. We observed reasonable interrater agreement for semiquantitative measures used by CERAD; we found significant differences among raters, however, for quantitative plaque and tangles counts. These differences reflected variations in stain sensitivity, staining technique (even when the same stain was used), and interpretation. This study suggested that greater attention to quality improvement is still needed for the neuropathological evaluation of Alzheimer's disease, particularly when data are pooled in multicenter studies such as CERADs.

Other investigators also have explored the reliability of neuropathological data derived from different centers. In a multicenter analysis under the auspices of EURAGE—a European organization that studies aging and dementia—Duykaerts et al. (1990) found poor agreement among centers with regard to plaque and tangle density but better concordance for ranking. Chui et al. (1993) observed moderate-to-substantial interrater reliability between two centers and two raters in a quantitative study of plaques and tangles in 35 cases of Alzheimer's disease, 9 healthy elderly control subjects, and 6 cases of non-Alzheimer's disease dementia.

Developments in Alzheimer's Disease Neuropathology

The foregoing studies confirm the need for continued reevaluation of diagnostic criteria for Alzheimer's disease. Berg et al. (1993) found that the frequency of senile plaques in the neocortex and hippocampus correlated weakly with the extent of dementia, although this result may have been related to methodology. In addition, researchers have challenged previous notions that plaques and amyloid burden accumulate with increasing age or duration of illness (Arriagada et al. 1992; Hyman et al. 1993; Kazee et al. 1993; McKeel et al. 1993). Hyman et al. (1993) found that amyloid burden in Alzheimer's disease and Down's syndrome eventually reaches a steady state; they suggested that disease progression may be associated with a process of continued deposition and degradation of amyloid.

Importance of Senile Plaque Subtype

With the advent of βA4 immunohistochemical and sensitive silver staining methods, investigators increasingly have recognized diffuse plaques—not only in the cerebral cortex of patients with Alzheimer's disease and other disorders (Mann and Jones 1990) and nondemented control subjects (Dickson et al. 1988) but also in subcortical locations such as the corpus striatum (Gearing et al. 1993), the cerebellum (Joachim et al. 1989), the diencephalon, and the hypothalamus (Standaert et al. 1991). The significance of diffuse plaques in the evolution of Alzheimer's disease and "normal aging" remains uncertain: do any or all diffuse plaques eventually evolve to neuritic forms, or are there region-specific differences? Does their presence in a cognitively healthy individual signal preclinical Alzheimer's disease?

Progression of Neurofibrillary Pathology

Another analysis with important implications for hierarchical change involves the neuroanatomical staging method advanced by Braak and Braak (1991). They examined autopsy brains from 83 individuals and found that whereas the distribution and frequency of amyloid deposits had limited significance for differentiating neuropathological stages, a characteristic distribution of neurofibrillary tangles and neuropil threads permitted differentiation of six stages exemplified by progression from transentorhinal/entorhinal layers to isocortex.

Synaptic Pathology in Alzheimer's Disease

Synaptic density has emerged as a key correlate with the severity of dementia. DeKosky and Scheff (1990), for example, found in an electron microscopic study that synapse loss paralleled the severity of cognitive decline. In a prospective clinical-pathological study of 15 patients with Alzheimer's disease and 9 neuropathologically healthy subjects in whom a series of neuropsychological batteries had been performed, Terry et al. (1991) assessed synaptic density using antibodies to the presynaptic marker, synaptophysin; they found a strong correlation between the density of neocortical synapses and cognitive alterations and concluded that synapse loss is the major correlate of cognitive impairment. Interestingly, however, synaptic numbers apparently are preserved in the entorhinal cortex (Scheff et al. 1993)—suggesting increased plasticity in this region and raising questions about the efficacy of such apparent sprouting (Terry 1993).

Apolipoprotein E and Alzheimer's Disease

The apolipoprotein E (ApoE) type 4 allele is a risk factor for the development of late-onset familial and sporadic forms of Alzheimer's disease (Corder et al. 1993; Poirier et al. 1993; Rebeck et al. 1993; Strittmatter et al. 1993). Several groups reported a protective effect of the ε2 allele (Corder et al. 1994; Talbot et al. 1994); this protective effect may vary, however, among ethnic groups (Maestre et al. 1995).

The *ApoE* gene is on the 19th chromosome, in the same genomic region that researchers have associated with familial late-onset Alzheimer's disease (Pericak-Vance et al. 1991). Investigators previously had linked the ε4 allele with hypercholesterolemia and increased risk of heart disease; its association with vascular dementia or ischemic cerebrovascular disease is controversial (Couderc et al. 1993; Frisoni et al. 1994; Saunders and Roses 1993). In the brain, *ApoE* is present in astrocytes and is upregulated following central or peripheral nervous system injury. *ApoE* has a high affinity to β-amyloid in colony-stimulating factor (Strittmatter et al. 1993; T. Wisniewski et al. 1993).

The mechanism by which the *ApoE* genotype influences the risk of developing Alzheimer's disease and age at onset remains unknown. Antibodies to *ApoE* label plaques and blood vessels (Figure 3–2) and co-localize with anti-βA4 in Alzheimer's disease (Namba et al. 1991; Rebeck et al. 1993; Schmechel et al. 1993); researchers observe more intense and frequent βA4 immunolabeling with the *ApoE*-ε4 allele than with other *ApoE* alleles (Schmechel et al. 1993). Strittmatter et al. (1994) reported isoform-specific differences in binding to tau in vitro and hypothesized that these differences may influence the development of neuropathological changes such as neurofibrillary tangles. They pointed out, however, that there appear to be no quantitative differences in tangles between cases with and without the ε4 allele. Moreover, aged nonhuman primates—in whom neuropathological changes consist predominantly of amyloid plaques (diffuse and neuritic) and amyloid angiopathy in the absence of tau-related neuropathology (neurofibrillary tangles or neuropil threads)—possess an ε4-like allele (Gearing et al. 1994; Poduri et al. 1994). Schneider et al. (1995) examined the *ApoE* genotype in 51 cases of diverse neurodegenerative disease; interestingly, they found an increased proportion of ε4 genotypes in certain disorders characterized by tau-related cytoskeletal pathology (Pick's disease, progressive supranuclear palsy, corticobasal ganglionic degeneration). Further studies must substantiate this finding with more well-characterized cases.

Vascular Dementia

The relationship between cerebrovascular disease and dementia has been controversial (Drachman 1993; Erkinjuntti and Hachinski 1993). Numerous factors have confounded clinical and pathological studies

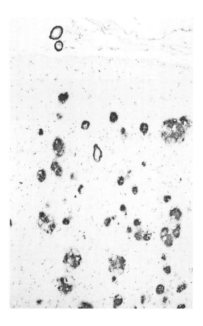

Figure 3–2. Apolipoprotein E immunoreactive senile plaques and blood vessels parallel Aβ label (ApoE immunohistochemistry).

designed to differentiate dementias of Alzheimer's disease and other primary neurodegenerative disorders from vascular dementia (Liston and LaRue 1983). Two groups of investigators proposed clinical criteria for the diagnosis of all vascular dementia and ischemic vascular dementia (Chui et al. 1992; Roman et al. 1993); these groups emphasized the importance of neuropathological correlation. Risks for the development of vascular disease vary among ethnic groups: Japanese American and African American populations, for example, are at greater risk than European Americans (Larson 1993).

In a recent clinical-neuropathological study by CERAD, approximately 25% of patients with a clinical diagnosis (at autopsy) of Alzheimer's disease not only met neuropathological criteria for Alzheimer's disease but also showed one or more vascular lesions of varying type, distribution, and magnitude (Gearing et al. 1995). Thus, comorbid Alzheimer's disease and vascular disease appears to be common. Researchers remain uncertain, however, about whether "pure" vascular dementia constitutes a significant subset of dementia cases. Neuropathologists rarely encounter such cases, although this pattern may reflect the predominantly white population in whom major medical centers perform autopsies. Standardized clinical-pathological study of well-characterized cases would clarify this issue.

Researchers have associated dementia with two major vascular disorders: multi-infarct dementia and Binswanger's disease. In addition, elderly nondemented and demented individuals with vascular disease and/or Alzheimer's disease exhibit white-matter hyperintensities—variously termed *leukoaraiosis, ubiquitous bright objects* (UBOs), or *nonspecific white-matter lesions*—on magnetic resonance imaging. The neuropathological correlates of these changes have been difficult to define; Grafton et al. (1991) reported white-matter pallor, gliosis, and dilated perivascular spaces. Deep subcortical intensities on imaging studies have been correlated at autopsy with white-matter pallor without clear abnormality of myelin or axons attributed to chronic vascular insufficiency (Braffman et al. 1988; Kirkpatrick and Hayman 1987); other investigators have attempted to distinguish ischemic and nonischemic changes (Fazekas et al. 1993).

Dementia and Lewy Body Diseases

About 40% of patients with idiopathic Parkinson's disease develop dementia (Mayeux et al. 1992). Although some patients apparently have coexistent Alzheimer's disease pathology (Boller et al. 1980; Sudarsky et al.

1989), researchers have not extensively studied the full range of neuro-pathology in Parkinson's disease with and without dementia. There are no gold standards for the neuropathological diagnosis of Parkinson's disease, and investigators have not thoroughly examined the specificity and sensitivity of Parkinson's disease pathology (Koller 1992).

Researchers encounter neuropathology typical of Parkinson's disease (nigral degeneration and Lewy bodies in nigra and other sites) and cortical Lewy bodies (Figure 3–3) in about 20% of neuropathologically confirmed cases of Alzheimer's disease (Ditter and Mirra 1987; Gearing et al. 1995). Investigators are still exploring methods of distinguishing the clinical-neuropathological features of such cases—variously termed *diffuse Lewy body disease, Lewy body variant of Alzheimer's disease, senile dementia of the Lewy body type, and Alzheimer's disease plus Parkinson's disease.* Fluctuating cognitive impairment, visual or auditory hallucinations and paranoid delusions, and the presence of extrapyramidal features in patients primarily presenting with dementia may suggest this disorder (McKeith et al. 1994).

Neuropathological features of Alzheimer's disease plus Parkinson's disease or Lewy body disease include a relative paucity of neurofibrillary tangles in the cortex (Hansen et al. 1993); the presence of ubiquitin-positive neurites in CA2-3 of the hippocampus (Dickson et al. 1991, 1994; Kim et al. 1995); and spongiform change in the entorhinal, superior temporal, and insular cortex, as well as the amygdala (Hansen et al. 1989). Cases of "pure" diffuse Lewy body disease are relatively uncommon,

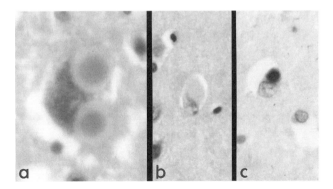

Figure 3–3.   Lewy bodies: a) Two Lewy bodies with peripheral halos in a pigmented neuron of the substantia nigra; b) A cortical Lewy body within a cortical neuron (Hematoxylin-eosin); c) A cortical Lewy body on ubiquitin immunohistochemistry.

however; most cases show combined neuropathological features of Alzheimer's disease and Parkinson's disease.

Other Disorders Clinically Diagnosed as Alzheimer's Disease

Hansen and Crain (1995) reviewed the neuropathology of non-Alzheimer's disease dementias and concluded that Alzheimer's disease—whether "pure" Alzheimer's disease or in combination with Lewy body or Parkinson's disease changes and/or vascular lesions—dominates the dementia landscape. CERAD data clearly support this conclusion (Gearing et al. 1995). However, 14 of 106 CERAD cases had primary diagnoses other than Alzheimer's disease. These diagnoses were subdivided into four general groups: Parkinson's disease and related disorders, hippocampal and/or entorhinal sclerosis, miscellaneous disorders such as adult polyglucosan body disease, and cases with no significant pathology.

Studies examining potentially detectable clinical differences in these cases are underway. Clinicians and neuropathologists clearly must allow for the possibility of other non-Alzheimer's disease dementias, including progressive supranuclear palsy, Creutzfeldt-Jakob disease, Pick's disease, and dementia lacking distinctive histopathological features.

References

Arriagada PV, Growdon JH, Hedley-Whyte ET, et al: Neurofibrillary tangles but not senile plaques parallel duration and severity of Alzheimer's disease. Neurology 42:631–639, 1992

Berg L, McKeel DW, Miller P, et al: Neuropathological indexes of Alzheimer's disease in demented and nondemented persons aged 80 years and older. Arch Neurol 50:349–358, 1993

Boller F, Mizutani T, Roessmann U, et al: Parkinson disease, dementia, and Alzheimer disease: clinicopathological correlations. Ann Neurol 7:329–335, 1980

Braak H, Braak E: Neuropathological staging of Alzheimer-related changes. Acta Neuropathol 82:239–259, 1991

Braffman BH, Zimmerman RA, Trojanowski JQ, et al: Brain MR: pathologic correlation with gross and histopathology, 2: hyperintense white-matter foci in the elderly. Amer J Roentgenol 151:559–566, 1988

Chui HC, Victoroff JI, Margolin D, et al: Criteria for the diagnosis of ischemic vascular dementia proposed by the state of California Alzheimer's Disease Diagnostic and Treatment Centers. Neurology 42:473–480, 1992

Chui HC, Tierney M, Zarow C, et al: Neuropathologic diagnosis of Alzheimer disease: interrater reliability in the assessment of senile plaques and neurofibrillary tangles. Alzheimer Dis Assoc Disord 7:48–54, 1993

Corder EH, Saunders AM, Strittmatter WJ, et al: Gene dose of apolipoprotein E type 4 allele and the risk of Alzheimer's disease in late onset families. Science 261:921–923, 1993

Corder EH, Saunders AM, Risch NJ, et al: Protective effect of apolipoprotein E type 2 allele for late onset Alzheimer disease. Nat Genet 7:180–184, 1994

Couderc R, Mahieux F, Bailleul S: Response to letter by A. M. Saunders and Allen D. Roses (letter). Stroke 24:1416, 1993

DeKosky ST, Scheff SW: Synapse loss in frontal cortex biopsies in Alzheimer's disease: correlation with cognitive severity. Ann Neurol 27:457–464, 1990

Dickson DW, Farlo J, Davies P, et al: Alzheimer's disease: a double-labeling immunohistochemical study of senile plaques. Am J Pathol 132:86–101, 1988

Dickson DW, Ruan D, Crystal H, et al: Hippocampal degeneration differentiates diffuse Lewy body disease (DLBD) from Alzheimer's disease. Neurology 41:1402–1409, 1991

Dickson DW, Schmidt ML, Lee VM-Y, et al: Immunoreactivity profile of hippocampal CA2/3 neurites in diffuse Lewy body disease. Acta Neuropathol 87: 269–276, 1994

Ditter SM, Mirra SS: Neuropathological and clinical features of Parkinson's disease in Alzheimer's disease patients. Neurology 37:754–760, 1987

Drachman DA: New criteria for the diagnosis of vascular dementia: do we know enough yet? (editorial). Neurology 43:243–245, 1993

Duykaerts C, Delaere P, Hauw J-J, et al: Rating of the lesions in senile dementia of the Alzheimer type: concordance between laboratories. J Neurol Sci 97: 295–323, 1990

Erkinjuntti T, Hachinski VC: Rethinking vascular dementia. Cerebrovascular Disease 3:3–23, 1993

Fazekas F, Kleinert R, Offenbacher H, et al: Pathologic correlates of incidental MRI white matter signal intensities. Neurology 43:1683–1689, 1993

Frisoni GB, Bianchetti A, Govoni S, et al: Association of apolipoprotein E E4 with vascular dementia (letter). JAMA 7:1317, 1994

Gearing M, Wilson RW, Unger ER, et al: Amyloid precursor protein (APP) in the striatum in Alzheimer's disease: an immunohistochemical study. J Neuropathol Exp Neurol 52:22–30, 1993

Gearing M, Rebeck W, Hyman BT, et al: Neuropathology of aged chimpanzees and apolipoprotein E: implications for Alzheimer's disease. Proc Natl Acad Sci U S A 91:9382–9386, 1994

Gearing M, Mirra SS, Hansen LA, et al: Neuropathology confirmation of the clinical diagnosis of Alzheimer's disease: CERAD (Consortium to Establish a Registry for Alzheimer's Disease) Part X. Neurology 45:461–466, 1995

Grafton ST, Sumi SM, Stimac GK, et al: Comparison of postmortem magnetic resonance imaging and neuropathologic findings in the cerebral white matter. Arch Neurol 48:293–298, 1991

Hansen LA, Crain BJ: Making the diagnosis of mixed and non-Alzheimer's dementias. Arch Pathol Lab Med 119:1023–1031, 1995

Hansen LA, Masliah E, Terry RD, et al: A neuropathological subset of Alzheimer's disease with concomitant Lewy body disease and spongiform change. Acta Neuropathol 78:194–201, 1989

Hansen LA, Masliah E, Galasko D, et al: Plaque-only Alzheimer disease is usually the Lewy body variant, and vice versa. J Neuropathol Exp Neurol 52:648–654, 1993

Hyman BT, Marzloff K, Arriagada PV: The lack of accumulation of senile plaques or amyloid burden in Alzheimer's disease suggests a dynamic balance between amyloid deposition and resolution. J Neuropathol Exp Neurol 52:594–600, 1993

Joachim CL, Morris JH, Selkoe DJ: Diffuse senile plaques occur commonly in the cerebellum in Alzheimer's disease. Am J Pathol 135:309–319, 1989

Kazee AM, Eskin TA, Lapham LW, et al: Clinicopathologic correlates in Alzheimer disease: assessment of clinical and pathologic diagnostic criteria. Alzheimer Dis Assoc Disord 7:152–164, 1993

Khachaturian ZS: Diagnosis of Alzheimer's disease. Arch Neurol 42:1097–1105, 1985

Kim H, Gearing M, Mirra SS: Ubiquitin immunoreactive CA2-3 neurites in hippocampus coexist with cortical Lewy bodies. Neurology 45:1768–1770, 1995

Kirkpatrick JB, Hayman LA: White-matter lesions in MR imaging of clinically healthy brains of elderly subjects: possible pathologic basis. Radiology 162:509–511, 1987

Koller WC: How accurately can Parkinson's disease be diagnosed? Neurology 42:6–16, 1992

Larson EB: Illnesses causing dementia in the very elderly (editorial). N Engl J Med 328:203–205, 1993

Liston E, LaRue A: Clinical differentiation of primary degenerative and multi-infarct dementia: a critical review of the evidence, II: pathological studies. Biol Psychol 18:1467–1484, 1983

Maestre G, Ottman R, Stern Y, et al: Apolipoprotein E and Alzheimer's disease: ethnic variation in genotypic risks. Ann Neurol 37:254–259, 1995

Mann DMA, Jones D: Deposition of amyloid (A4) protein within the brains of persons with dementing disorders other than Alzheimer's disease and Down's syndrome. Neurosci Lett 109:68–75, 1990

Mayeux R, Denaro J, Hemenegildo N, et al: A population-based investigation of Parkinson's disease with and without dementia. Relationship to age and gender. Arch Neurol 49:492–497, 1992

McKeel DW Jr, Ball MJ, Price JL, et al: Interlaboratory histopathological assessment of Alzheimer neuropathology: different methodologies yield comparable diagnostic results. Alzheimer Dis Assoc Disord 7:121–131, 1993

McKeith IG, Fairbairn AF, Bothwell RA, et al: An evaluation of the predictive validity and inter-rater reliability of clinical diagnostic criteria for senile dementia of Lewy body type. Neurology 44:872–877, 1994

McKhann G, Drachman D, Folstein M, et al: Clinical diagnosis of Alzheimer's disease: report of the NINCDS-ADRDA Work Group under the auspices of the Department of Health and Human Services Task Force on Alzheimer's disease. Neurology 34:939–944, 1984

Mendez MF, Mastri AR, Sung JH, et al: Clinically diagnosed Alzheimer disease: neuropathologic findings in 650 cases. Alzheimer Dis Assoc Disord 6:35–43, 1992

Mirra SS, Heyman A, McKeel D, et al: The Consortium to Establish a Registry for Alzheimer's Disease (CERAD), II: standardization of the neuropathological assessment of Alzheimer's disease. Neurology 41:479–486, 1991

Mirra SS, Hart MN, Terry RD: Making the diagnosis of Alzheimer's disease: a primer for practicing pathologists. Arch Pathol Lab Med 117:132–144, 1993

Mirra SS, Gearing M, Hughes J, et al: Inter-laboratory comparison of neuropathology assessments in Alzheimer's disease: a multicenter study of the Consortium to Establish a Registry for Alzheimer's Disease (CERAD). Erratum in J Neuropathol Exp Neurol 53:305–315, 1995

Namba Y, Tomonaga M, Kawasaki H, et al: Apolipoprotein E immunoreactivity in cerebral amyloid deposits and neurofibrillary tangles in Alzheimer's disease. Brain Res 541:163–166, 1991

Pericak-Vance MA, Bebout JL, Gaskell PC, et al: Linkage studies in familial Alzheimer disease: evidence for chromosome 19 linkage. Am J Hum Genet 48:1034–1050, 1991

Poduri A, Gearing M, Rebeck GW, et al: Apolipoprotein ε4 and beta-amyloid in senile plaques and cerebral blood vessels of aged rhesus monkeys. Am J Pathol 144:1183–1187, 1994

Poirier J, Davignon J, Bouthillier D, et al: Apolipoprotein E polymorphism and Alzheimer's disease. Lancet 342:697–699, 1993

Rebeck GW, Reiter JS, Strickland DK, et al: Apolipoprotein E in sporadic Alzheimer's disease: allelic variation and receptor interactions. Neuron 11:575–580, 1993

Roman GC, Tatemichi TK, Erkinjuntti T, et al: Vascular dementia: diagnostic criteria for research studies: report of the NINDS-AIREN International Workshop. Neurology 43:250–260, 1993

Saunders AM, Roses AD: Apolipoprotein E4 allele frequency, ischemic cerebrovascular disease, and Alzheimer's disease (letter). Stroke 24:1416–1417, 1993

Scheff SW, Sparks DL, Price DA: Quantitative assessment of synaptic density in the entorhinal cortex in Alzheimer's disease. Ann Neurol 34:356–361, 1993

Schmechel DE, Saunders AM, Strittmatter WJ, et al: Increased amyloid β-peptide deposition in cerebral cortex as a consequence of apolipoprotein E genotype in late-onset Alzheimer disease. Proc Natl Acad Sci U S A 90:9649–9653, 1993

Schneider JA, Gearing M, de l'Aune W, et al: The apolipoprotein E e4 allele in diverse neurodegenerative disorders. Ann Neurol 38:131–135, 1995

Standaert DG, Lee VM-Y, Greenberg BD, et al: Molecular features of hypothalamic plaques in Alzheimer's disease. Am J Pathol 139:681–691, 1991

Strittmatter WJ, Saunders AM, Schmechel D, et al: Apolipoprotein E: high-avidity binding to β-amyloid and increased frequency of type 4 allele in late-onset familial Alzheimer disease. Proc Natl Acad Sci U S A 90:1977–1981, 1993

Strittmatter WJ, Saunders AM, Goedert M, et al: Isoform-specific interactions of apolipoprotein E with microtubule-associated protein tau: implications for Alzheimer's disease. Proc Natl Acad Sci U S A 91:11183–11186, 1994

Sudarsky L, Morris J, Romero J, et al: Dementia in Parkinson's disease: the problem of clinicopathological correlation. J Neuropsychiatry Clin Neurosci 1: 159–166, 1989

Talbot C, Lendon C, Craddock N, et al: Protection against Alzheimer's disease with apoE e2 (letter). Lancet 343:1432–1433, 1994

Terry RD: Synaptic plasticity in Alzheimer's disease (editorial). Ann Neurol 34:321, 1993

Terry RD, Masliah E, Salmon DP, et al: Physical basis of cognitive alterations in Alzheimer's disease: synapse loss in the major correlate of cognitive impairment. Ann Neurol 30:572–580, 1991

Tierney MC, Fisher RH, Lewis AJ, et al: The NINCDS-ADRDA Work Group criteria for the clinical diagnosis of probable Alzheimer's disease: a clinicopathologic study of 57 cases. Neurology 38:359–364, 1988

Whitehouse PJ: Autopsy (editorial). Gerontologist 33:436–439, 1993

Wisniewski HM, Rabe A, Zigman W, et al: Neuropathological diagnosis of Alzheimer disease (editorial). J Neuropathol Exp Neurol 48:606–609, 1989

Wisniewski T, Golabek A, Matsubara E, et al: Apolipoprotein E: binding to soluble Alzheimer's β-amyloid. Biochem Biophys Res Commun 193:359–365, 1993

Chapter 4

Multimodal In Vivo Brain Imaging in Alzheimer's Disease

Diagnosis, Characteristics, and Mechanisms

Stanley I. Rapoport, M.D.

———◆———

Before the introduction of in vivo brain imaging, information about metabolic and anatomic brain abnormalities that underlie the signs and symptoms of Alzheimer's disease in a given individual, as well as diagnostic accuracy for Alzheimer's disease and other dementias, was limited. Indeed, structural imaging in the form of computed tomography (CT), which was introduced just 20 years ago (Hounsfield 1973), was accompanied by an increase in diagnostic accuracy for Alzheimer's disease from 43% to more than 70% (Boller et al. 1989).

With regard to functional imaging, a low-resolution ^{133}Xe clearance technique first established a relationship between reduced regional cerebral blood flow (rCBF) and dementia severity in Alzheimer's disease (Hagberg and Ingvar 1976). This procedure was replaced in the early 1980s by the more quantitative and higher-resolution positron-emission tomography (PET), which provided values for rCBF, regional cerebral metabolic rates for glucose ($rCMR_{glc}$) and for O_2 ($rCMRO_2$), and regional oxygen extraction fractions (rOEF) in Alzheimer's disease (Duara et al. 1986; Frackowiak et al. 1981; Malison et al. 1994). Researchers also have used PET to examine blood-brain barrier integrity, dopamine metabolism, and receptor density in the brains of Alzheimer's disease patients (Mueller-Gaertner et al. 1991; Nordberg et al. 1992; Schlageter et al. 1987; Tyrrell et al. 1990).

Researchers also use single photon emission computed tomography (SPECT) to study Alzheimer's disease. SPECT is a semiquantitative imaging tool that is less expensive and more readily available than PET (Holman et al. 1991; Malison et al. 1994).

In vivo brain imaging is especially informative in relation to cognitive profiles of Alzheimer's disease patients. Imaging with PET, for example, has demonstrated that resting-state metabolic reductions in specific neocortical areas predict and reflect altered neuropsychological abilities that appear to be subserved by these areas (Haxby et al. 1985, 1988, 1990). Investigators must take individual profiles into account because Alzheimer's disease is heterogeneous with regard to the severity and pattern of neuropsychological deficits (Haxby et al. 1992; Mayeux et al. 1985), as well as with regard to genetic factors involving chromosomes 14, 19, or 21 (Small et al. 1995; van Broeckhoven 1995).

Quantifying dementia severity—for example, through scores on the Mini-Mental State Exam (MMSE) (Folstein et al. 1975)—is important in studies of Alzheimer's disease. Table 4–1 presents comparisons of mean cognitive profiles for mild or moderate dementia severity (Haxby et al. 1990). Patients with moderate dementia had significantly reduced mean scores on each neuropsychological test, whereas patients with mild dementia had reduced mean scores only on measures of memory, attention, and planning.

Computed Tomography and Magnetic Resonance Imaging

Quantitative Volumetric Imaging

Computed tomography.   Cross-sectional CT measurements cannot reliably distinguish Alzheimer's disease patients with mild or moderate dementia from healthy, age-matched control subjects when causes of dementia other than Alzheimer's disease are excluded (DeCarli et al. 1990; Luxenberg et al. 1986). This lack of sensitivity largely reflects a marked similarity of brain atrophy between Alzheimer's disease patients and

Table 4–1.   Cognitive profiles for Alzheimer's disease patients with mild or moderate dementia

Neuropsychological test	Control subjects (*n* = 21–29)	Mild Alzheimer's disease (*n* = 11)	Moderate Alzheimer's disease (*n* = 13)
Omnibus tests			
Wechsler Adult			
Intelligence Scale			
Full-scale IQ	126 ± 10	117 ± 8	92 ± 17[a]
Deviation quotients			
Verbal comprehension	129 ± 10	123 ± 9	102 ± 17[a]
Memory and			
distractibility	116 ± 13	113 ± 8	9 ± 15[a]
Perceptual			
organization	119 ± 13	109 ± 13	84 ± 26[a]
Memory			
Wechsler Memory Scale			
Immediate story recall	22 ± 15	11 ± 5[a]	5 ± 3[a]
Immediate figure recall	10 ± 3	7 ± 4[b]	1 ± 2[a]
Delayed story recall	17 ± 5	2 ± 4[a]	1 ± 1[a]
Delayed figure recall	7 ± 3	1 ± 1[a]	0 ± 1[a]
Attention, planning,			
and abstract reasoning			
Trailmaking (trail A)	40 ± 17	54 ± 30	153 ± 98[a]
Trailmaking (trail B)	82 ± 40	192 ± 155[b]	428 ± 139[a]
Stroop color-word			
interference, no/45s	37 ± 8	24 ± 8[b]	12 ± 8[a]
Porteus mazes, age in			
years	15.4 ± 1.6	12.8 ± 3.9	7.7 ± 3.8[a]
Language			
Syntax comprehension	24 ± 2	23 ± 2	17 ± 5[a]
Controlled word			
association	42 ± 2	34 ± 13	25 ± 12[a]
Boston naming	37 ± 4	35 ± 7	25 ± 8[a]
Visuospatial function			
Extended range drawing	21 ± 2	19 ± 4	13 ± 5[a]
Hiskey-Nebraska block			
patterns	15 ± 4	11 ± 5	4 ± 3[a]
Benton facial recognition	44 ± 4	42 ± 5	9 ± 5[b]

Note.   Neuropsychological tests classified by cognitive sphere they are considered to evaluate.
[a]Mean ± SD differs from control mean (*P* < .001).
[b]Mean ± SD differs from control mean (*P* < .05).
Source.   Haxby JV, Grady CL, Koss E, et al: "Longitudinal Study of Cerebral Metabolic Asymmetries and Associated Neuropsychological Patterns in Early Dementia of the Alzheimer Type." *Archives of Neurolology* 47:753–760, 1990.

healthy elderly individuals (Creasey et al. 1986; Drayer 1988; Kaye et al. 1992). Nevertheless, mean differences obtained with cross-sectional CT have confirmed that brain atrophy—implying neuronal loss—characterizes Alzheimer's disease. Patients with Alzheimer's disease have statistically significant reductions in mean gray-matter volume and mean gray-matter/white-matter volume ratio and increases in lateral ventricular volume, in relation to dementia severity (Creasey et al. 1986).

Longitudinal morphometric studies have demonstrated progressive brain atrophy in Alzheimer's disease. In one study, the mean rate of enlargement of lateral ventricular volume on CT (cm^3/year) completely separated a group of 12 men with Alzheimer's disease (including 8 with mild dementia) examined during a mean interval of 1.4 years from control subjects examined during a mean interval of 3.3 years (Luxenberg et al. 1987). In addition, rates of enlargement in individual patients correlated with rates of decline on a composite neuropsychological test battery. In a follow-up study (DeCarli et al. 1992), the rate of lateral ventricular enlargement differed significantly between patients and control subjects—with a 94% specificity (ability to make a correct positive diagnosis) and a 90% sensitivity (ability to correctly exclude Alzheimer's disease). The diagnostic power of volumetric measurements from two CT scans taken 1 year apart was only 33% in patients with mild dementia, however.

Magnetic resonance imaging (MRI).   The limitations of CT include low spatial resolution and low tissue contrast differences as well as artifactual elevation of brain density adjacent to the skull ("bone hardening artifact"), which renders CT unreliable for quantifying subarachnoid cerebrospinal fluid (CSF) and cortical atrophy. MRI can overcome some of these limitations because it requires no ionizing radiation, repeated measures carry no known risk, and images are free of bone-hardening artifacts (although MRI scans do contain spectral inhomogeneities) (Drayer 1988; Murphy et al. 1993b). MRI—but not CT—can quantify lobar and cortical atrophy as well as volumes of CSF. Diagnosticians should use MRI, which is more costly than CT, only when CT is inadequate for diagnosis.

A cross-sectional volumetric CT study of the brain demonstrated no significant difference between Alzheimer's disease patients with mild dementia and control subjects (Creasey et al. 1986). A comparable cross-sectional MRI study, however, showed that Alzheimer's disease patients with mild dementia had smaller mean cerebral brain matter and temporal lobe volumes and larger volumes of lateral ventricles and temporal lobe CSF than control subjects (Murphy et al. 1993b)—suggesting that MRI is more sensitive than CT for early diagnosis.

Discriminant analysis is a statistical procedure involving a linear combination of observed variables that best describes group differences and can classify group membership of any individual. A discriminant analysis applied to MRI volumetric data distinguished each of 31 Alzheimer's disease patients with mild dementia from sex- and age-matched control subjects (DeCarli et al. 1995b). Age and brain volume were the most significant discriminators for men, whereas temporal lobe and CSF volumes were most significant for women. In this study, 10 patients had a diagnosis of "possible" Alzheimer's disease, with impaired memory as the only apparent cognitive deficit; a discriminant analysis using volumetric MRI variables may add diagnostic certainty in "possible" Alzheimer's disease patients with mild dementia using NINCDS-ADRDA (National Institute of Communicative Disorders and Stroke-Alzheimer's Disease and Related Disorders Association) criteria (McKhann et al. 1984).

CT and MRI Densities to Distinguish Alzheimer's Disease From Vascular Dementia

Distinguishing vascular dementia from Alzheimer's disease is crucial in diagnosis. Boller et al. (1989) reported on 2,143 patients with a diagnosis of Alzheimer's disease and/or vascular dementia with 15% pathological confirmation; of these 2,143 patients, 51% had a diagnosis of Alzheimer's disease alone, 23% had vascular dementia alone, and 15% had Alzheimer's disease plus cerebrovascular disease. Thus, vascular disease contributed to 38% of reported dementias.

Causes of vascular dementia include arteriosclerotic encephalopathy (lacunar state, multiple small infarcts, large cerebral infarcts), hypertensive arteriosclerosis (including mixed cortical and subcortical leukoencephalopathy of Binswanger), and congophilic angiopathy (Chui et al. 1992; Jellinger 1976). In subcortical disease (leukoencephalopathy), CT and T_2-weighted MRI images demonstrate periventricular and deep white-matter changes, referred to as *leukoaraiosis*. To date, however, investigators have not formally incorporated diagnostic criteria to distinguish vascular dementia from Alzheimer's disease into neuroimaging, although published studies demonstrate that such criteria can be helpful (Chui et al. 1992; McKhann et al. 1984; Rosen et al. 1980).

The relationship between white-matter hyperintensities on CT or MRI images and cognitive or brain metabolic function is unclear. Studies indicate that 30%–80% of elderly individuals without neurological symptoms have focal density abnormalities in cerebral white matter; the frequency of these abnormalities increases with systolic blood pressure (Chui et al. 1992). Such abnormalities may include small focal or confluent areas of increased signal intensity on T_2-weighted MRI images, which demonstrate them more frequently than CT images (Drayer 1988)

In one study, cognitive testing failed to demonstrate differences between healthy elderly adults with and without white-matter hyperintensities (Almkvist et al. 1992). In another study, leukoencephalopathy on MRI images in normotensive healthy subjects ages 19–91 years correlated with increased lateral ventricular volume, reduced brain volume, reduced cognitive scores, lower whole brain and frontal lobe glucose metabolism, and decreased systolic blood pressure (DeCarli et al. 1995a). These findings strongly suggest that leukoencephalopathy represents significant neuropathologicity that adds to the Alzheimer's disease insult.

Kozachuk et al. (1990) found that prevalence of grade 2–3 white-matter abnormalities in elderly normotensive control subjects (17%) was statistically the same as in normotensive Alzheimer's disease patients (27%). At autopsy, three normotensive Alzheimer's disease patients with leukoencephalopathy in life demonstrated, in addition to the senile plaques and tangles of Alzheimer's disease, extensive myelin pallor in the distributions of white-matter hyperintensities (DeCarli et al., unpublished data). In each patient, Congo-red staining revealed striking amyloid deposition (amyloid angiopathy) in meningeal and cerebral perforating arteries but normal-appearing arteries in white matter and lenticulostriate vasculature; there was no evidence of hypertensive lipohyalinosis or atherosclerosis in these vessels. Thus, white-matter changes in normotensive Alzheimer's disease patients may reflect the amyloid angiography that frequently appears in the brains of patients with Alzheimer's disease (which is severe in 30% of cases).

Grading of white-matter lesions on MRI images to distinguish Alzheimer's disease from vascular dementia has had limited success. In one study, the extent of periventricular lesions could not distinguish the two conditions; scores of subcortical lesions, although somewhat better, showed too much overlap to be useful (Bowen et al. 1990). Forty percent of Alzheimer's disease patients did not have subcortical white-matter changes, whereas such changes were present in all vascular dementia patients. In another study, vascular dementia patients had more frequent infarcts and lacunae ($P < .001$) and focal signal hyperintensities ($P < .05$)

in the basal ganglia and thalamus than Alzheimer's disease patients (Lechner and Bertha 1991).

Magnetic Resonance Spectroscopy

In vivo magnetic resonance spectroscopy (MRS) produces spectra of relatively weak magnetic signals from phosphorus, carbon, or nonwater hydrogen nuclei (the signals are weak because of the small concentrations of these nuclei). These spectra provide information about chemical compounds and the energy state within the brain; they can be localized to specific brain regions (Shulman et al. 1993).

Phosphomonoesters (e.g., phosphoethanolamine and phosphocholine) are considered anabolic precursors of membrane phospholipids, whereas phosphodiesters (e.g., glycerol-3-phospho-ethanolamine and glycerol-3-phosphocholine) represent catabolic products from the breakdown of phospholipids (Pettegrew et al. 1988). Using in vivo ^{31}P MRS, Brown et al. (1989) found that Alzheimer's disease patients had larger-than-normal concentrations of phosphomonoesters in the temporoparietal cortex. This observation, along with postmortem evidence that phosphomonoesters and phosphodiesters were abnormal in the brains of patients with Alzheimer's disease (Pettegrew et al. 1988; Smith et al. 1993), suggests that regenerative processes involving phospholipids occur early in Alzheimer's disease, whereas degenerative processes occur later on. Brown et al. (1989) also reported that the phosphocreatine-to-inorganic phosphorus ratio distinguished patients with Alzheimer's disease from vascular dementia patients. A subsequent in vivo ^{31}P MRS study also indicated increased concentrations of phosphomonoesters in Alzheimer's disease (Cuenod et al. 1995).

Other findings also suggest disturbed phospholipid metabolism in Alzheimer's disease. For example, a study with ^{1}H MRS found a 50% increase in the concentration of myoinositol in the parietal and occipital cortices of Alzheimer's disease patients, compared with control subjects, but an 11% decrease in the concentration of the neuronal marker N-acetylaspartate (Moats et al. 1994). Because myoinositol is part of phosphatidylinositol and participates in the phosphatidylinositide cycle during signal transduction (Berridge and Irvine 1984), its increased brain concentration may reflect accelerated breakdown of phosphatidylinositol. Additional evidence for abnormal phospholipid metabolism in Alzheimer's disease includes reduced critical temperature for membrane lipid stability in association but not in primary neocortical areas of post-mortem Alzheimer's disease brains (Ginsberg et al. 1993). This defect may be related to a deficiency of the phospholipid ethanolamine plasmalogen (Ginsberg et al. 1992, 1995); it suggests instability of neuronal membranes.

However, one study that used ^{31}P MRS to quantitate phosphorus metabolites with internal standards in large areas of the brain found no significant difference between Alzheimer's disease patients and control subjects in absolute concentrations of adenosine triphosphate, phosphocreatine, inorganic phosphate, phosphomonoesters, or phosphodiesters (Murphy et al. 1993a). Furthermore, neither absolute concentration nor concentration ratio in Alzheimer's disease was related to dementia severity or to $rCMR_{glc}$ (as measured independently with PET). The researchers concluded that reduced $rCMR_{glc}$ in Alzheimer's disease (see "PET Methods") was unrelated to rate-limited delivery of glucose or oxygen to the brain and that normal levels of high-energy phosphorus metabolites are maintained even with severe dementia. MRS study using these quantitative methods but localized only to the association neocortex would be necessary to determine conclusively whether abnormal phosphorus metabolism can be demonstrated in vivo in Alzheimer's disease.

Functional Imaging: Positron-Emission Tomography

PET Methods

With PET, a positron-emitting compound that is administered intravenously is taken up by the brain, where it releases positrons (positively charged electrons). These positrons collide with electrons and are annihilated, releasing two gamma rays at 180° to each other. Radiation detectors surrounding the head identify by coincidence counting the quantities and locations of radioactivity within the brain. Researchers have used ^{18}F-2-fluoro-2-deoxy-D-glucose (^{18}F-FDG; radioactive half-life of ^{18}F = 110 minutes) or ^{11}C-deoxy-D-glucose (^{11}C-DG; radioactive half-life of ^{11}C = 20 minutes) to measure $rCMR_{glc}$ with PET, whereas $H_2^{15}O$ and $^{15}O_2$ or ^{15}O-CO_2 (radioactive half-life of ^{15}O = 2.03 minutes) have generated $rCMRO_2$ and rCBF images, respectively.

In the absence of acute functional activation or an acute pathological condition, rCBF generally is proportional (coupled) to $rCMR_{glc}$ and

$rCMRO_2$, with a stoichiometry of 5.0 to 6.0 between $rCMRO_2$ and $rCMR_{glc}$ (Raichle et al. 1976; Sokoloff 1989). Fox et al. (1988) reported that during focal transient activation, coupling was maintained between rCBF and $rCMR_{glc}$ but disrupted between each of these measures and $rCMRO_2$—implying glycolytic metabolism at the expense of oxidative metabolism of glucose.

Other investigators, however, have argued cogently that the PET model used to determine $rCMRO_2$ during functional activation (Mintun et al. 1984) was oversimplified and was based on steady-state assumptions, whereas transient functional changes do not occur at a steady state (Sokoloff 1992). This line of reasoning concludes that coupling among rCBF, $rCMR_{glc}$, and $rCMRO_2$ (stoichiometry of 5.0 to 6.0) is maintained even during functional activation, although transient dissociation between the time courses of glycolytic and respiratory responses is likely.

Resting Cerebral Metabolism in Alzheimer's Disease

Data from more than 20 cross-sectional PET studies have demonstrated reductions in resting-state metabolism or rCBF throughout the neocortex in Alzheimer's disease patients—more so in association areas than in primary areas (Rapoport 1991). These reductions were more severe in relation to dementia severity—ranging from –17% in the prefrontal association cortex of patients with mild dementia to –54% in the parietal association cortex of patients with severe dementia. Reductions in frontal association cortex correlated with atrophy of the anterior corpus callosum on MRI images, whereas those in the parietal-occipital association cortex correlated with atrophy of the posterior corpus callosum (Yamauchi et al. 1993). These correlations suggest dropout in the cortical layer III pyramidal neurons that supply the myelinated fibers within the corpus callosum (Rapoport 1990).

Table 4–2 presents representative $rCMR_{glc}$ data on 47 carefully screened patients with Alzheimer's disease of differing dementia severity and 30 control subjects from the most complete study with a high-resolution multislice PET scanner (Kumar et al. 1991). With the exception of the caudate nucleus, mean metabolic rates even in Alzheimer's disease patients with mild dementia were significantly lower than in control subjects. Involvement of the posterior but not anterior cingulate cortex early in disease likely represents limbic dysfunction (Minoshima et al. 1994). At each level of dementia severity, $rCMR_{glc}$ was lower in association than primary neocortices or subcortical nuclei, consistent with reported gradients in neuropathology

Table 4–2. Glucose metabolism in Alzheimer's disease patients with differing dementia severity, in relation to metabolism in age-matched healthy control subjects

Region	Control subjects (n = 30)	Mild Alzheimer's disease (n = 17)	Moderate Alzheimer's disease (n = 19)	Severe Alzheimer's disease (n = 11)
Association neocortex				
Prefrontal	7.96 ± 1.09	6.59 ± 1.34(83)[a,b]	6.22 ± 1.40(78)[b]	4.69 ± 1.64(59)[b]
Premotor	8.69 ± 1.16	6.90 ± 1.46(79)[b]	6.26 ± 1.43(72)[b]	4.70 ± 1.74(54)[b]
Parietal	8.27 ± 1.13	6.09 ± 1.37(74)[b]	5.36 ± 1.28(65)[b]	3.83 ± 1.46(46)[b]
Temporal	7.53 ± 0.79	5.98 ± 0.91(79)[b]	5.63 ± 1.23(75)[b]	3.97 ± 1.28(52)[b]
Occipital	7.72 ± 0.94	6.65 ± 1.28(86)[b]	6.13 ± 1.23(79)[b]	5.00 + 1.83(65)[b]
Allocortex				
Anterior cingulate	7.72 ± 1.24	6.71 ± 1.15(87)	6.53 ± 1.41(85)[b]	5.38 ± 1.72(80)[b]
Primary neocortex				
Sensorimotor	8.31 ± 1.00	7.27 ± 1.03(87)[b]	6.75 ± 1.14(82)[b]	5.61 ± 1.71(68)[b]
Calcarine	8.06 ± 1.12	7.02 ± 1.09(87)[b]	7.09 ± 1.12(88)[b]	6.52 ± 1.89(81)[b]
Subcortical nuclei				
Caudate	9.24 ± 1.64	8.35 ± 1.26(90)	7.72 ± 1.87(84)[b]	6.45 ± 1.21(70)[b]
Lenticular	9.41 ± 1.37	8.76 ± 1.45(93)[b]	8.71 ± 1.85(93)[b]	6.87 ± 1.48(73)[b]
Thalamus	8.99 ± 1.37	8.27 ± 1.46(92)[b]	8.15 ± 0.94(91)[b]	6.42 ± 2.05(71)[b]

Note. Numbers reflect rCMR$_{glc}$ (mg/100 g/minute).
[a]Mean ± SD (% of control mean)
[b]Differs significantly from control mean ($P < .05$), corrected for six comparisons.
Source. Kumar A, Schapiro MB, Grady C, et al: "High-Resolution PET Studies in Alzheimer's Disease." *Neuropsychopharmacology* 4:35–46, 1991.

(Lewis et al. 1987). Figure 4–1 illustrates that the association neocortex is metabolically spared relative to the primary neocortex and subcortical basal ganglia and thalamic regions, regardless of the pattern of metabolic deficits in Alzheimer's disease.

In patients with dementia found at autopsy to have Alzheimer's disease, neurofibrillary tangle densities were common in cortical association areas that had the greatest reductions in $rCMR_{glc}$ before death but were much less common in primary cortical areas (DeCarli et al. 1992). This correlation was consistent with other reports on gradients of tangle distribution and atrophy associated with loss of layer III and layer V pyramidal neurons in the neocortex in Alzheimer's disease (Rapoport 1988, 1991) and with a report that atrophy of the corpus callosum—reflecting dropout of axons from layer III pyramidal neurons—correlated with appropriate cortical reductions in $rCMR_{glc}$ (Yamauchi et al. 1993). Because cortical atrophy in Alzheimer's disease may artificially reduce PET metabolic values as a result of partial voluming, future PET studies will have to

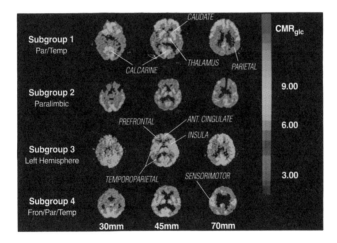

Figure 4–1.   PET scan images from four Alzheimer's disease patients that best characterize four independent subgroups of metabolic patterns ($rCMR_{glc}$ scale in mg/ 100 g/minutes). Three planes are shown for each subject: left, at level of orbitofrontal cortex 30 mm above inferior orbitomeatal (IOM) line; middle, at level of basal ganglia 45 mm above IOM line; right, at level of centrum ovale 70 mm above IOM line. *Source.*   Grady CL, Haxby JV, Schapiro MB, et al: "Subgroups in Dementia of the Alzheimer Type Identified Using Positron Emission Tomography." *Journal of Neuropsychiatry and Clinical Neurosciences* 2:373–384, 1990.

include anatomic registration to obtain true estimates of cortical metabolism or flow per gram tissue (Lim et al. 1994; Malison et al. 1994).

A discriminant function of PET-derived $rCMR_{glc}$ values in frontal and parietal association areas correctly identified 87% of Alzheimer's disease patients with mild to moderate dementia and control subjects (Azari et al. 1993). Thus, this function converted a "possible" to a "probable" Alzheimer's disease diagnosis in patients with mild dementia. It also identified one individual with isolated memory impairment and a family history of autosomal dominant Alzheimer's disease, whose PET scan had normal absolute and ratio values of $rCMR_{glc}$ (Pietrini et al. 1993). This patient subsequently developed severe dementia and reduced parietal $rCMR_{glc}$.

Kennedy et al. (1995) reported that focal reductions in parietotemporal $rCMR_{glc}$ identified asymptomatic, at-risk individuals from Alzheimer's disease families, whereas Small et al. (1995) used hypometabolism and left-right metabolic asymmetries to identify at-risk patients who had mild memory complaints, at least two relatives with Alzheimer's disease, and the apolipoprotein type ε4 allele coded by a gene on chromosome 19. This allele occurs more frequently in late-onset Alzheimer's disease families, as well as in sporadic cases (Corder et al. 1993). Each of these reports was cross-sectional, and the second may have included symptomatic patients; thus, they do not conclusively determine if abnormal PET patterns in completely unaffected (no memory complaints) but at-risk individuals exist. Longitudinal studies would help to clarify this issue.

In this regard, longitudinal studies on older Down's syndrome (trisomy 21) patients with no dementia may be useful. Down's syndrome patients older than 40 years often develop the neuropathology of Alzheimer's disease and frequently exhibit dementia; the age at onset of their dementia is earlier if they have the apolipoprotein type ε4 allele than if they do not (Schapiro et al. 1988, 1995). Other studies assessed two older Down's syndrome patients (initially ages 49 and 50 years) with PET repeatedly over 8 years (Dani et al. 1995; Schapiro et al. 1989). Before the appearance of dementia—in the sixth year in each case— $rCMR_{glc}$ in parietotemporal areas remained stable or declined slowly, whereas memory scores fell significantly. Only when overt dementia appeared did $rCMR_{glc}$ begin to decline sharply, in association with progressive ventricular dilatation. Thus, memory defects precede neocortical reductions in brain metabolism and brain atrophy in this model for Alzheimer's disease.

Can PET distinguish Alzheimer's disease from vascular dementia?   Independent of clinical history and evaluation of CT or MRI, PET—like

SPECT (see "SPECT in Alzheimer's Disease: Comparison With PET and Utility for Clinical Diagnosis")—cannot easily distinguish Alzheimer's disease from vascular dementia. Both syndromes demonstrate global reductions in brain metabolism and flow in relation to dementia severity (Frackowiak et al. 1981), as well as heterogeneity of cognitive and local metabolic deficits. Large asymmetric metabolic or flow reductions that correspond to CT or MRI abnormalities or reductions in the basal ganglia or thalamus suggest vascular dementia, whereas sparing of primary compared with association cortical areas suggests Alzheimer's disease (Benson et al. 1983).

Neither Alzheimer's disease nor vascular dementia is accompanied by elevated rOEF (Frackowiak et al. 1981; Fukuyama et al. 1994); rOEF may be elevated, however, before the appearance of dementia in some patients with leukoaraiosis and hypertension (a major risk factor for vascular dementia) (Yao et al. 1992)—suggesting that hypoperfusion may precede vascular dementia (O'Brien and Mallett 1970). Using PET, Kuwabara et al. (1992) demonstrated that the rCBF response to hypercapnia was normal in Alzheimer's disease but defective in vascular dementia of the Binswanger type.

Metabolic and Cognitive-Behavioral Correlations in Alzheimer's Disease

Group Patterns

As Figure 4–1 illustrates, a principal component analysis of high-resolution $rCMR_{glc}$ data from 16 regions of 36 Alzheimer's disease patients with mild to severe dementia identified four statistically significant patterns (Grady et al. 1990). The most common pattern (Group 1, 15 of 36 patients) entailed reduced $rCMR_{glc}$ in superior and inferior parietal lobules and the posterior medial temporal lobe. Group 2 (paralimbic) patients (8 of 36) had reduced metabolism in orbitofrontal and anterior cingulate gyri, whereas parietal regions were relatively spared. Group 3 patients (5 of 36) showed reduced left hemisphere metabolism; Group 4 patients (5 of 36) had reductions in frontal, parietal, and temporal cortices. In each group, the association neocortex was metabolically spared compared with the primary neocortex, thalamus, and caudate nucleus.

Each patient group had a characteristic neuropsychological-behavioral profile, consistent with the principle that a profile in an individual patient is related to the patient's pattern of brain metabolic deficits (Table 4–3).

Group 2 patients had poorer verbal performance and fluency but better visuospatial performance and spatial memory than Group 1 (parietal/temporal) patients. Group 3 patients (left hemisphere) had worse verbal memory, verbal fluency, and calculating ability but better visuoperceptual performance and drawing ability than Group 1 patients. Group 1 patients were likely to be depressed, whereas Group 4 patients tended to show inappropriate behavior and psychotic symptoms. Group 2 patients demonstrated agitation, inappropriate behavior, and personality change; those in Group 3 frequently had depressive symptoms (Grady et al. 1990).

Different PET metabolic patterns do not appear to be related to etiology in Alzheimer's disease. No relationship exists between metabolic asymmetry and early- or late-onset Alzheimer's disease (Grady et al. 1988), and PET cannot distinguish familial from sporadic Alzheimer's disease (Hoffman et al. 1989). Whereas biparietotemporal hypometabolism in the appropriate clinical setting indicates a high likelihood of Alzheimer's disease, it is not necessarily specific for this dementia. Schapiro et al. (1993), for example, reported this syndrome in a patient with clinical signs of slowly progressive dementia and Parkinson's disease whose autopsy showed pathological findings of Parkinson's disease only.

Table 4–3. Percentage of Alzheimer's disease patients in each subgroup (see Figure 4–1) showing behavioral disturbances

| | Subgroup | | | |
| | 1 | 2 | 3 | 4 |
Symptom	Parietal-temporal ($n = 15$)	Paralimbic ($n = 8$)	Left hemisphere ($n = 5$)	Frontal/parietal/temporal ($n = 5$)
Anxiety/agitation	13	25	20	20
Inappropriate behavior	7	25	0	40
Personality change	13	25	0	20
Depression	33	0	60	20
Psychosis	20	0	0	40
At least one symptom	67	50	60	100

Note. Numbers represent percent of subgroup. Subgroup is defined by predominant pattern of metabolic deficits.
Source. Adapted from Grady CL, Haxby JV, Schapiro MB: "Subgroups in Dementia of the Alzheimer Type Identified Using Positron Emission Tomography." *Journal of Neuropsychiatry and Clinical Neurosciences* 2:373–384, 1990.

Metabolic-Cognitive Correlations in Individual Patients

According to Haxby et al. (1990), extended-range drawing and visual recall tests reflect right neocortical function, and syntax comprehension and verbal recall tests reflect left neocortical function. This study ranked Alzheimer's disease patients and control subjects separately on these test scores and classified differences between ranks as "drawing/comprehension discrepancies" or "visual recall/verbal recall discrepancies" to reflect hemispheric functional asymmetry. They then correlated discrepancies with a metabolic asymmetry index (where $rCMR_{glc,right}$ is metabolic rate in a right hemisphere region and $rCMR_{glc,left}$ is the rate in the homologous left hemisphere region):

$$\text{Metabolic asymmetry index } (\%) = \frac{_rCMR_{glc,right} - {_r}CMR_{glc,left}}{_rCMR_{glc,right} + {_r}CMR_{glc,left}/2} \quad (1)$$

Figure 4–2 illustrates asymmetry indices for four association and two primary cortical areas for Alzheimer's disease patients with mild to severe

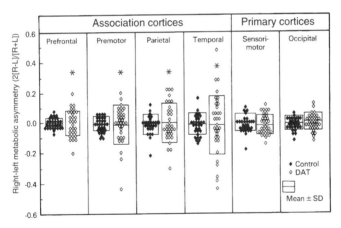

Figure 4–2. Right-left metabolic asymmetries [see equation (1)] in association and primary cortical regions in Alzheimer's disease patients with mild to severe dementia and control subjects (right, $rCMR_{glc,right}$; left, $rCMR_{glc,left}$); * = coefficient of variation differs from control value ($P < .05$). *Source.* High-resolution Scanditronix PC 1024-7B data from Haxby JV, Grady CL, Koss E, et al: "Longitudinal Study of Cerebral Metabolic Asymmetries and Associated Neuropsychological Patterns in Early Dementia of the Alzheimer Type." *Archives of Neurology* 47:753–760, 1990.

dementia and control subjects. Patients had significantly greater variances (SD^2) than control subjects in association but not in primary cortices. Distinct metabolic asymmetries were visually evident in PET scans of individual patients (Figure 4–1, Group 3).

Abnormal variances of metabolic asymmetry were present at each dementia severity (Table 4–4); the asymmetry correlated significantly and in expected directions with cognitive discrepancy in patients with moderate but not mild dementia (Table 4–5). In patients with moderate dementia, lower right-sided metabolism corresponded to worse drawing and visual recall test scores, compared with syntax comprehension and verbal recall test scores, respectively. The opposite was true for left-sided hypometabolism (Haxby et al. 1990).

PET scans of Alzheimer's disease patients frequently display gradients in metabolism between parietal and frontal lobes (Figure 4–1, Groups 1 and 3). Accordingly, Haxby et al. (1988) compared cognitive tests of parietal lobe function—such as the arithmetic subtest of the Wechsler Adult Intelligence Scale (WAIS), syntax comprehension test, extended-range drawing test, block-tapping span test—in terms of rank ordering and cognitive discrepancies (see above) with tests of prefrontal integrity—such as controlled word association (FAS) and trailmaking (trail A) tests. As Table 4–6 shows, statistically significant correlations in expected directions were evident between cognitive discrepancies and the parietal/prefrontal metabolic ratios in patients with moderate but not mild dementia.

Indeed, longitudinal PET studies of 11 Alzheimer's disease patients demonstrated retention of the initial direction of right/left metabolic asymmetry and parietal/frontal metabolic ratios for up to 4 years (Figure 4–3) (Grady et al. 1988). Likewise, Spearman correlations between initial and follow-up metabolic ratios at least 1.5 years later ranged from 0.67 to 0.86 ($P < .01$) (Haxby et al. 1988).

This consistency explains why metabolic asymmetries in Alzheimer's disease patients with mild dementia initially were significant predictors of expected cognitive discrepancies that appeared 1–3 years later (language worse with initial left-sided hypometabolism, visuospatial function worse with initial right-sided hypometabolism) and why parietal compared with frontal hypometabolism in patients with mild dementia more accurately predicted worst scores on cognitive tests of parietal than frontal integrity (Grady et al. 1988; Haxby et al. 1990). Thus, in Alzheimer's disease patients with mild dementia initially in whom the direction of metabolic asymmetry

Table 4–4. Right/left metabolic asymmetries [see equation (1)] in control subjects and in Alzheimer's disease patients with differing dementia severity

| | | Right/left metabolic asymmetries | | |
Brain regions	Control subjects (n = 31)	Mild Alzheimer's disease (n = 11)	Moderate Alzheimer's disease (n = 13)	Severe Alzheimer's disease (n = 8)
Association cortex				
Prefrontal	.01 ± .03	−.01 ± .07[a]	−.01 ± .08[b]	.05 ± .10[b]
Premotor	.01 ± .05	−.01 ± .10[c]	−.02 ± .16[b]	.05 ± .11[c]
Orbitofrontal	−.01 ± .06	−.03 ± .08	−.03 ± .11[c]	.00 ± .11[a]
Parietal	−.01 ± .06	−.01 ± .11[a]	−.03 ± .13[c]	.08 ± .13[a]
Lateral temporal	−.01 ± .07	−.05 ± .17[b]	−.03 ± .18[b]	.08 ± .23[b]
Primary cortex				
Sensorimotor	−.02 ± .05	−.01 ± .07	.00 ± .06	.01 ± .06
Occipital[d]	−.01 ± .04	.00 ± .05	−.01 ± .03	.03 ± .08[a]

Note. Values are means ± SD (number of subjects)
[a]Variance greater than in control subjects: $P < .05$
[b]Variance greater than in control subjects: $P < .001$
[c]Variance greater than in control subjects: $P < .01$
[d]Primary and unimodal association cortex
Source. Scanditronix PC 1024-7B data from Haxby JV, Grady CL, Koss E, et al: "Longitudinal Study of Cerebral Metabolic Asymmetries and Associated Neuropsychological Patterns in Early Dementia of the Alzheimer Type." *Archives of Neurology* 47:753–760, 1990.

Table 4–5. Spearman rank-sum correlations between right/left metabolic asymmetries [see equation (1)] and drawing/syntax comprehension or visual recall/verbal recall discrepancies in Alzheimer's disease patients with varying dementia severity

Neuropsychological discrepancy	Right/left metabolic asymmetry			
	Prefrontal	Premotor	Parietal	Lateral temporal
Control subjects (*n* = 15–16)				
Drawing versus comprehension	−.10	−.33	.00	.12
Visual versus verbal recall	−.30	−.39	−.40	−.17
Alzheimer's disease with mild dementia (*n* = 10)				
Drawing versus comprehension	.04	−.15	.04	−.24
Visual versus verbal recall	−.22	−.21	−.16	−.18
Alzheimer's disease with moderate dementia (*n* = 13)				
Drawing versus comprehension	.76[a]	.76[a]	.79[a]	.53
Visual versus verbal recall	.49	.55[b]	.69[a]	.48

Note. Numbers indicate correlation coefficient. Positive correlation indicates that better drawing capacity or better visual recall is associated with relative high right-sided metabolism.
[a]Spearman rank-sum correlation differs from zero: $P < .01$.
[b]Spearman rank-sum correlation differs from zero: $P < .05$.
Source. Scanditronix PC 1024-7B data from Haxby JV, Grady CL, Koss E, et al: "Longitudinal Study of Cerebral Metabolic Asymmetries and Associated Neuropsychological Patterns in Early Dementia of the Alzheimer Type." *Archives of Neurology* 47:753–760, 1990.

was maintained (Figure 4–3), Spearman rank-sum correlations between asymmetries and appropriate neuropsychological discrepancies were significant at the last but not at the first evaluation (Table 4–5) (Haxby et al. 1990).

According to NINCDS-ADRDA criteria, a patient presenting with a history of memory decline and a singular memory disorder would

Table 4–6.   Spearman correlations between parietal/prefrontal rCMR$_{glc}$ ratios and parietal/prefrontal neuropsychological test score discrepancies in Alzheimer's disease patients

Neuropsychological discrepancy	Parietal/prefrontal metabolic ratio					
	Control subjects (14–17)		Mild Alzheimer's disease (10)		Moderate Alzheimer's disease (14)	
	Right	Left	Right	Left	Right	Left
Arithmetic versus						
Verbal fluency	–.02	.00	–.14	–.04	.63[a]	.57[a]
Attention (trail A)	–.34	–.08	–.02	–.21	.43	.46
Verbal comprehension versus						
Verbal fluency	.00	.03	–.30	–.06	.66[a]	.67[a]
Attention (trail A)	–.12	.11	.04	–.01	.51	.56[a]
Drawing versus						
Verbal fluency	–.02	.11	–.02	.22	.66[a]	.57
Attention (trail A)	–.21	.20	.42	.32	.44	.43
Immediate memory span for visuospatial location (block tapping) versus						
Verbal fluency	.16	.05	–.25	–.11	.62[a]	.54
Attention (trail A)	.14	.32	.26	.11	.73[b]	.72[b]

Note.   Numbers indicate correlation coefficient. Neuropsychological discrepancy = rank on test of arithmetic, syntax comprehension, extended range drawing – rank on controlled word association or attentional trailmaking (trail A) test score.
[a]Spearman correlation coefficient in Alzheimer's disease differs from control: $P < .05$.
[b]Spearman correlation coefficient in Alzheimer's disease differs from control: $P < .01$.
Source.   Scanditronix PC 1024-7B data from Haxby JV, Grady CL, Koss E, et al: "Heterogeneous Anterior-Posterior Metabolic Patterns in Dementia of the Alzheimer Type." *Neurology* 38:1853–1863, 1988.

receive a diagnosis of "possible" Alzheimer's disease (McKhann et al. 1984). However, if this patient also had an abnormal metabolic asymmetry (2 SD from mean; see Figure 4–2) or an abnormal parietal/frontal metabolic gradient—each of which predicts patterns of later cognitive dysfunction that would lead to a "probable" diagnosis—the early metabolic abnormalities might convert the "possible" diagnosis to a "probable" diagnosis. One way to statistically identify an abnormal metabolic PET pattern in an individual with only a memory deficit and make a reliable early "probable" diagnosis of Alzheimer's disease is to use a discriminant function of rCMR$_{glc}$ values from the frontal and parietal association cortices (Azari et al. 1993).

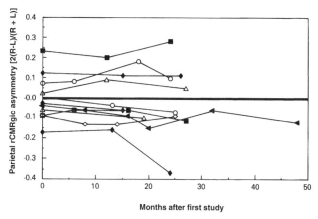

Months after first study

Figure 4–3.   Stability over time of right/left metabolic asymmetries in parietal association cortex of 11 Alzheimer's disease patients with mild initial dementia. *Source:*   Haxby JV, Grady CL, Koss E, et al: "Longitudinal Study of Cerebral Metabolic Asymmetries and Associated Neuropsychological Patterns in Early Dementia of the Alzheimer Type." *Archives of Neurology* 47:753–760, 1990.

Brain Activation in Alzheimer's Disease

Postmortem examination of brain tissue reveals reduced synaptic markers in patients with Alzheimer's disease (Terry et al. 1991); presynaptic elements are reduced in number in biopsy tissue representing middle-stage disease, with remaining elements hypertrophied to maintain a normal area of apposition with postsynaptic elements (DeKosky and Scheff 1990). These and other findings suggest that metabolic reductions early in Alzheimer's disease reflect reduced efficacy of synaptic transmission, which appropriate cognitive or pharmacological stimulation might overcome (Rapoport and Grady 1993). In vitro evidence that $rCMR_{glc}$ represents functional activity of terminal synapses and their postsynaptic dendritic connections (Malison et al. 1994) and that patients with Alzheimer's disease have fewer significant positive correlations between pairs of PET-derived resting $rCMR_{glc}$ values than control subjects (Horwitz et al. 1987) supports this hypothesis.

To examine the hypothesis of reversible synaptic failure, my colleagues and I used $H_2^{15}O$ and PET to measure rCBF in occipitotemporal visual association regions that subserve object recognition among patients with Alzheimer's disease and in healthy control subjects while they performed a control or face-matching task (Figure 4–4) (Grady et al. 1993; Rapoport and Grady 1993). We subtracted rCBF during the control task (in which

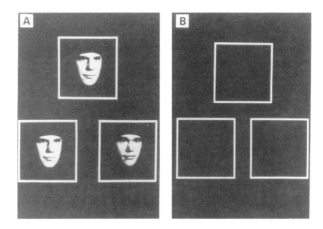

Figure 4–4.   Sample items from face-matching (A) and control (B) tasks. Responses during face matching involved pressing buttons with the right or left thumb, depending on which of the two choice items below (right or left) was a correct match to the top face; right and left button presses were alternated during the control task. *Source.*   Grady CL, Haxby JV, Horwitz B, et al: "Activation of Cerebral Blood Flow During a Visuoperceptual Task in Patients With Alzheimer-Type Dementia." *Neurobiology of Aging* 14:35–44, 1993.

the subject pressed a button alternately with right and left thumbs in response to a neutral visual stimulus) from rCBF during the face-matching task (in which the subject pressed the button with the appropriate thumb after deciding whether the right or left face was to be matched) to produce a "difference" image (Figure 4–5). We selected Alzheimer's disease patients with mild to moderate dementia who were capable of performing the face-matching task as accurately (85% ± 8 SD correct choices) as control subjects (92% ±5, respectively); reaction times during the task, however, were more variable in the Alzheimer's disease patients than in the control subjects—3.34 seconds ± 1.46 (SD) compared with 2.07 seconds ± 0.54.

In the control task, rCBF was lower in occipitotemporal regions (Brodmann areas 17, 19, and 37) in Alzheimer's disease patients than in control subjects, consistent with functional activity in these areas (Table 4–7). During face matching, however, the mean incremental ΔrCBF (mL/100 g/minute) did not differ significantly or differed only minimally between patients and control subjects. Thus, the association areas affected by Alzheimer's disease were capable of being fully activated by a given face-recognition task—suggesting a degree of reversibility of

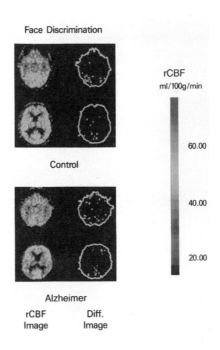

Figure 4–5. rCBF and ΔrCBF (difference between face-discrimination and control rCBF) images in control and Alzheimer's disease patient. Note reduced parietal-temporal flow in lower rCBF image from the Alzheimer's patient. Difference image identifies pixels in which flow was increased by more than 30% above baseline (rCBF in units of mL/100 g/minutes). *Source.* Grady CL, Haxby JV, Horwitz B, et al: "Activation of Cerebral Blood Flow During a Visuoperceptual Task in Patients With Alzheimer-Type Dementia." *Neurobiology of Aging* 14:35–44, 1993.

functional failure (Rapoport and Grady 1993). Pietrini et al. (1995) subsequently confirmed the brain's ability to respond to activation in Alzheimer's disease patients with mild to moderate dementia by showing that temporoparietal regions with resting-state reductions in $rCMR_{glc}$ showed marked increases in $rCMR_{glc}$ during combined auditory and visual stimulation.

In clinical pharmacology, administration of drugs at different doses helps to establish dose-response and toxicity relationships and estimate maximal effect and drug concentrations (K_D) that provide half-maximal effect (Ross 1993). Similarly, stimulation-response relations in hippocampal slices and other in vitro synaptic preparations suggest that a wide range of measurable (parameterized) stimulus intensities is required to

Table 4–7.   rCBF in occipitotemporal visual association areas in Alzheimer's disease patients and control subjects performing control or face-matching tasks

Parameter	Control subjects (n = 13)	Alzheimer's disease (n = 11)
Baseline control task	48.4 ± 0.9	40.1 ± 1.1[a]
Face-matching task	53.1 ± 0.9	44.1 ± 1.2[a]
Difference (ΔrCBF = face matching – control task)	4.7 ± 0.2	4.0 ± 0.4

Note.   Numbers reflect $rCMR_{glc}$ (mg/100 g/minute). rCBF measured in occipitotemporal visual association areas (Brodmann 19 and part of 37).
[a]Mean ± SE differs significantly from control mean; $P < .001$.
Source.   From Van Meter J, Rapoport SI, Grady C (unpublished results) and Rapoport SI, Grady CL: "Parametric In Vivo Brain Imaging During Activation to Examine Pathological Mechanisms of Functional Failure in Alzheimer Disease." *International Journal of Neuroscience* 70:39–56, 1993.

determine synaptic responsiveness under a variety of conditions (Pellmar 1986). Accordingly, to further elucidate the Alzheimer's disease process, my colleagues and I proposed to vary cognitive or other stimulation in intensity or difficulty in a measurable manner while measuring rCBF (Rapoport and Grady 1993).

Using this parametric approach, we measured rCBF in Alzheimer's disease patients with mild to moderate dementia and in control subjects during a patterned flash stimulus at different frequencies (Mentis et al. 1994, 1996). In control subjects, striate cortex rCBF increased linearly as the stimulus frequency increased from 0 to 7 Hz, then decreased at higher stimulus frequencies. In Alzheimer's disease patients, rCBF increased with stimulus frequency from 0 Hz only to 4 Hz, then declined—although ΔrCBF values at frequencies up to 4 Hz did not differ quantitatively from control increments. Furthermore, in a middle temporal association region (V5/MT) that subserves motion perception and is dominated by magnocellular visual input, ΔrCBF at 1 Hz was significant in control subjects but not in Alzheimer's disease patients.

We concluded that the magnocellular visual system, which can respond to visual stimulation at frequencies above 8 Hz (Livingstone and Hubel 1988), is more dysfunctional in early Alzheimer's disease than the parvocellular system, which responds to frequencies at 8 Hz and below. These results imply selective vulnerability of high-frequency synapses early in Alzheimer's disease and confirm that parametric activation can elucidate brain changes in Alzheimer's disease.

Pharmacology

Limited data are available with regard to PET images and drug effects. In one study in patients with Alzheimer's disease, scans before and during physostigmine infusion demonstrated increments as well as decrements of normalized (related to global) $rCMR_{glc}$ (Tune et al. 1991). In another study of six patients with Alzheimer's disease, acutely administered physostigmine (5 µg/kg/hour) reduced $rCMR_{glc}$ below its already reduced value in the neocortex (Blin et al. 1994).

With regard to cholinergic therapy, PET studies show that Alzheimer's disease patients with mild to moderate dementia, treated orally with the cholinesterase inhibitor tetrahydroaminoacridine for several months, had improved neuropsychological performance and increased $rCMR_{glc}$ but unchanged rCBF (Nordberg 1993a). These observations are difficult to explain in view of established coupling between blood flow and metabolism, as well as increased uptake of $(+)$-^{11}C-nicotine in frontal and temporal cortices, suggesting partial restoration of nicotinic cholinergic receptors (Nordberg 1993b). In another study, phosphatidylserine administered to 18 Alzheimer's disease patients over a 6-month period did not affect $rCMR_{glc}$ at rest or during visual stimulation; it also did not affect cognitive performance (Heiss et al. 1994).

Although PET researchers have developed positron-emitting ligands—including $(+)$-^{11}C-nicotine—for receptors, few studies have applied these compounds to Alzheimer's disease. Mueller-Gaertner et al. (1991), for example, used ^{11}C-carfentanil to demonstrate early loss of mµ opiate receptors in the amygdaloid complex of patients with Alzheimer's disease. Blin et al. (1993) found that ^{18}F-setoperone—a 5-HT_2 antagonist whose regional binding was quantitated by subtraction using cerebellum as reference—reduced binding by 31%–46% in association cortical areas of nine patients with Alzheimer's disease, consistent with postmortem evidence.

SPECT in Alzheimer's Disease: Comparison With PET and Utility for Clinical Diagnosis

Researchers introduced SPECT into clinical settings to estimate rCBF and receptor densities because it is less expensive than PET and requires fewer personnel and less technical support. In some cases, SPECT uses high-sensitivity gamma cameras with ^{133}Xe gas to image single slices during 4- to 7.5-minute scans, with a resolution approaching 8 mm (Malison et al. 1994). Alternatively, low-sensitivity, rotating gamma cameras—using commercially available long-lived [123]I- or ^{99m}Tc-labeled radiopharmaceuticals—can provide volumetric information (Holman et al. 1991, 1992). The use of long-lived isotopes with a need for long signal acquisition times extends scanning time to 30–60 minutes and allows only one scan per day.

SPECT is not truly quantitative because its reconstruction paradigms have not adequately addressed photon scatter and attenuation compensation. Investigators using SPECT usually determine ratios of radioactivity between one brain region and another; they usually do not obtain arterial input functions for absolute flow calculations.

Whereas PET researchers have reported four statistically distinct patterns of $rCMR_{glc}$ in Alzheimer's disease (Grady et al. 1990), investigators using ^{99m}Tc-hexamethyl-propyleneamine oxime (^{99m}Tc-HMPAO) SPECT have identified seven qualitative rCBF patterns in a prospective study of 132 consecutive patients with varying dementia severity (Holman et al. 1992). The probability of Alzheimer's disease was 82% for bilateral temporoparietal defects, 72% for bilateral temporoparietal plus additional defects, 57% for unilateral temporoparietal defects, 43% for frontal defects, 18% for large focal defects, and 0% for multiple small cortical defects. Other studies have reported a normal SPECT pattern in 45% of patients with mild dementia (Reed et al. 1989); therefore, ^{99m}Tc-HMPAO SPECT has minimal diagnostic utility in Alzheimer's disease patients with mild dementia, except those for whom considerable diagnostic doubt exists (Claus et al. 1993).

A temporoparietal reduction in SPECT rCBF is more likely with Alzheimer's disease, whereas a patchy whole brain reduction involving the motor cortex and thalamus is more likely with vascular dementia (Kawabata et al. 1993; Lechner and Bertha 1991). However, normal SPECT images occur in Alzheimer's disease patients with mild dementia and in vascular dementia patients, and asymmetric presentation in Alzheimer's disease may be indistinguishable from a pattern of cerebral infarction in another patient (Holman et al. 1991). In a study of Alzheimer's disease and vascular dementia patients matched for dementia severity, ^{99m}Tc-HMPAO ratios of temporoparietal cortex, parietal cortex, or frontal cortex to cerebellar radioactivity did not distinguish between the two groups (Weinstein et al. 1991). A discriminant analysis of ^{99m}Tc-HMPAO-derived flows, however, correctly identified 100% of control subjects and 87% of Alzheimer's disease patients with mild dementia (O'Mahony et al. 1994).

The muscarinic M_2 presynaptic receptor subtype is selectively lost in Alzheimer's disease, leaving the M_1 postsynaptic subtype in place (Mash et al. 1985). Intravenous physostigmine (0.5 mg) increased rCBF in the left posterior parietotemporal region of Alzheimer's disease patients whose baseline rCBF was reduced but not in healthy control subjects, suggesting upregulation of postsynaptic cholinergic sensitivity (Geaney et al. 1990). Furthermore, the radioligand ^{123}I-3-quinuclidinyl-4-iodobenzilate (^{123}I-QNB) has different pharmacokinetic properties for M_1 receptors than for M_2 receptors, which may enable SPECT imaging with this tracer to quantitate loss of the M_2 subtype in the Alzheimer's disease brain. Such results, however, are unlikely in the parietal cortex, where M_1 = 88 nM and M_2 = 12 nM in healthy brains (Zeeberg et al. 1992). Researchers have reported focal reductions of ^{123}I-QNB binding by SPECT—in excess of reductions in $rCMR_{glc}$ by PET—in the thalamus and frontal cortex of patients with Alzheimer's disease; these reductions suggest selective loss of M_2 receptors in these regions (Weinberger et al. 1992).

References

Almkvist O, Wahlund L-O, Andersson-Lundman G, et al: White-matter hyperintensity and neuropsychological functions in dementia and healthy aging. Arch Neurol 49:626–632, 1992

Azari NP, Pettigrew KD, Schapiro MB, et al: Early detection of Alzheimer's disease: a statistical approach using positron emission tomographic data. J Cereb Blood Flow Metab 13:438–447, 1993

Benson DF, Kuhl DE, Hawkins RA, et al: The fluorodeoxyglucose ^{18}F scan in Alzheimer's disease and multi-infarct dementia. Arch Neurol 40:711–714, 1983

Berridge MJ, Irvine RF: Inositol trisphosphate: a novel second messenger in cellular signal transduction. Nature 312:315–321, 1984

Blin J, Baron JC, Dubois B, et al: Loss of brain 5-HT$_2$ receptors in Alzheimer's disease. Brain 116:497–510, 1993

Blin J, Piercey MF, Giuffra MA, et al: Metabolic effects of scopolamine and physostigmine in human brain measured by positron emission tomography. J Neurol Sci 123:44–51, 1994

Boller F, Lopez OL, Moossy J: Diagnosis of dementia: clinicopathologic correlations. Neurology 39:76–79, 1989

Bowen BC, Barker WW, Loewenstein DA, et al: MR signal abnormalities in memory disorder and dementia. Am J Roentgenol 154:1285–1292, 1990

Brown GG, Levine SR, Gorell JM, et al: In vivo ^{31}P NMR profiles of Alzheimer's disease and multiple subcortical infarct dementia. Neurology 39:1423–1427, 1989

Chui HC, Victoroff JI, Margolin D, et al: Criteria for the diagnosis of ischemic vascular dementia proposed by the state of California Alzheimer's disease diagnostic and treatment centers. Neurology 42:473–480, 1992

Claus JJ, Hasan D, van Harskamp FH, et al: SPECT with ^{99m}Tc-HMPAO is of limited diagnostic value in mild Alzheimer's disease: a population-based study (abstract). Presented at the annual meeting of the American Academy of Neurology, New York, April 24–May 1, 1993. Neurology 43(suppl 2):A406, 1993

Corder EH, Saunders AM, Strittmatter WJ, et al: Gene dose of apolipoprotein E type 4 allele and the risk of Alzheimer's disease in late onset families. Science 261:921–923, 1993

Creasey H, Schwartz M, Frederickson H, et al: Quantitative computed tomography in dementia of the Alzheimer type. Neurol 36:1563–1568, 1986

Cuenod CA, Kaplan DB, Michot JL, et al: Phospholipid abnormalities in early Alzheimer's disease: in vivo phosphorus 31 magnetic resonance spectroscopy. Arch Neurol 52:89–94, 1995

Dani A, Pietrini P, Furey M, et al: Transition to dementia in Down syndrome adults: bilinear trajectories of cerebral metabolic decline. Presented at the XVII International Symposium on Cerebral Blood Flow and Metabolism, July 2–6, 1995. J Cereb Blood Flow Metab 15(suppl 1):S787, 1995

DeCarli C, Kaye JA, Horwitz B, et al: Critical analysis of the use of computer-assisted transverse axial tomography to study human brain in aging and dementia of the Alzheimer type. Neurology 40:872–883, 1990

DeCarli C, Haxby JV, Gillette JA, et al: Longitudinal changes in lateral ventricular volume in patients with dementia of the Alzheimer type. Neurology 42: 2029–2036, 1992

DeCarli C, Murphy DGM, McIntosh AR, et al: Discriminant analysis of MRI measures determines the presence of dementia of the Alzheimer type in males and females. Psych Res 57:119–130, 1995a

DeCarli C, Murphy DGM, Tran M, et al: The effect of white matter hyperintensity volume on brain structure, cognitive performance and cerebral metabolism of glucose in very healthy adults. Neurology 45:2077–2084, 1995b

DeKosky ST, Scheff SW: Synapse loss in frontal cortex biopsies in Alzheimer's disease: correlation with cognitive severity. Ann Neurol 27:457–464, 1990

Drayer BP: Imaging of the aging brain, II: pathologic conditions. Radiology 166:797–806, 1988

Duara R, Grady C, Haxby J, et al: Positron emission tomography in Alzheimer's disease. Neurology 36:879–887, 1986

Folstein MF, Folstein SE, McHugh PR: Mini-Mental State: a practical method for grading the cognitive state of patients for the clinician. J Psychiatr Res 12: 189–198, 1975

Fox PT, Raichle ME, Mintun MA, et al: Nonoxidative glucose consumption during focal physiologic neural activity. Science 241:462–464, 1988

Frackowiak RSJ, Pozzilli C, Legg NJ, et al: Regional cerebral oxygen supply and utilization in dementia: a clinical and physiological study with oxygen-15 and positron tomography. Brain 104:753–778, 1981

Fukuyama H, Ogawa M, Yamauchi H, et al: Altered cerebral energy metabolism in Alzheimer's disease: a PET study. J Nucl Med 35:1–6, 1994

Geaney DP, Soper N, Shepstone BJ, et al: Effect of central cholinergic stimulation on regional cerebral blood flow in Alzheimer's disease. Lancet 335:1484–1487, 1990

Ginsberg L, Atack JR, Rapoport SI, et al: Plasmalogen deficit parallels membrane bilayer instability selectively in Alzheimer's disease cortex. Paper presented to the third meeting of the European Neurological Society, Lausanne, Switzerland, June 27–July 1, 1992

Ginsberg L, Atack JR, Rapoport SI, et al: Regional specificity of membrane instability in Alzheimer's disease brain. Brain Res 615:355–357, 1993

Ginsberg L, Rafique S, Xuereb JH, et al: Disease and anatomic specificity of ethanolamine plasmalogen deficiency in Alzheimer's disease brain. Brain Res 698:223–226, 1995

Grady CL, Haxby JV, Horwitz B, et al: Longitudinal study of the early neuropsychological and cerebral metabolic changes in dementia of the Alzheimer type. J Clin Exp Neuropsychol 10:576–596, 1988

Grady CL, Haxby JV, Schapiro MB, et al: Subgroups in dementia of the Alzheimer type identified using positron emission tomography. J Neuropsychiatry Clin Neurosci 2:373–384, 1990

Grady CL, Haxby JV, Horwitz B, et al: Activation of cerebral blood flow during a visuoperceptual task in patients with Alzheimer-type dementia. Neurobiol Aging 14:35–44, 1993

Hagberg BO, Ingvar DH: Cognitive reduction in presenile dementia related to regional abnormalities of the cerebral blood flow. Br J Psychiatry 128: 209–222, 1976

Haxby JV, Duara R, Grady CL, et al: Relations between neuropsychological and cerebral metabolic asymmetries in early Alzheimer's disease. J Cereb Blood Flow Metab 5:193–200, 1985

Haxby JV, Grady CL, Koss E, et al: Heterogeneous anterior-posterior metabolic patterns in dementia of the Alzheimer type. Neurology 38:1853–1863, 1988

Haxby JV, Grady CL, Koss E, et al: Longitudinal study of cerebral metabolic asymmetries and associated neuropsychological patterns in early dementia of the Alzheimer type. Arch Neurol 47:753–760, 1990

Haxby JV, Raffaele K, Gillette J, et al: Individual trajectories of cognitive decline in patients with dementia of the Alzheimer type. J Clin Exp Neuropsychol 14:575–592, 1992

Heiss W-D, Kessler J, Mielke R, et al: Long-term effects of phosphatidylserine, pyritinol, and cognitive training in Alzheimer's disease. Dementia 5:88–98, 1994

Hoffman JM, Guze BH, Baxter L, et al: Metabolic homogeneity in familial and sporadic Alzheimer's disease: an FDG-PET study. Presented at the 41st Annual Meeting of the American Academy of Neurology, Chicago, IL, April 13–19, 1989. Neurology 39(suppl 1):167, 1989

Holman BL, Nagel JS, Johnson KA, et al: Imaging dementia with SPECT. Ann N Y Acad Sci 620:165–174, 1991

Holman BL, Johnson KA, Gerada B, et al: The scintigraphic appearance of Alzheimer's disease: a prospective study using technetium-99m-HMPAO SPECT. J Nucl Med 33:181–185, 1992

Horwitz B, Grady CL, Schlageter NL, et al: Intercorrelations of regional cerebral glucose metabolic rates in Alzheimer's disease. Brain Res 407:294–306, 1987

Hounsfield GN: Computerized transverse axial scanning (tomography), I: description of system. Br J Radiol 46:1016–1022, 1973

Jellinger K: Neuropathological aspects of dementias resulting from abnormal blood and cerebrospinal fluid dynamics. Acta Neurol Belg 76:83–102, 1976

Kawabata K, Tachibana H, Sugita M, et al: A comparative I-123 IMP SPECT study in Binswanger's disease and Alzheimer's disease. Clin Nucl Med 18:329–336, 1993

Kaye JA, DeCarli C, Luxenberg JS, et al: The significance of age-related enlargement of the cerebral ventricles in healthy men and women measured by quantitative computed X-ray tomography. J Am Geriatr Soc 40:225–231, 1992

Kennedy AM, Frackowiak RSJ, Newman SK, et al: Deficits in cerebral glucose metabolism demonstrated by positron emission tomography in individuals at risk of familial Alzheimer's disease. Neurosci Lett 186:17–20, 1995

Kozachuk WE, DeCarli C, Schapiro MB, et al: White matter hyperintensities in dementia of Alzheimer's type and in healthy subjects without cerebrovascular risk factors: a magnetic resonance imaging study. Arch Neurol 47:1306–1310, 1990

Kumar A, Schapiro MB, Grady C, et al: High-resolution PET studies in Alzheimer's disease. Neuropsychopharmacology 4:35–46, 1991

Kuwabara Y, Ichiya Y, Otsuka M, et al: Cerebrovascular responsiveness to hypercapnia in Alzheimer's dementia and vascular dementia of the Binswanger type. Stroke 23:594–598, 1992

Lechner H, Bertha G: Multiinfarct dementia. J Neural Transm 33(suppl):49–52, 1991

Lewis DA, Campbell MJ, Terry RD, et al: Laminar and regional distributions of neurofibrillary tangles and neuritic plaques in Alzheimer's disease: a quantitative study of visual and auditory cortices. J Neurosci 7:1799–1808, 1987

Lim KO, Rosenbloom M, Pfefferbaum A: In vivo structural brain assessment, in Psychopharmacology: The Fourth Generation of Progress. Edited by Bloom FE, Kupfer DJ. New York, Raven, 1994, pp 881–894

Livingstone M, Hubel D: Segregation of form, color, movement, and depth: anatomy, physiology, and perception. Science 240:740–749, 1988

Luxenberg JS, Friedland RP, Rapoport SI: Quantitative X-ray computed tomography (CT) in dementia of the Alzheimer type (DAT). Can J Neurol Sci 13: 570–572, 1986

Luxenberg JS, Haxby JV, Creasey H, et al: Rate of ventricular enlargement in dementia of the Alzheimer type correlates with rate of neuropsychological deterioration. Neurology 37:1135–1140, 1987

Malison RT, Laruelle M, Innis RB: Positron and single photon emission tomography: principles and applications in psychopharmacology, in Psychopharmacology: The Fourth Generation of Progress. Edited by Bloom FE, Kupfer DJ. New York, Raven, 1994, pp 865–880

Mash DC, Flynn DD, Potter LT: Loss of M_2 muscarine receptors in the cerebral cortex in Alzheimer's disease and experimental cholinergic denervation. Science 228:1115–1117, 1985

Mayeux R, Stern Y, Spanton S: Heterogeneity in dementia of the Alzheimer type: evidence of subgroups. Neurology 35:453–461, 1985

McKhann G, Drachman D, Folstein M, et al: Clinical diagnosis of Alzheimer's disease: report of the NINCDS-ADRDA work group under the auspices of Department of Health and Human Services task force on Alzheimer's disease. Neurology 34:939–944, 1984

Mentis MJ, Stoll J, Grady C, et al: Reduction in area 17 blood flow to high but not low frequency flashing lights in dementia of the Alzheimer type. Abstr Soc Neurosci 20:1778, 1994

Mentis MJ, Horwitz B, Grady C, et al: Visual cortical dysfunction evaluated with a temporally graded "stress test" during PET. Am J Psychiatry 153:32–40, 1996

Minoshima S, Foster NL, Kuhl DE: Posterior cingulate cortex in Alzheimer's disease (letter). Lancet 344:895, 1994

Mintun MA, Raichle ME, Martin WRW, et al: Brain oxygen utilization measured with O-15 radiotracers and positron emission tomography. J Nucl Med 25: 177–187, 1984

Moats RA, Ernst T, Shonk TK, et al: Abnormal cerebral metabolite concentrations in patients with probably Alzheimer disease. Magn Reson Med 32: 110–115, 1994

Mueller-Gaertner HW, Mayberg HS, Tune L, et al: Mu opiate receptor binding in amygdala in Alzheimer's disease: in vivo quantification by 11C carfentanil and PET (abstract). J Cereb Blood Flow Metab 11(suppl 2):S20, 1991

Murphy DGM, Bottomley PA, Salerno JA, et al: An in vivo study of phosphorus and glucose metabolism in Alzheimer's disease using magnetic resonance spectroscopy and PET. Arch Gen Psychiatry 50:341–349, 1993a

Murphy DGM, DeCarli C, Daly E, et al: Volumetric magnetic resonance imaging in men with dementia of the Alzheimer type: correlations with disease severity. Biol Psychiatry 34:612–621, 1993b

Nordberg A: Clinical studies in Alzheimer patients with positron emission tomography. Behav Brain Res 57:215–224, 1993a

Nordberg A: Effect of long-term treatment with tacrine (THA) in Alzheimer's disease as visualized by PET. Acta Neurol Scand 149(suppl):62–65, 1993b

Nordberg A, Lilja A, Lundqvist H, et al: Tacrine restores cholinergic nicotinic receptors and glucose metabolism in Alzheimer patients as visualized by positron emission tomography. Neurobiol Aging 13:747–758, 1992

O'Brien MD, Mallett BL: Cerebral cortex perfusion rates in dementia. J Neurol Neurosurg Psychiatry 33:497–500, 1970

O'Mahony D, Coffey J, Murphy J, et al: The discriminant value of semiquantitative SPECT data in mild Alzheimer's disease. J Nucl Med 35:1450–1455, 1994

Pellmar T: Electrophysiological correlates of peroxide damage in guinea pig hippocampus in vitro. Brain Res 364:377–381, 1986

Pettegrew JW, Moossy J, Withers G, et al: ^{31}P nuclear magnetic resonance study of the brain in Alzheimer's disease. J Neuropathol Exp Neurol 47:235–248, 1988

Pietrini P, Azari NP, Grady CL, et al: Pattern of cerebral metabolic interactions in a subject with isolated amnesia at risk for Alzheimer's disease: a longitudinal evaluation. Dementia 4:94–101, 1993

Pietrini P, Furey ML, Horwitz B, et al: Regional cerebral glucose metabolism (rCMR$_{glc}$) at rest and during sensory stimulation in patients with Alzheimer disease (AD). Paper presented at the annual meeting of the American Neurological Association, Washington, DC, October 1995

Raichle ME, Grubb RL Jr, Gado MH, et al: Correlation between regional cerebral blood flow and oxidative metabolism. Arch Neurol 33:523–526, 1976

Rapoport SI: Brain evolution and Alzheimer's disease. Rev Neurol (Paris) 144: 79–90, 1988

Rapoport SI: Integrated phylogeny of the primate brain, with special reference to humans and their diseases. Brain Res 15:267–294, 1990

Rapoport SI: Positron emission tomography in Alzheimer's disease in relation to disease pathogenesis: a critical review. Cerebrovasc Brain Metab Rev 3: 297–335, 1991

Rapoport SI, Grady CL: Parametric in vivo brain imaging during activation to examine pathological mechanisms of functional failure in Alzheimer disease. Int J Neurosci 70:39–56, 1993

Reed BR, Jagust WJ, Seab JP, et al: Memory and regional cerebral blood flow in mildly symptomatic Alzheimer's disease. Neurology 39:1537–1539, 1989

Rosen WG, Terry RD, Fuld PA, et al: Pathological verification of ischemic score in differentiation of dementias. Ann Neurol 7:486–488, 1980

Ross EM: Pharmacodynamics: mechanism of drug action and the relationship between drug concentration and effect, in The Pharmacological Basis of Therapeutics, 8th Edition. Edited by Gilman AG, Rall TW, Nies AS, et al. New York, McGraw-Hill, 1993, pp 33–48

Schapiro MB, Ball MJ, Grady CL, et al: Dementia in Down syndrome: cerebral glucose utilization, neuropsychological assessment and neuropathology. Neurology 38:938–942, 1988

Schapiro MB, Luxenberg JS, Kaye JA, et al: Serial quantitative CT analysis of brain morphometrics in adult Down's syndrome at different ages. Neurology 39: 1349–1353, 1989

Schapiro MB, Pietrini P, Grady CL, et al: Reductions in parietal and temporal cerebral metabolic rates for glucose are not specific for Alzheimer's disease. J Neurol Neurosurg Psychiatry 56:859–864, 1993

Schapiro MB, Saunders AM, Simon E, et al: Survival and dementia in Down syndrome (DS) is related to APOE allele type. Abstract presented at the 47th annual meeting of the American Academy of Neurology, Seattle, WA, May 6–13, 1995

Schlageter NL, Carson RE, Rapoport SI: Examination of blood-brain barrier permeability in dementia of the Alzheimer type with [68-Ga]EDTA and positron emission tomography. J Cereb Blood Flow Metab 77:1–8, 1987

Shulman RG, Blamire AM, Rothman DL, et al: Nuclear magnetic resonance imaging and spectroscopy of human brain function. Proc Natl Acad Sci U S A 90:3127–3133, 1993

Small GW, Mazziotta JC, Collins MT, et al: Apolipoprotein E type 4 allele and cerebral glucose metabolism in relatives at risk for familial Alzheimer disease. JAMA 273:942–947, 1995

Smith CD, Gallenstein LG, Layton WJ, et al: ^{31}P magnetic resonance spectroscopy in Alzheimer's and Pick's disease. Neurobiol Aging 14:85–92, 1993

Sokoloff L: Circulation and energy metabolism of the brain, in Basic Neurochemistry, 4th Edition. Edited by Siegel G, Agranoff B, Albers RW, et al. New York, Raven, 1989, pp 565–590

Sokoloff L: Energy metabolism and effects of energy depletion or exposure to glutamate. Can J Physiol Pharmacol 70:S107–S112, 1992

Terry RD, Masliah E, Salmon DP, et al: Physical basis of cognitive alterations in Alzheimer's disease: synapse loss is the major correlate of cognitive impairment. Ann Neurol 30:572–580, 1991

Tune L, Brandt J, Frost JJ, et al: Physostigmine in Alzheimer's disease: effects on cognitive functioning, cerebral glucose metabolism analyzed by positron emission tomography and cerebral blood flow analyzed by single photon emission tomography. Acta Psychiatr Scand Suppl 366:61–65, 1991

Tyrrell PJ, Sawle GV, Ibanez V, et al: Clinical and positron emission tomography studies in the "extrapyramidal syndrome" of dementia of the Alzheimer type. Arch Neurol 47:1318–1323, 1990

van Broeckhoven CL: Molecular genetics of Alzheimer disease: identification of genes and gene mutations. Eur Neurol 35:8–19, 1995

Weinberger DR, Jones D, Reba RC, et al: A comparison of FDG PET and IQNB SPECT in normal subjects and in patients with dementia. J Neuropsychiatry Clin Neurosci 4:239–248, 1992

Weinstein HC, Haan J, van Royen EO, et al: SPECT in the diagnosis of Alzheimer's disease and multi-infarct-dementia. Clin Neurol Neurosurg 93:39–43, 1991

Yamauchi H, Fukuyama H, Harada K, et al: Callosal atrophy parallels decreased cortical oxygen metabolism and neuropsychological impairment in Alzheimer's disease. Arch Neurol 50:1070–1074, 1993

Yao H, Sadoshima S, Ibayashi S, et al: Leukoaraiosis and dementia in hypertensive patients. Stroke 23:1673–1677, 1992

Zeeberg BR, Kim H-J, Reba RC: Pharmacokinetic simulations of SPECT quantitation of the M_2 muscarinic neuroreceptor sybtype in disease states using radioiodinated (R,R)-4IQNB. Life Sci 51:661–670, 1992

Chapter 5
Hoch Award Lecture

Prion Biology and Diseases

Sporadic, Inherited, and Infectious Degenerative Illnesses of Humans and Animals

Stanley B. Prusiner, M.D.

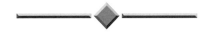

Prions cause a variety of human and animal neurodegenerative diseases; epidemiologists now classify these diseases together because their etiology and pathogenesis involve modification of the prion protein (PrP) (Prusiner 1991). Prion diseases manifest as infectious, genetic, and sporadic disorders (Table 5–1). These diseases may be transmitted among mammals by the infectious particle designated "prion" (Prusiner 1982).

I thank M. Baldwin, D. Borchelt, G. Carlson, F. Cohen, C. Cooper, S. DeArmond, R. Fletterick, M. Gasset, R. Gabizon, D. Groth, R. Koehler, L. Hood, K. Hsiao, Z. Huang, V. Lingappa, K.-M. Pan, D. Riesner, M. Scott, A. Serban, N. Stahl, G. Telling, A. Taraboulos, M. Torchia, and D. Westaway for their help in these studies. This work was supported by grants from the National Institutes of Health (NS14069, AG08967, AG02132, NS22786, and AG10770) and the American Health Assistance Foundation, as well as by gifts from the Sherman Fairchild Foundation and Bernard Osher Foundation.

Table 5–1. Human prion diseases

Disease	Etiology
Kuru	Infection
Creutzfeldt-Jakob disease	
Iatrogenic	Infection
Sporadic	Unknown
Familial	PrP mutation
Gerstmann-Sträussler-Scheinker disease	PrP mutation
Fatal familial insomnia	PrP mutation

Despite intensive searches over the past three decades, researchers have found no nucleic acid within prions (Alper et al. 1966, 1967; G. D. Hunter 1972; Riesner et al. 1992); nevertheless, a modified isoform of host-encoded PrP—designated PrP^{Sc}—is essential for infectivity (Büeler et al. 1993; Prusiner 1991; Prusiner et al. 1983, 1993a, 1993b). In fact, considerable experimental data indicate that prions are composed exclusively of PrP^{Sc}. Earlier researchers described prion diseases as transmissible encephalopathies, spongiform encephalopathies, and slow virus diseases (Gajdusek 1977, 1985; Sigurdsson 1954).

Human Prion Diseases

The human (Hu) prion diseases form a quartet: kuru, Creutzfeldt-Jakob disease (CJD), Gerstmann-Sträussler-Scheinker (GSS) disease, and fatal familial insomnia (FFI). Cerebellar deficits produced by kuru often are associated with uncontrollable and inappropriate episodes of laughter, giving rise to the term *laughing death*. Investigators suggested that kuru spread among the Fore people of Papua New Guinea by ritualistic cannibalism (Gajdusek 1977; Gajdusek et al. 1966). Indeed, kuru once was the most common cause of death among New Guinea women in the Fore region of the Highlands (Gajdusek and Zigas 1957, 1959; Gajdusek et al. 1966); it has virtually disappeared with the cessation of ritualistic cannibalism (Alpers 1987). Kuru was the first human prion disease that researchers transmitted to experimental animals; the experimental and presumed human-to-human transmission of kuru led to the hypothesis that prion diseases are infectious disorders caused by unusual viruses similar to those that cause scrapie in sheep and goats.

CJD has a worldwide incidence of approximately one case per million persons (Masters et al. 1978). Less than 1% of CJD cases are infectious; all of those cases appear to be iatrogenic. Between 10%–15% of prion disease cases are inherited; the remaining cases are sporadic. Patients with CJD frequently present with dementia, although approximately 10% of patients initially exhibit cerebellar dysfunction. Patients with kuru or GSS usually present with ataxia, whereas those with FFI manifest insomnia and autonomic dysfunction (Brown 1992; Hsiao and Prusiner 1990; Medori et al. 1992b).

The occurrence of CJD in families—first reported almost 70 years ago (Kirschbaum 1924; Meggendorfer 1930)—perplexed researchers (to say the least). The significance of familial CJD remained unappreciated until researchers discovered mutations in the protein coding region of the PrP gene on the short arm of chromosome 20 (Hsiao et al. 1989; Prusiner 1994; Sparkes et al. 1986). Findings that brain tissue from patients who had died of familial prion diseases, inoculated into experimental animals, often transmitted disease posed a conundrum that researchers resolved through genetic linkage of these diseases to mutations of the PrP gene (Masters et al. 1981; Prusiner 1989; Tateishi et al. 1992).

Sporadic CJD is the most common form of human prion disease. Many attempts to show that sporadic prion diseases are caused by infection have been unsuccessful (Brown et al. 1987; Cousens et al. 1990; Harries-Jones et al. 1988; Malmgren et al. 1979). The discovery that inherited prion diseases are caused by germ-line mutation of the PrP gene raised the possibility that sporadic forms of these diseases might result from a somatic mutation (Prusiner 1989). However, the discovery that PrP^{Sc} is formed from the cellular isoform of the prion protein, PrP^{C}, by a post-translational process (Borchelt et al. 1990) and that overexpression of wild-type (wt) PrP transgenes produces spongiform degeneration and infectivity de novo (Westaway et al. 1994b) raised the possibility that sporadic prion diseases result from the spontaneous conversion of PrP^{C} into PrP^{Sc}.

Researchers have found PrP^{CJD} in the brains of most patients who died of prion disease. Although some investigators prefer the term PrP^{CJD} when referring to the abnormal isoform of HuPrP in the human brain, I use PrP^{Sc} interchangeably with PrP^{CJD} in this chapter. PrP^{Sc} is always used after human CJD prions have been passaged into an experimental animal because the nascent PrP^{Sc} molecules are produced from host PrP^{C}, and the PrP^{CJD} in the inoculum only serves to initiate the process.

Detection of PrP^{Sc} in the brains of some patients with inherited prion diseases, as well as in transgenic (Tg) mice expressing mouse (Mo) PrP with the human GSS point mutation (Pro→Leu), has been problematic despite clinical and neuropathological hallmarks of neurodegeneration (Hsiao et al. 1990, 1994). Presumably, neurodegeneration is caused, at least in part, by the abnormal metabolism of mutant PrP (Hsiao et al. 1990). Notably, horizontal transmission of neurodegeneration from the brains of patients with inherited prion diseases to inoculated rodents has been less frequent than from the brains of patients with sporadic prion diseases (Tateishi et al. 1992). Researchers have not determined whether this distinction between transmissible and nontransmissible inherited prion diseases will persist.

Researchers have found that Tg mice expressing a chimeric Hu/Mo PrP gene are susceptible to Hu prions from sporadic and iatrogenic CJD cases (Telling et al. 1994). These Tg(MHu2M) mice should make the use of apes and monkeys for the study of human prion diseases unnecessary and allow researchers to tailor PrP^C translated from the transgene to match the sequence of PrP^{CJD} in the inoculum. Other Tg mouse studies have demonstrated that PrP^{Sc} in the inoculum interacts preferentially with homotypic PrP^C during the propagation of prions (Prusiner et al. 1990; Scott et al. 1993). PrP^C is the cellular isoform of the prion protein, which has been identified in all mammals and birds examined to date. PrP^C is anchored to the external surface of cells by a glycolipid moiety; its function is unknown (Stahl et al. 1987).

Scrapie

Scrapie is the most common natural prion disease of animals. An investigation into the etiology of scrapie (Gordon 1946) followed the vaccination of sheep for looping ill virus with formalin-treated extracts of ovine lymphoid tissue unknowingly contaminated with scrapie prions; 2 years later, more than 1,500 sheep had developed scrapie from this vaccine.

Although researchers established the transmissibility of experimental scrapie, the spread of natural scrapie within and among flocks of sheep remained puzzling. Parry (1962, 1983) argued that host genes were responsible for the development of scrapie in sheep. He was convinced that natural scrapie was a genetic disease that could be eradicated by proper breeding protocols. Parry considered scrapie transmission by inoculation important primarily for laboratory studies; he regarded communicable infection as inconsequential in nature. Other investigators, however, viewed natural scrapie as an infectious disease and argued that host genetics only modulate susceptibility to an endemic infectious agent (Dickinson et al. 1965).

Mad Cow Disease

Epidemiologists believe that the offal of scrapied sheep in Great Britain is responsible for the current epidemic of bovine spongiform encephalopathy (BSE), or "mad cow disease" (Wilesmith et al. 1992). Prions in the offal from scrapie-infected sheep appear to have survived rendering that produced meat and bone meal (MBM). After researchers recognized BSE, authorities banned from further use MBM produced from domestic animals. Since 1986, when BSE was first recognized, more than 150,000 cattle have died of BSE. Many people have expressed considerable concern about whether humans might develop CJD after consuming beef from cattle with BSE prions.

PrP^{Sc} Formation

The fundamental event in prion diseases seems to be a conformational change in PrP. To date, all attempts to identify a post-translational chemical modification that distinguishes PrP^{Sc} from PrP^C have been unsuccessful (Stahl et al. 1993). PrP^C contains approximately 45% α-helix and is virtually devoid of β-sheet (Pan et al. 1993). Conversion to PrP^{Sc} creates a protein that contains approximately 30% α-helix and 45% β-sheet (Pan et al. 1993; Safar et al. 1993). The mechanism by which PrP^C is converted into PrP^{Sc} remains unknown, but PrP^C appears to bind to PrP^{Sc} to form an intermediate complex during the formation of nascent PrP^{Sc} (Prusiner et al. 1990; Scott et al. 1993; Telling et al. 1995).

Scientific Heresy?

The concept of prions initially met with great skepticism. Nevertheless, a growing body of experimental data convinced most skeptics of the existence of prions. The results of many studies have converged to show that prions differ from all other known infectious pathogens in several respects. First, prions do not contain a nucleic acid genome that codes for their progeny; viruses, viroids, bacteria, fungi, and parasites all have nucleic acid genomes that code for their progeny. Second, the only known component of the prion is a modified protein encoded by a cellular gene.

Third, the major—and possibly only—component of the prion is PrP^{Sc}, which is a pathogenic conformer of PrP^{C}.

As knowledge about prion diseases increases and researchers learn more about the molecular and genetic characteristics of prion proteins, the classification of these disorders undoubtedly will undergo modification. Indeed, the discovery of the PrP gene and the identification of pathogenic PrP gene mutations already have forced investigators to view these illnesses from previously unimagined perspectives.

Transgenetics and Gene Targeting

Transgenetic studies have yielded a wealth of new knowledge about infectious, genetic, and sporadic prion diseases. Unfortunately, however, the laborious production of Tg mice limits the number of studies that researchers can perform. The relatively long gestation period of mice and the need to microinject fertilized embryos prevent the creation of large numbers of different Tg mice; such large numbers would yield the greatest amount of new information. Assays that entail screening of a multitude of possible phenotypes in genetic experiments generally are the most informative.

Although the limited number of mice expressing different transgenes clearly is a liability, experiments with Tg mice expressing foreign and mutant PrP molecules have been extraordinarily useful in advancing investigators' understanding of prion biology. Importantly, however, transgenetic studies can readily yield an incomplete and sometimes erroneous interpretation of data if the number of lines of mice examined expressing a particular construct is inadequate. Defining an adequate number of lines is difficult; comparisons of lines expressing high and low levels of a given PrP transgene have proved to be quite helpful (Hsiao et al. 1994; Prusiner et al. 1990).

Transmission of Human Prions to Transgenic Mice

For three decades, epidemiologists studied the transmission of human prion diseases primarily with apes and monkeys; researchers believed that more than 90% of cases are transmissible (Brown et al. 1994; Gajdusek et al. 1966). Inoculations of mice, rats, and hamsters produced variable results (Manuelidis et al. 1978; Tateishi and Kitamoto 1995; Tateishi et al. 1983).

In our experience, only approximately 10% of intracerebrally inoculated mice developed central nervous system (CNS) dysfunction with incubation times of more than 500 days (Prusiner 1987; Telling et al. 1994). Other investigations showed that expression of a SHa PrP transgene in mice can abrogate the "species barrier" between mice and Syrian hamsters (SHa) for the transmission of prions (Scott et al. 1989); therefore, we constructed transgenic (Tg) mice expressing HuPrP. These Tg(HuPrP) mice expressed levels of HuPrP^C that were four to eight times higher than those of endogenous MoPrP^C. On inoculation with Hu prions, however, they failed to develop CNS dysfunction more frequently than non-Tg control subjects (Telling et al. 1994).

Because of the resistance of Tg(HuPrP) mice to Hu prions, we constructed mice expressing a chimeric Hu/Mo PrP transgene designated MHu2M. Earlier studies showed that chimeric SHa/Mo PrP transgenes supported transmission of either Mo or SHa prions (Scott et al. 1992, 1993). We found that Tg(MHu2M) mice expressing the chimeric transgene at a level slightly below that of endogenous MoPrP^C were highly susceptible to Hu prions—suggesting that Tg(HuPrP) mice have considerable difficulty converting HuPrP^C into PrP^{Sc} (Telling et al. 1994). Although MoPrP and HuPrP differ at 28 residues, only nine or perhaps fewer amino acids in the region between codons 96 and 167 feature in the species barrier in the transmission of Hu prions into mice, as demonstrated by the susceptibility of Tg(MHu2M) mice to Hu prions.

To explore why Hu prions transmitted disease to Tg(MHu2M) mice expressing chimeric PrP but not to Tg(HuPrP) mice, we crossed Tg(HuPrP)FVB mice with those in which the MoPrP gene had been ablated, designated Prnp$^{0/0}$ (Büeler et al. 1992). The resulting Tg(HuPrP)Prnp$^{0/0}$ mice were susceptible to Hu prions, whereas Tg(MHu2M)Prnp$^{0/0}$ mice were only slightly more susceptible (Telling et al. 1995). These observations suggested that MoPrP^C inhibited the conversion of HuPrP^C into PrP^{Sc}; once MoPrP^C was removed by gene ablation, inhibition was abolished.

Protein X and Prion Propagation

The results of our studies suggested that two separate domains of HuPrP^C participate in the formation of PrP^{Sc}: the central domain delimited by codons 96 and 167, as defined by the Hu sequence in chimeric MHu2MPrP^C that binds to PrP^{Sc}, and an additional domain through which HuPrP^C binds to a macromolecule other than PrP^{Sc} (Telling et al. 1995).

We assumed that this macromolecule was a protein and provisionally designated it "protein X."

Our chimeric transgene studies indicated that the second domain of PrP^C must be at the N- or C-terminus (i.e., outside the central region of PrP). Similar to the binding of PrP^C to PrP^{Sc}—which is most efficient when the two isoforms have the same sequence (Prusiner et al. 1990)—the binding of PrP^C to protein X seems to exhibit the highest affinity when these two proteins are from the same species. Although the level of MoPrP^C is only 10%–20% of the transgene product HuPrP^C in the brains of the Tg(HuPrP) mice, it prevented the conversion of HuPrP^C into PrP^{Sc}. These findings suggested that MoPrP^C binds to Mo protein X with a considerably higher affinity than does HuPrP^C, which provides an explanation for why MoPrP^C inhibits the transmission of Hu prions in Tg(HuPrP) mice.

Truncation of the N-terminus of recombinant PrP expressed in cultured cells still permitted the formation of PrP^{Sc}-like molecules (Rogers et al. 1993). Therefore, the site at which PrP^C binds to another protein probably is at the C-terminal end of PrP^C. Mature HuPrP differs from MoPrP at only five positions at the C-terminus, which lie between residues 215 and 230—some of which are likely to form the protein X binding site for PrP^C (Telling et al. 1995).

Studies on an inherited form of prion disease modeled in mice supported our proposed model for prion propagation involving protein X. Hsiao et al. (1994) found spontaneous CNS disease in uninoculated mice expressing the P102L point mutation of GSS when this substitution was introduced into MoPrP. The P102L mutation expressed in chimeric MHu2MPrP but not HuPrP produced CNS dysfunction in Tg mice. These findings suggested that inherited prion disease, like the transmissible disorder, requires protein X for the conversion of mutant PrP^C into a pathological isoform.

Modeling of GSS in Tg(MoPrP-P101L) Mice

We introduced the codon 102 point mutation found in GSS patients into the MoPrP gene and created Tg(MoPrP-P101L)H mice expressing high (H) levels of the mutant transgene product. The two lines of Tg(MoPrP-P101L)H mice, designated 174 and 87, spontaneously developed CNS degeneration characterized by clinical signs indistinguishable from experimental murine scrapie and neuropathology consisting of widespread spongiform morphology and astrocytic gliosis (Hsiao et al. 1990) and PrP amyloid plaques (Figure 5–1) (Hsiao et al. 1994). These results implied that PrP gene mutations cause GSS, familial CJD, and FFI.

Brain extracts prepared from spontaneously ill Tg(MoPrP-P101L)H mice transmitted CNS degeneration to Tg196 mice expressing low levels of the mutant transgene product, as well as some Syrian hamsters (Hsiao et al. 1994). Many Tg196 mice and some Syrian hamsters developed CNS degeneration between 200 and 700 days after inoculation; inoculated CD-1 Swiss mice remained healthy. Serial transmission of CNS degeneration in Tg196 mice required about 1 year, whereas serial transmission in Syrian hamsters occurred after approximately 75 days (Hsiao et al. 1994).

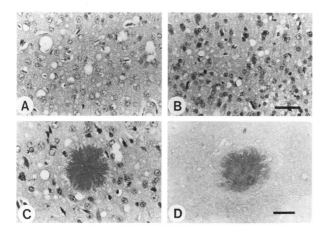

Figure 5–1. Neuropathology of Tg(MoPrP-P101L) mice developing neurodegeneration spontaneously. A: Vacuolation in cerebral cortex of Swiss CD-1 mouse that exhibited signs of neurological dysfunction at 138 days after intracerebral inoculation with approximately 10^6 ID_{50} units of RML scrapie prions; B: Vacuolation in cerebral cortex of Tg(MoPrP-P101L) mouse that exhibited signs of neurological dysfunction at age 252 days; C: Kuru-type PrP amyloid plaque stained with periodic acid Schiff in caudate nucleus of Tg(MoPrP-P101L) mouse that exhibited signs of neurological dysfunction; D: PrP amyloid plaques stained with a-PrP antiserum (RO73) in caudate nucleus of Tg(MoPrP-P101L) mouse that exhibited signs of neurological dysfunction. Bar in B (also applies to A) = 50 μm. Bar in D (also applies to C) = 25 μm.

Although brain extracts prepared from Tg(MoPrP-P101L)H mice transmitted CNS degeneration to some inoculated recipients, immunoassays detected little or no PrP^{Sc} after limited proteolysis. Undetectable or low levels of PrP^{Sc} in the brains of these Tg(MoPrP-P101L)H mice are consistent with the results of our transmission experiments, which suggest low titers of infectious prions. Although immunoassays after limited proteolysis detected no PrP^{Sc} in the brains of inoculated Tg196 mice exhibiting neurological dysfunction, we frequently found PrP amyloid plaques and spongiform degeneration (Table 5–2).

The neurodegeneration found in inoculated Tg196 mice seems likely to result from a modification of mutant PrP^{C} initiated by mutant PrP^{Sc} in brain extracts prepared from ill Tg(MoPrP-P101L)H mice. Findings from studies of inherited human prion diseases support this explanation: neither protease-resistant PrP (Brown et al. 1992; Medori et al. 1992a) nor transmission to experimental rodents (Tateishi et al. 1992) could be demonstrated. Furthermore, transmission of disease from Tg(MoPrP-P101L)H mice to Tg196 mice but not to Swiss mice is consistent with findings that demonstrate that homotypic interactions between PrP^{C} and PrP^{Sc} feature in the formation of PrP^{Sc}.

Modification of the expression of mutant and wtPrP genes in Tg mice facilitated experimental manipulation of the pathogenesis of inherited and infectious prion diseases. Although eightfold overexpression of the wtPrP-A transgene was not deleterious to the mice, it did shorten scrapie incubation times from approximately 145 days to approximately 45 days after inoculation with Mo scrapie prions (Telling et al., unpublished data). In contrast, overexpression at the same level of a PrP-A transgene mutated at codon 101 produced spontaneous, fatal neurodegeneration at ages 150–300 days in two new lines of Tg(MoPrP-P101L) mice designated 2866 and 2247.

Genetic crosses of Tg(MoPrP-P101L)2866 mice with gene-targeted mice lacking both PrP alleles (Prnp$^{0/0}$) produced animals with a highly synchronous onset of illness at ages 150–160 days. Tg(MoPrP-P101L)2866/Prnp$^{0/0}$ mice had numerous PrP plaques and widespread spongiform degeneration—in contrast to Tg2866 and 2247 mice, which exhibited spongiform degeneration but only a few PrP amyloid plaques. Another line of mice, designated Tg2862, overexpressed the mutant transgene approximately 32-fold and developed fatal neurodegeneration at ages 200–400 days. Tg2862 mice exhibited the most severe spongiform degeneration and had numerous large PrP amyloid plaques.

Table 5–2. Species-specific prion inocula determine the distribution of spongiform change and deposition of PrP amyloid plaques in transgenic mice

Animal	SHa prions					Mo prions				
	Spongiform change[a]		PrP plaques[b]		Diameter[d]	Spongiform change[a]			PrP plaques[b]	
	n[c]	Grey	Wht	Frequency		n[c]	Grey	Wht	Wht	Frequency
Non-Tg	6	N.D.[e]		N.D.		10	+	+	+	+
Tg 69	5	+[f]	−	Numerous	6.5 ± 3.1 (389)	2	+	+	+	−
Tg 71	7	+	−	Numerous	8.1 ± 3.6 (345)	2	+	+	+	−
Tg 81	7	+	−	Numerous	8.3 ± 3.0 (439)	3	+	+	+	Few
Tg 7	3	+[g]	−	Numerous	14.0 ± 8.3 (19)	4	+	+	+	−
SHa	3	+	−	Numerous	5.7 ± 2.7 (247)		N.D.			N.D.

[a] Spongiform change evaluated in hippocampus, thalamus, cerebral cortex, and brain stem for grey matter and deep cerebellum for white matter.

[b] Plaques in subcallosal region stained with SHaPrP mAb 13A5, anti-PrP rabbit antisera R073, and trichrome stain.

[c] n = number of brains examined.

[d] Mean diameter of PrP plaques in microns ± standard error (number of observations in parentheses).

[e] N.D. = not determined.

[f] + = present; − = not found.

[g] Focal; confirmed to dorsal nucleus of raphe.

Source. Prusiner SB: "Molecular Biology and Genetics of Neurodegenerative Diseases Caused by Prions." *Advances in Virus Research* 41:241–280, 1992.

Whereas mutant PrP^C(P101L) clearly produces neurodegeneration, wtPrP^C profoundly modifies the age at onset of illness and the neuropathology for a given level of transgene expression. These findings and those from other studies (e.g., Telling et al. 1994) suggest that mutant and wtPrP interact—perhaps through a chaperone-like protein—to modify the pathogenesis of dominantly inherited prion diseases.

Overexpression of wtPrP Transgenes

During transgenetic studies, we discovered that uninoculated older mice harboring high copy-numbers of wtPrP transgenes derived from Syrian hamsters, sheep, and PrP-B mice spontaneously developed truncal ataxia, hind-limb paralysis, and tremors (Westaway et al. 1994a). These Tg mice exhibited a profound necrotizing myopathy involving skeletal muscle, a demyelinating polyneuropathy, and focal vacuolation of the CNS.

Development of disease was dependent on transgene dosage. For example, Tg(SHaPrP$^{+/+}$)7 mice homozygous for the SHaPrP transgene array regularly developed disease at ages 400–600 days; hemizygous Tg(SHaPrP$^{+/0}$)7 mice also developed disease but after more than 650 days.

Attempts to demonstrate PrP^{Sc} in muscle or brain tissue were unsuccessful, although transmission of disease with brain extracts from Tg(SHaPrP$^{+/+}$)7 mice inoculated into Syrian hamsters did occur. These Syrian hamsters had PrP^{Sc}, as detected by immunoblotting and spongiform degeneration (Groth and Prusiner, unpublished data). We observed serial passage with brain extracts from these animals to recipients. De novo synthesis of prions in Tg(SHaPrP$^{+/+}$)7 mice overexpressing wtSHaPrP^C provided support for the hypothesis that sporadic CJD results not from infection but from spontaneous, albeit rare, conversion of PrP^C into PrP^{Sc}. Alternatively, a somatic mutation in which mutant SHaPrP^C is spontaneously converted into PrP^{Sc}—as in the inherited prion diseases—also could explain sporadic CJD. These findings, coupled with those described later for Tg(MoPrP-P101L) mice, suggest that prions are devoid of foreign nucleic acid, in accord with many earlier studies that used other experimental approaches.

Ablation of the PrP Gene

Surprisingly, ablation of the PrP gene in Tg (Prnp$^{0/0}$) mice did not affect the development of these animals (Büeler et al. 1992; Manson et al. 1994a).

In fact, they were healthy at age 2 years. Some investigators have presented data suggesting that synaptic transmission and neuronal excitability in these mice are abnormal (Collinge et al. 1994; Manson et al. 1995; Whittington et al. 1995); we have been unable to confirm these findings, however. $Prnp^{0/0}$ mice are resistant to prions (Figure 5–2) and do not propagate scrapie infectivity (Büeler et al. 1993; Prusiner et al. 1993a).

$Prnp^{0/0}$ mice crossed with Tg(SHaPrP) mice were susceptible to SHa prions but remained resistant to Mo prions (Büeler et al. 1993; Prusiner et al. 1993a). Because the absence of PrP^C expression does not provoke disease, scrapie and other prion diseases probably result from PrP^{Sc} accumulation rather than inhibition of PrP^C function (Büeler et al. 1992).

Mice heterozygous ($Prnp^{+/0}$) for ablation of the PrP gene had prolonged incubation times when inoculated with Mo prions (Figure 5–2) (Büeler et al. 1994; Manson et al. 1994b; Prusiner et al. 1993a). These $Prnp^{+/0}$ mice developed signs of neurological dysfunction at 400–460 days after inoculation. These findings are in accord with studies on Tg(SHaPrP) mice in which diminished incubation times accompanied increased SHaPrP expression (Prusiner et al. 1990).

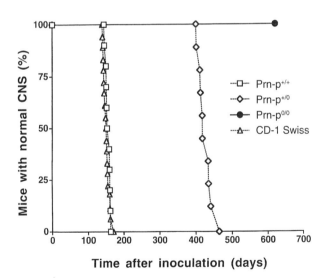

Figure 5–2. Incubation times in PrP gene-ablated Prn-p$^{0/+}$ and Prn-p$^{0/0}$ mice, as well as wt Prn-p$^{+/+}$ and CD-1 mice inoculated with RML mouse prions. RML prions were heated and irradiated at 254 nm before intracerebral inoculation into CD-1 Swiss mice (open triangles), Prn-p$^{+/+}$ mice (open squares), Prn-p$^{0/+}$ mice (open diamonds), or Prn-p$^{0/0}$ mice (filled circle).

Because Prnp$^{0/0}$ mice do not express PrP^C, we reasoned that they might more readily produce α-PrP antibodies. Prnp$^{0/0}$ mice immunized with Mo or SHa prion rods produced α-PrP antisera that bound Mo, SHa, and HuPrP (Prusiner et al. 1993a). These findings contrasted with earlier studies in which α-MoPrP antibodies could not be produced in mice—presumably because the mice had been rendered tolerant by the presence of MoPrP^C (Barry and Prusiner 1986; Kascsak et al. 1987; Rogers et al. 1991). Production of α-PrP antibodies by Prnp$^{0/0}$ mice is consistent with the hypothesis that the absence of an immune response in prion diseases relates to the fact that PrP^C and PrP^{Sc} share many epitopes. Future research must determine whether Prn-p$^{0/0}$ mice produce α-PrP antibodies that specifically recognize conformational dependent epitopes present on PrP^{Sc} but absent from PrP^C.

Protein Y and the Neuropathology of Prion Disease

We produced four lines of congenic mice by crossing the PrP gene of the ILn/J mouse onto C57BL. We designated these four lines of congenic mice B6.I-4 for B6.I-*B2m*^{a}, B6.I-1 for B6.I-*Prn-p*^{b}, B6.I-2 for B6.I-*Il-1a*^{d} *Prn-p*^{b}, B6.I-3 for B6.I-*B2m*^{a} *Prn-p*^{b} (Carlson et al. 1993).

Neuropathological examination of B6.I-1, B6.I-2, I/LnJ, and VM/Dk mice inoculated with 87V prions showed numerous PrP amyloid plaques, in agreement with an earlier report on VM/Dk mice (Bruce et al. 1976). We found intense spongiform degeneration, gliosis, and PrP immunostaining in the ventral posterior lateral (VPL) nucleus of the thalamus, the habenula, and the raphe nuclei of the brain stem in B6.I-1 mice (Carlson et al. 1994); these same regions showed intense immunoreactivity for PrP^{Sc} on histoblots. Unexpectedly, B6.I-2 and ILn/J mice exhibited only mild vacuolation of the thalamus and brain stem. These findings suggested that a locus near *Prn-p* influences the deposition of PrP^{Sc}—and thus vacuolation—in the thalamus, the habenula, and raphe nuclei. We provisionally designated the product of this gene "protein Y."

Identification of the gene that encodes protein Y that is distinct from but near *Prn-p* will be important. The gene Y product appears to control, at least in part, neuronal vacuolation and presumably PrP^{Sc} deposition in mice inoculated with scrapie prions. Isolation of protein Y should help researchers to dissect the molecular events that feature in the pathogenesis of prion diseases.

Prion Diversity

Prion Strains and Variations in Patterns of Disease

For many years, researchers performed studies of experimental scrapie exclusively with sheep and goats. They transmitted the disease first by intraocular inoculation (Cuillé and Chelle 1939) and later by intracerebral, oral, subcutaneous, intramuscular, and intravenous injections of brain extracts from sheep developing scrapie. Incubation periods of 1–3 years were common; many of the inoculated animals failed to develop disease (Dickinson and Stamp 1969; Hadlow et al. 1980, 1982). Different breeds of sheep exhibited markedly different susceptibilities to scrapie prions inoculated subcutaneously, suggesting that genetic background might influence host permissiveness (Gordon 1966).

Researchers first appreciated the diversity of scrapie prions in goats inoculated with "hyper" and "drowsy" isolates (Pattison and Millson 1961). Subsequent studies in mice demonstrated the existence of many scrapie "strains" (Bruce and Dickinson 1987; Dickinson and Fraser 1979; Dickinson and Outram 1988; Kimberlin et al. 1987). This diversity continues to pose a fascinating conundrum: what is the macromolecule that carries the information required for each strain to manifest a unique set of biological properties—if it is not a nucleic acid?

Investigators have found evidence for multiple "strains" or distinct isolates of prions as defined by specific incubation times, distribution of vacuolar lesions, and patterns of PrP^{Sc} accumulation (Bruce et al. 1989; Dickinson et al. 1968; Fraser and Dickinson 1973; Hecker et al. 1992). Researchers have used the lengths of incubation times to distinguish prion strains inoculated into sheep, goats, mice, and hamsters.

Dickinson and his colleagues developed a system for "strain typing" by which mice with genetically determined short and long incubation times were used in combination with the F1 cross (Dickinson and Meikle 1971; Dickinson et al. 1968, 1984). For example, C57BL mice exhibited short incubation times—approximately 150 days—when inoculated with either the Me7 or Chandler isolates; VM mice inoculated with these same isolates had prolonged incubation times—approximately 300 days. The mouse gene controlling incubation times was labeled *Sinc*; long incubation times were considered to be a dominant trait because of prolonged incubation times in F1 mice. Prion strains were categorized into two groups, based on their incubation times: those causing disease more rapidly in "short" incubation time C57BL mice and those causing disease more rapidly in "long" incubation time VM mice.

PrP Gene Dosage Controls the Length of Scrapie Incubation Time

More than a decade of study was required to unravel the mechanism responsible for the "dominance" of long incubation times; not unexpectedly, investigators found that long incubation times were not dominant traits. Instead, the apparent dominance of long incubation times relates to a gene dosage effect (Carlson et al. 1994).

Our own studies began with the identification of a widely available mouse strain with long incubation times. ILn/J mice inoculated with RML prions had incubation times exceeding 200 days (Kingsbury et al. 1983)— a finding confirmed by other investigators (Carp et al. 1987). Once molecular clones of the PrP gene were available, we wondered whether the PrP genes of short and long mice segregate with incubation times. We used a restriction fragment length polymorphism (RFLP) of the PrP gene to follow the segregation of MoPrP genes (*Prn-p*) from short NZW or C57BL mice with long ILn/J mice in F1 and F2 crosses. This approach demonstrated genetic linkage between a *Prn-p* and a gene modulating incubation times (*Prn-i*) (Carlson et al. 1986). Other investigators confirmed the genetic linkage; one group showed that the incubation time gene *Sinc* also was linked to PrP (N. Hunter et al. 1987; Race et al. 1990).

The evidence suggests that the genes for PrP, *Prn-i*, and *Sinc* probably are congruent; as a result, researchers no longer use the term *Sinc* (Ziegler 1993). The PrP sequences of NZW with short and long scrapie incubation times, respectively, differ at codons 108 (L→F) and 189 (T→V) (Westaway et al. 1987).

Although the amino acid substitutions in PrP that distinguish *Prn-p^a* from *Prn-p^b* mice argued for the congruency of *Prn-p* and *Prn-i*, experiments with *Prn-p^a* mice expressing *Prn-p^b* transgenes demonstrated an apparently paradoxical shortening of incubation times (Westaway et al. 1991). We had predicted that these Tg mice would exhibit a prolongation of incubation time after inoculation with RML prions based on (*Prn-p^a* x *Prn-p^b*) F1 mice, which do exhibit long incubation times. We described those findings as a "paradoxical shortening" because we and others had believed for many years that long incubation times were dominant traits (Carlson et al. 1986; Dickinson et al. 1968).

Studies of congenic and transgenic mice expressing different numbers of the a and b alleles of $Prn-p$, however (Table 5–3), led us to realize that these findings were not paradoxical; indeed, they resulted from increased PrP gene dosage (Carlson et al. 1994). When we inoculated the RML isolate into congenic and transgenic mice, we found that an increase in the number of copies of the a allele was the major determinant in reducing the incubation time; increasing the number of copies of the b allele also reduced the incubation time, but not to the same extent as with the a allele (Table 5–3).

In fact, studies of Tg(SHaPrP) mice in which the length of the incubation time after inoculation with SHa prions was inversely proportional to the transgene product SHaPrP^C (Prusiner et al. 1990) foreshadowed the discovery that incubation times are controlled by the relative dosage of $Prn-p^a$ and $Prn-p^b$ alleles. The PrP gene dose determines not only the length of the incubation time but also the passage history of the inoculum, particularly in $Prn-p^b$ mice (Table 5–4). The PrP^{Sc} allotype in the inoculum produced the shortest incubation times when it was the same as the allotype of PrP^C in the host (Carlson et al. 1989). (The term *allotype* describes allelic variants of PrP.)

To address the issue of whether gene products other than PrP might be responsible for these findings, we inoculated B6 and B6.I-4 mice carrying $Prn-p^{a/a}$, as well as I/Ln, and B6.I-2 mice (Carlson et al. 1993, 1994) with RML prions passaged in mice homozygous for either the a or b allele of $Prn-p$ (Table 5–4). CD-1 and NZW/LacJ mice produced prions containing PrP^{Sc}-A encoded by $Prn-p^a$; I/LnJ mice produced PrP^{Sc}-B prions. The incubation times in the congenic mice reflected the PrP allotype rather than other factors acquired during prion passage. The effect of the allotype barrier was small when measured in $Prn-p^{a/a}$ mice but clearly demonstrable in $Prn-p^{b/b}$ mice. B6.I-2 congenic mice inoculated with prions from I/Ln mice had an incubation time of 237 ± 8 days, compared with 360 ± 16 days and 404 ± 4 days for mice inoculated with prions passaged in CD-1 and NZW mice, respectively. Thus, previous passage of prions in $Prn-p^b$ mice shortened the incubation time by approximately 40% when assayed in $Prn-p^b$ mice, compared with those inoculated with prions passaged in $Prn-p^a$ mice (Carlson et al. 1989).

Overdominance

The phenomenon of "overdominance"—in which incubation times in F1 hybrids are longer than those of either parent (Dickinson and Meikle

Table 5–3. MoPrP-A expression is a major determinant of incubation times in mice inoculated with the RML scrapie prions

Mice	Prn-p genotype (copies)	Prn-p transgenes (copies)	Alleles		Incubation time[a] (days ± SEM)	n
			a	b		
Prn-p$^{0/0}$	0/0		0	0	>600	4
Prn-p$^{+/0}$	a/0		1	0	426 ± 18	9[a]
B6.I-1	b/b		0	2	360 ± 16	7[b]
B6.I-2	b/b		0	2	379 ± 8	10[b]
B6.I-3	b/b		0	2	404 ± 10	20
(B6 x B6.I-1)F1	a/b		1	1	268 ± 4	7
B6.I-1 x Tg(MoPrP-B$^{0/0}$)15	a/b		1	1	255 ± 7	11[c]
B6.I-1 x Tg(MoPrP-B$^{0/0}$)15	a/b		1	1	274 ± 3	9[d]
B6.I-1 x Tg(MoPrP-B$^{+/0}$)15	a/b	bbb/0	1	4	166 ± 2	11[c]
B6.I-1 x Tg(MoPrP-B$^{+/0}$)15	a/b	bbb/0	1	4	162 ± 3	8[d]
C57BL/6J (B6)	a/a		2	0	143 ± 4	8
B6.I-4	a/a		2	0	144 ± 5	8
Non-Tg(MoPrP-B$^{0/0}$)15	a/a		2	0	130 ± 3	10
Tg(MoPrP-B$^{+/0}$)15	a/a	bbb/0	2	3	115 ± 2	18
Tg(MoPrP-B$^{+/+}$)15	a/a	bbb/bbb	2	6	111 ± 5	5
Tg(MoPrP-B$^{+/0}$)94	a/a	>30b	2	>30	75 ± 2	15[e]
Tg(MoPrP-A$^{+/0}$)B4053	a/a	>30a	>30	0	50 ± 2	16

[a] *Source.* Data from Prusiner SB, Groth D, Serban A, et al: "Ablation of the Prion Protein (PrP) Gene in Mice Prevents Scrapie and Facilitates Production of Anti-PrP Antibodies." *Proceedings of the National Academy of Sciences of the United States of America* 90:10608–10612, 1993a.

[b] *Source.* Data from Carlson GA, Ebeling C, Torchia M, et al: "Delimiting the Location of the Scrapie Prion Incubation Time Gene on Chromosome 2 of the Mouse." *Genetics* 133:979–988, 1993.

[c] Homozygous Tg(MoPrP-B$^{+/+}$)15 mice were maintained as a distinct subline selected for transgene homozygosity two generations removed from (B6 x LT/Sv)F2 founder. Hemizygous Tg(MoPrP-B$^{+/0}$)15 mice were produced by crossing the Tg(MoPrP-B$^{+/+}$)15 line with B6 mice.

[d] Tg(MoPrP-B$^{+/0}$)15 mice were maintained by repeated backcrossing to B6 mice.

[e] *Source.* Data from Westaway D, Mirenda CA, Foster D, et al: "Paradoxical Shortening of Scrapie Incubation Times by Expression of Prion Protein Transgenes Derived From Long Incubation Period Mice." *Neuron* 7:59–68, 1991.

Table 5–4. Mismatching of PrP allotypes between PrP^{Sc} in inoculum and PrP^{C} in inoculated host extends prion incubation times in congenic mice

Donor inoculum		Recipient host			
Mouse	Genotype	Mouse	Genotype	Incubation time	n
CD-1	a/a	C57BL/6J (B6)	a/a	143 ± 4	8
NZW	a/a	B6.I-4	a/a	144 ± 5	8
I/Ln	b/b	B6.I-4	a/a	150 ± 6	6
CD-1	a/a	B6.I-2	b/b	360 ± 16	8
NZW	a/a	B6.I-2	b/b	404 ± 4	20
I/Ln	b/b	B6.I-2	b/b	237 ± 8	17
CD-1	a/a	I/LnJ[a]	b/b	314 ± 13	11
NZW	a/a	I/LnJ	b/b	283 ± 21	8
I/Ln	b/b	I/LnJ	b/b	193 ± 6	16

[a]*Source.* I/LnJ results previously reported (Carlson GA, Ebeling C, Yang S-L: "Prion Isolate Specified Allotypic Interactions Between the Cellular and Scrapie Prion Proteins in Congenic and Transgenic Mice." *Proceedings of the National Academy of Sciences of the United States of America* 91:5690–5694, 1994).

1969)—contributed to confusion surrounding control of scrapie incubation times. We observed overdominance when we inoculated the 22A scrapie isolate into B6, B6.I-1, and (B6 × B6.I-1)F1: The scrapie incubation time in B6 mice was 405 ± 2 days, in B6.I mice 194 ± 10 days, and in (B6 × B6.I-1)F1 mice 508 ± 14 days (Table 5–5). We observed shorter incubation times in Tg(MoPrP-B)15 mice that were either homozygous or hemizygous for the *Prn-p^b* transgene. Hemizygous Tg(MoPrP-B$^{+/0}$)15 mice exhibited a scrapie incubation time of 395 ± 12 days; homozygous mice had an incubation time of 286 ± 15 days.

As with the results with the RML isolate (Table 5–4), the findings with the 22A isolate can be explained on the basis of gene dosage. The relative effects of the *a* and *b* alleles differ in two respects, however. First, the *b* allele—not the *a* allele—is the major determinant of the scrapie incubation time with the 22A isolate. Second, increasing the number of copies of the *a* allele prolongs rather than diminishes the incubation: the *a* allele is inhibitory with the 22A isolate (Table 5–5). The inhibitory effect of the *Prn-p^a* allele is even more pronounced with the 87V prion isolate; only a few *Prn-p^a* and (*Prn-p^a* × *Prn-p^b*)F1 mice developed scrapie after more than 600 days postinoculation (Carlson et al. 1994).

The most interesting feature of the incubation time profile for 22A is the overdominance of the *a* allele of *Prn-p* in prolonging incubation period. Dickinson and Outram (1979) proposed the replication site hypothesis on the basis of overdominance; they postulated that dimers of the *Sinc* gene product feature in the replication of the scrapie agent. The results presented in Table 5–5 are compatible with the interpretation that the target for PrP^{Sc} may be a PrP^C dimer or multimer. This model assumes that PrP^C-B dimers are more readily converted to PrP^{Sc} than are PrP^C-A dimers and that PrP^C-A:PrP^C-B heterodimers are even more resistant to conversion to PrP^{Sc} than PrP^C-A dimers. Increasing the ratio of PrP-B to PrP-A would favor the formation of PrP^C-B homodimers and lead to shorter incubation times (Table 5–5). A similar mechanism may account for the relative paucity of individuals heterozygous for the Met/Val polymorphism at codon 129 of the human PrP gene in spontaneous and iatrogenic CJD (Palmer et al. 1991).

Alternatively, PrPC-PrP^{Sc} interaction may be broken down to two distinct aspects: binding affinity and efficacy of conversion to PrP^{Sc}. If PrP-A has a higher affinity for 22A PrP^{Sc} than does PrP^C-B but is inefficiently converted to PrP^{Sc}, the exceptionally long incubation time of *Prn-p$^{a/b}$* heterozygotes might reflect reduction in the supply of 22A prions available for interaction with the PrP^C-B product of the single *Prn-p^b* allele. Additionally, PrP^C-A may inhibit the interaction of 22A PrP^{Sc} with PrP^C-B, leading to prolongation of the incubation time. This interpretation is supported by prolonged incubation times in Tg(SHaPrP) mice inoculated with mouse

Table 5–5.   MoPrPC-A inhibits synthesis of 22A scrapie prions

Mice	Prn-p genotype	Prn-p transgenes (copies)	Alleles *a* (copies)	*b*	Incubation time (days ± SEM)	*n*
B6.I-1	b/b		0	2	194 ± 10	7
(B6 x B6.I-1)F1	a/b		1	1	508 ± 14	7
C57BL/6J (B6)	a/a		2	0	405 ± 2	8
Non-Tg(MoPrP-B$^{0/0}$)15		a/a	2	0	378 ± 8	3[a]
Tg(MoPrP-B$^{+/0}$)15	a/a	bbb/0	2	3	318 ± 14	15[a]
Tg(MoPrP-B$^{+/0}$)15	a/a	bbb/0	2	3	395 ± 12	6[b]
Tg(MoPrP-B$^{+/+}$)15	a/a	bbb/bbb	2	6	266 ± 1	6[a]
Tg(MoPrP-B$^{+/+}$)15	a/a	bbb/bbb	2	6	286 ± 15	5[b]

[a]Homozygous Tg(MoPrP-B$^{+/+}$)15 mice were maintained as a distinct subline selected for transgene homozygosity two generations removed from (B6 x LT/Sv)F2 founder. Hemizygous Tg(MoPrP-B$^{+/0}$)15 mice were produced by crossing the Tg(MoPrP-B$^{+/+}$)15 line with B6 mice.

[b]Tg(MoPrP-B$^{+/0}$)15 mice were maintained by repeated backcrossing to B6 mice.

prions in which SHaPrP^C is thought to inhibit the binding of MoPrP^{Sc} to the substrate MoPrP^C (Prusiner et al. 1990).

Patterns of PrP^{Sc} Deposition

In addition to measuring the length of the incubation time, researchers have used profiles of spongiform degeneration to characterize different prion strains (Fraser 1979; Fraser and Dickinson 1973). The development of a new procedure for in situ detection of PrP^{Sc}—namely, histoblotting (Taraboulos et al. 1992)—allowed researchers to localize and quantify PrP^{Sc}, as well as to determine whether different strains produce different, reproducible patterns of PrP^{Sc} accumulation (DeArmond et al. 1993; Hecker et al. 1992).

Histoblotting overcame two obstacles that plagued standard immuno-histochemical techniques for PrP^{Sc} detection in brain tissue: the presence of PrP^C and weak antigenicity of PrP^{Sc} (DeArmond et al. 1987). A histoblot is made by pressing 10 μm-thick cryostat sections of fresh frozen brain tissue to nitrocellulose paper. To localize protease-resistant PrP^{Sc} in brain tissue, the histoblot is digested with proteinase K to eliminate PrP^C; this step is followed by denaturation of the undigested PrP^{Sc} to enhance binding of PrP antibodies. Researchers can localize PrP^C in histoblots of normal brain tissue by eliminating the proteinase K digestion step.

Immunohistochemical staining yields a far more intense, specific, and reproducible PrP signal than immunohistochemistry on standard tissue sections. The intensity of immunostaining correlates well with neurochemical estimates of PrP^{Sc} concentration in homogenates of dissected brain regions.

Comparisons of PrP^{Sc} accumulation on histoblots with histological sections showed that PrP^{Sc} deposition preceded vacuolation; only regions with PrP^{Sc} underwent degeneration. Microdissection of individual brain regions confirmed the conclusions of histoblot studies: regions with high levels of PrP 27–30 had intense vacuolation (Casaccia-Bonnefil et al. 1993). Thus, we concluded that the deposition of PrP^{Sc} is responsible for the neuropathological changes in prion diseases.

Although studies with mice and Syrian hamsters established that each isolate has a specific signature, as defined by a specific pattern of PrP^{Sc} accumulation in the brain (Carlson et al. 1994; DeArmond et al. 1993; Hecker et al. 1992), further studies must do comparisons on an isogenic background (Hsiao et al. 1994; Scott et al. 1993). Variations in the patterns of PrP^{Sc} accumulation were as large as those variations between two strains when a single strain is inoculated in mice expressing different PrP genes. Based on initial studies in animals of a single genotype, we suggested that PrP[Sc] synthesis occurs in specific populations of cells for a given distinct prion isolate.

Are Prion Strains Different PrP[Sc] Conformers?

Multiple PrP[Sc] conformers that act as templates for the folding of de novo synthesized PrP[Sc] molecules during prion "replication" might account for the problem of multiple distinct prion isolates. Although passage history clearly may be responsible for prolongation of incubation time when prions are passed between mice expressing different PrP allotypes (Carlson et al. 1989) or between species (Prusiner et al. 1990), many scrapie strains show distinct incubation times in the same inbred host (Bruce et al. 1991).

We inoculated three strains of prions into congenic and Tg mice harboring various numbers of the *a* and *b* alleles of *Prn-p* (Carlson et al. 1994). The number of *Prn-p^a* genes was the major determinant of incubation times in mice inoculated with the RML prion isolate; the number of *Prn-p^a* genes was inversely related to the length of the incubation time (Table 5–3). In contrast, the *Prn-p^a* allele prevented scrapie in mice inoculated with 87V prions. *Prn-p^b* genes were permissive for 87V prions and shortened incubation times in most mice inoculated with 22A prions (Table 5–5).

Experiments with the 87V isolate suggested that a genetic locus encoding protein Y—distinct from *Prn-p*—controls the deposition of PrP[Sc] and attendant neuropathology. Although each prion isolate produced distinguishable patterns of PrP[Sc] accumulation in brain tissue, comparison of these patterns showed that patterns with RML and 22A prions in congenic *Prn-p^b* mice were more similar than those with RML prions in *Prn-p^a* and *Prn-p^b* congenic mice. Thus, the PrP genotype and the prion isolate both modify the distribution of PrP[Sc] and the length of incubation time. These findings suggested that prion strain-specified properties result from different affinities of PrP[Sc] in the inocula for PrP[C]-A and PrP[C]-B allotypes encoded by the host.

Although the proposal regarding multiple PrP[Sc] conformers is unorthodox, we already know that PrP can assume at least two profoundly different conformations: PrP[C] and PrP[Sc] (Pan et al. 1993). Notably, two different isolates from mink dying of transmissible mink encephalopathy exhibit different sensitivities of PrP[Sc] to proteolytic digestion, supporting the suggestion that PrP[Sc] might carry isolate-specific information (Bessen and Marsh 1992a, 1992b, 1994; Bessen et al. 1995; Marsh et al. 1991). Researchers do not know how many conformations PrP[Sc] can assume. The molecular weight of a PrP^{Sc} homodimer is consistent with the ionizing radiation target size of 55,000 ± 9,000 daltons, as determined for infectious prion particles independent of their polymeric form (Bellinger-Kawahara et al. 1988). If prions are oligomers of PrP^{Sc} (which seems likely), this model offers another level of complexity—which, in turn, generates additional diversity.

Conclusion

Prions Are Not Viruses

The study of prions has taken several unexpected directions over the past several years. The discovery that prion diseases in humans are uniquely genetic and infectious has greatly strengthened and extended the prion concept. Researchers have found 18 different mutations in the human PrP gene—all resulting in nonconservative substitutions—that are genetically linked to or segregate with inherited prion diseases.

However, the transmissible prion particle is composed largely, if not entirely, of an abnormal isoform of the prion protein designated PrP^{Sc} (Prusiner 1991). These findings suggest that epidemiologists should consider prion diseases to be pseudoinfections because the particles transmitting disease appear to be devoid of a foreign nucleic acid and thus differ from all known microorganisms, as well as from viruses and viroids. Researchers continue to use terms such as *infection, incubation period, transmissibility,* and *endpoint titration* in studies of prion diseases because investigators have derived a great deal of information—especially about scrapie of rodents—using experimental protocols adapted from virology.

Do Prions Exist in Lower Organisms?

Lacroute (1971) described ure2 and [URA3⁺] mutants in *S. cervisiae* that can grow on ureidosuccinate under conditions of nitrogen repression such as glutamic acid and ammonia. Mutants of URE2 exhibit Mendelian inheritance, whereas [URE3⁺] is cytoplasmically inherited (Wickner 1994). The [URE3⁺] phenotype can be induced by UV irradiation and overexpression of ure2p, the gene product of ure2; deletion of ure2 abolishes [URE3⁺]. The function of ure2p is unknown, but it has substantial homology with glutathione-S-transferase; attempts to demonstrate this enzymic activity with purified ure2p have not been successful (Coschigano and Magasanik 1991). Researchers have not yet established whether the [URE3+] protein is a post-translationally modified form of ure2p that acts on unmodified ure2p to produce more of itself.

The [PSI+] phenotype is another possible yeast prion (Wickner 1994). [PSI+] is a non-Mendelian inherited trait that can be induced by expression of Sup35 (Cox et al. 1988). [PSI+] and [URE3+] can be cured by exposure of the yeast to 3 mM GdnHCl. The mechanism responsible for abolishing [PSI+] and [URE3+] with a low concentration of GdnHCl is unknown; it may be mediated by inducing high levels of Hsp104. Intermediate levels of Hsp104 are required for maintenance of [PSI+] (Chernoff et al. 1995).

In the filamentous fungus *Podospora anserina*, the het-s locus controls vegetative incompatibility. Conversion from the S^s to the s state seems to be a post-translational, autocatalytic process (Deleu et al. 1993).

Research demonstrating that any of these examples functions similarly to prions in animals would facilitate new, more rapid, and more economical approaches to prion diseases.

Common Neurodegenerative Diseases

Knowledge accrued from the study of prion diseases may provide an effective strategy for defining the etiologies and dissecting the molecular pathogenesis of more common neurodegenerative disorders such as Alzheimer's disease, Parkinson's disease, and amyotrophic lateral sclerosis (ALS). Advances in the molecular genetics of Alzheimer's disease and ALS suggest that—as with prion diseases—an important subset is caused by mutations that result in nonconservative amino acid substitutions in proteins expressed in the CNS (Goate et al. 1991; Levy et al. 1990; Mullan et al. 1992; Rosen et al. 1993; Schellenberg et al. 1992; St. George-Hyslop et al. 1992; Van Broeckhoven et al. 1990, 1992). Because clinicians can now identify people at risk for inherited prion diseases decades before neurological dysfunction is evident, development of effective therapies is imperative.

Future Studies

Tg mice expressing foreign or mutant PrP genes now enable researchers to study virtually all facets of prion diseases; this work has created a framework for future investigations. Furthermore, the structure and organization of the PrP gene suggests that PrP^{Sc} is derived from PrP^C or a precursor by a post-translational process. Studies with scrapie-infected cultured cells have provided evidence that the conversion of PrP^C to PrP^{Sc} is a post-translational process that probably occurs within a subcellular compartment bounded by cholesterol-rich membranes. Although researchers have not yet elucidated the molecular mechanism of PrP^{Sc} formation, chemical and physical studies have shown that the conformations of PrP^{C} and PrP^{Sc} are profoundly different.

The study of prion biology and diseases is an emerging area of biomedical investigation. Although prion biology has its roots in virology, neurology, and neuropathology, its relationships to molecular and cell biology—as well as to protein chemistry—have become evident only recently. Learning how prions multiply and cause disease is likely to open new vistas in biochemistry and genetics.

References

Alper T, Haig DA, Clarke MC: The exceptionally small size of the scrapie agent. Biochem Biophys Res Commun 22:278–284, 1966

Alper T, Cramp WA, Haig DA, et al: Does the agent of scrapie replicate without nucleic acid? Nature 214:764–766, 1967

Alpers M: Epidemiology and clinical aspects of kuru, in Prions—Novel Infectious Pathogens Causing Scrapie and Creutzfeldt-Jakob Disease. Edited by Prusiner SB, McKinley MP. Orlando, FL, Academic Press, 1987, pp 451–465

Barry RA, Prusiner SB: Monoclonal antibodies to the cellular and scrapie prion proteins. J Infect Dis 154:518–521, 1986

Bellinger-Kawahara CG, Kempner E, Groth DF, et al: Scrapie prion liposomes and rods exhibit target sizes of 55,000 Da. Virology 164:537–541, 1988

Bessen RA, Marsh RF: Biochemical and physical properties of the prion protein from two strains of the transmissible mink encephalopathy agent. J Virol 66:2096–2101, 1992a

Bessen RA, Marsh RF: Identification of two biologically distinct strains of transmissible mink encephalopathy in hamsters. J Gen Virol 73:329–334, 1992b

Bessen RA, Marsh RF: Distinct PrP properties suggest the molecular basis of strain variation in transmissible mink encephalopathy. J Virol 68:7859–7868, 1994

Bessen RA, Kocisko DA, Raymond GJ, et al: Non-genetic propagation of strain-specific properties of scrapie prion protein. Nature 375:698–700, 1995

Borchelt DR, Scott M, Taraboulos A, Stahl N, et al: Scrapie and cellular prion proteins differ in their kinetics of synthesis and topology in cultured cells. J Cell Biol 110:743–752, 1990

Brown P: The phenotypic expression of different mutations in transmissible human spongiform encephalopathy. Rev Neurol 148:317–327, 1992

Brown P, Cathala F, Raubertas RF, et al: The epidemiology of Creutzfeldt-Jakob disease: conclusion of 15-year investigation in France and review of the world literature. Neurology 37:895–904, 1987

Brown P, Goldfarb LG, Kovanen J, et al: Phenotypic characteristics of familial Creutzfeldt-Jakob disease associated with the codon 178[Asn] *PRNP* mutation. Ann Neurol 31:282–285, 1992

Brown P, Gibbs CJ Jr, Rodgers-Johnson P, et al: Human spongiform encephalopathy: the National Institutes of Health series of 300 cases of experimentally transmitted disease. Ann Neurol 35:513–529, 1994

Bruce ME, Dickinson AG: Biological evidence that the scrapie agent has an independent genome. J Gen Virol 68:79–89, 1987

Bruce ME, Dickinson AG, Fraser H: Cerebral amyloidosis in scrapie in the mouse: effect of agent strain and mouse genotype. Neuropathol Appl Neurobiol 2: 471–478, 1976

Bruce ME, McBride PA, Farquhar CF: Precise targeting of the pathology of the sialoglycoprotein, PrP, and vacuolar degeneration in mouse scrapie. Neurosci Lett 102:1–6, 1989

Bruce ME, McConnell I, Fraser H, et al: The disease characteristics of different strains of scrapie in *Sinc* congenic mouse lines: implications for the nature of the agent and host control of pathogenesis. J Gen Virol 72:595–603, 1991

Büeler H, Fischer M, Lang Y, et al: Normal development and behaviour of mice lacking the neuronal cell-surface PrP protein. Nature 356:577–582, 1992

Büeler H, Aguzzi A, Sailer A, et al: Mice devoid of PrP are resistant to scrapie. Cell 73:1339–1347, 1993

Büeler H, Raeber A, Sailer A, et al: High prion and PrP[Sc] levels but delayed onset of disease in scrapie-inoculated mice heterozygous for a disrupted PrP gene. Mol Med 1:19–30, 1994

Carlson GA, Kingsbury DT, Goodman PA, et al: Linkage of prion protein and scrapie incubation time genes. Cell 46:503–511, 1986

Carlson GA, Westaway D, DeArmond SJ, et al: Primary structure of prion protein may modify scrapie isolate properties. Proc Natl Acad Sci U S A 86:7475–7479, 1989

Carlson GA, Ebeling C, Torchia M, et al: Delimiting the location of the scrapie prion incubation time gene on chromosome 2 of the mouse. Genetics 133: 979–988, 1993

Carlson GA, Ebeling C, Yang S-L, et al: Prion isolate specified allotypic interactions between the cellular and scrapie prion proteins in congenic and transgenic mice. Proc Natl Acad Sci U S A 91:5690–5694, 1994

Carp RI, Moretz RC, Natelli M, et al: Genetic control of scrapie: incubation period and plaque formation in mice. J Gen Virol 68:401–407, 1987

Casaccia-Bonnefil P, Kascsak RJ, Fersko R, et al: Brain regional distribution of prion protein PrP27-30 in mice stereotaxically microinjected with different strains of scrapie. J Infect Dis 167:7–12, 1993

Chernoff YO, Lindquist SL, Ono B, et al: Role of the chaperone protein Hsp104 in propagation of the yeast prion-like factor [*psi+*]. Science 268:880–884, 1995

Collinge J, Whittington MA, Sidle KC, et al: Prion protein is necessary for normal synaptic function. Nature 370:295–297, 1994

Coschigano PW, Magasanik B: The *URE2* gene product of *Saccharomyces cerevisiae* plays an important role in the cellular response to the nitrogen source and has homology to glutathione *S*-transferases. Mol Cell Biol 11:822–832, 1991

Cousens SN, Harries-Jones R, Knight R, et al: Geographical distribution of cases of Creutzfeldt-Jakob disease in England and Wales 1970–84. J Neurol Neurosurg Psychiatry 53:459–465, 1990

Cox BS, Tuite MF, McLaughlin CS: The psi factor of yeast: a problem in inheritance. Yeast 4:159–178, 1988

Cuillé J, Chelle PL: Experimental transmission of trembling to the goat. C.R. Seances Acad. Sci. 208:1058–1060, 1939

DeArmond SJ, Mobley WC, DeMott DL, et al: Changes in the localization of brain prion proteins during scrapie infection. Neurology 37:1271–1280, 1987

DeArmond SJ, Yang S-L, Lee A, et al: Three scrapie prion isolates exhibit different accumulation patterns of the prion protein scrapie isoform. Proc Natl Acad Sci U S A 90:6449–6453, 1993

Deleu C, Clave C, Begueret J: A single amino acid difference is sufficient to elicit vegetative incompatibility in the fungus *Podospora anserina*. Genetics 135: 45–52, 1993

Dickinson AG, Fraser H: An assessment of the genetics of scrapie in sheep and mice, in Slow Transmissible Diseases of the Nervous System, Vol 1. Edited by Prusiner SB, Hadlow WJ. New York, Academic Press, 1979, pp 367–386

Dickinson AG, Meikle VM: A comparison of some biological characteristics of the mouse-passaged scrapie agents, 22A and ME7. Genet Res 13:213–225, 1969

Dickinson AG, Meikle VMH: Host-genotype and agent effects in scrapie incubation: change in allelic interaction with different strains of agent. Mol Gen Genet 112:73–79, 1971

Dickinson AG, Outram GW: The scrapie replication-site hypothesis and its implications for pathogenesis, in Slow Transmissible Diseases of the Nervous System, Vol 2. Edited by Prusiner SB, Hadlow WJ. New York, Academic Press, 1979, pp 13–31

Dickinson AG, Outram GW: Genetic aspects of unconventional virus infections: the basis of the virino hypothesis, in Novel Infectious Agents and the Central Nervous System: Ciba Foundation Symposium 135. Edited by Bock G, Marsh J. Chichester, England, John Wiley and Sons, 1988, pp 63–83

Dickinson AG, Stamp JT: Experimental scrapie in Cheviot and Suffolk sheep. J Comp Pathol 79:23–26, 1969

Dickinson AG, Young GB, Stamp JT, et al: An analysis of natural scrapie in Suffolk sheep. Heredity 20:485–503, 1965

Dickinson AG, Meikle VMH, Fraser H: Identification of a gene which controls the incubation period of some strains of scrapie agent in mice. J Comp Pathol 78:293–299, 1968

Dickinson AG, Bruce ME, Outram GW, et al: Scrapie strain differences: the implications of stability and mutation, in Proceedings of Workshop on Slow Transmissible Diseases. Edited by Tateishi J. Tokyo, Japan, Japanese Ministry of Health and Welfare, 1984, pp 105–118

Fraser H: Neuropathology of scrapie: the precision of the lesions and their diversity, in Slow Transmissible Diseases of the Nervous System, Vol 1. Edited by Prusiner SB, Hadlow WJ. New York: Academic Press, 1979, pp 387–406

Fraser H, Dickinson AG: Scrapie in mice. Agent-strain differences in the distribution and intensity of grey matter vacuolation. J Comp Pathol 83:29–40, 1973

Gajdusek DC: Unconventional viruses and the origin and disappearance of kuru. Science 197:943–960, 1977

Gajdusek DC: Subacute spongiform virus encephalopathies caused by unconventional viruses, in Subviral Pathogens of Plants and Animals: Viroids and Prions. Edited by Maramorosch K, McKelvey JJ Jr. Orlando, FL, Academic Press, 1985, pp 483–544

Gajdusek DC, Zigas V: Degenerative disease of the central nervous system in New Guinea—the endemic occurrence of "kuru" in the native population. N Engl J Med 257:974–978, 1957

Gajdusek DC, Zigas V: Clinical, pathological and epidemiological study of an acute progressive degenerative disease of the central nervous system among natives of the eastern highlands of New Guinea. Am J Med 26:442–469, 1959

Gajdusek DC, Gibbs CJ Jr, Alpers M: Experimental transmission of a kuru-like syndrome to chimpanzees. Nature 209:794–796, 1966

Goate A, Chartier-Harlin M-C, Mullan M, et al: Segregation of a missense mutation in the amyloid precursor protein gene with familial Alzheimer's disease. Nature 349:704–706, 1991

Gordon WS: Advances in veterinary research. Vet Res 58:516–520, 1946

Gordon WS: Variation in susceptibility of sheep to scrapie and genetic implications, in Report of Scrapie Seminar, ARS 91-53. Washington, DC, U.S. Department of Agriculture, 1966, pp 53–67

Hadlow WJ, Kennedy RC, Race RE, et al: Virologic and neurohistologic findings in dairy goats affected with natural scrapie. Vet Pathol 17:187–199, 1980

Hadlow WJ, Kennedy RC, Race RE: Natural infection of Suffolk sheep with scrapie virus. J Infect Dis 146:657–664, 1982

Harries-Jones R, Knight R, Will RG, et al: Creutzfeldt-Jakob disease in England and Wales, 1980–1984: a case-control study of potential risk factors. J Neurol Neurosurg Psychiatry 51:1113–1119, 1988

Hecker R, Taraboulos A, Scott M, et al: Replication of distinct prion isolates is region specific in brains of transgenic mice and hamsters. Genes Dev 6:1213–1228, 1992

Hsiao KK, Prusiner SB: Inherited human prion diseases. Neurology 40:1820–1827, 1990

Hsiao KK, Baker HF, Crow TJ, et al: Linkage of a prion protein missense variant to Gerstmann-Straussler syndrome. Nature 338:342–345, 1989

Hsiao KK, Scott M, Foster D, et al: Spontaneous neurodegeneration in transgenic mice with mutant prion protein. Science 250:1587–1590, 1990

Hsiao KK, Groth D, Scott M, et al: Serial transmission in rodents of neurodegeneration from transgenic mice expressing mutant prion protein. Proc Natl Acad Sci U S A 91:9126–9130, 1994

Hunter GD: Scrapie: a prototype slow infection. J Infect Dis 125:427–440, 1972

Hunter N, Hope J, McConnell I, et al: Linkage of the scrapie-associated fibril protein (PrP) gene and Sinc using congenic mice and restriction fragment length polymorphism analysis. J Gen Virol 68:2711–2716, 1987

Kascsak RJ, Rubenstein R, Merz PA, et al: Mouse polyclonal and monoclonal antibody to scrapie-associated fibril proteins. J Virol 61:3688–3693, 1987

Kimberlin RH, Cole S, Walker CA: Temporary and permanent modifications to a single strain of mouse scrapie on transmission to rats and hamsters. J Gen Virol 68:1875–1881, 1987

Kingsbury DT, Kasper KC, Stites DP, et al: Genetic control of scrapie and Creutzfeldt-Jakob disease in mice. J Immunol 131:491–496, 1983

Kirschbaum WR: Zwei eigenartige Erkrankungen des Zentralnervensystems nach Art der spastischen Pseudosklerose (Jakob). Zeitschrift für die Gesamte Neurologie und Psychiatrie 92:175–220, 1924

Lacroute F: Non-Mendelian mutation allowing ureidosuccinic acid uptake in yeast. J Bacteriol 106:519–522, 1971

Levy E, Carman MD, Fernandez-Madrid IJ, et al: Mutation of the Alzheimer's disease amyloid gene in hereditary cerebral hemorrhage, Dutch type. Science 248:1124–1126, 1990

Malmgren R, Kurland L, Mokri B, et al: The epidemiology of Creutzfeldt-Jakob disease, in Slow Transmissible Diseases of the Nervous System, Vol 1. Edited by Prusiner SB, Hadlow WJ. New York, Academic Press, 1979, pp 93–112

Manson JC, Clarke AR, Hooper ML, et al: 129/Ola mice carrying a null mutation in PrP that abolishes mRNA production are developmentally normal. Mol Neurobiol 8:121–127, 1994a

Manson JC, Clarke AR, McBride PA, et al: PrP gene dosage determines the timing but not the final intensity or distribution of lesions in scrapie pathology. Neurodegeneration 3:331–340, 1994b

Manson JC, Hope J, Clarke AR, et al: PrP gene dosage and long term potentiation (letter). Neurodegeneration 4:113–114, 1995

Manuelidis E, Gorgacz EJ, Manuelidis L: Interspecies transmission of Creutzfeldt-Jakob disease to Syrian hamsters with reference to clinical syndromes and strains of agent. Proc Natl Acad Sci U S A 75:3422–3436, 1978

Marsh RF, Bessen RA, Lehmann S, et al: Epidemiological and experimental studies on a new incident of transmissible mink encephalopathy. J Gen Virol 72: 589–594, 1991

Masters CL, Harris JO, Gajdusek DC, et al: Creutzfeldt-Jakob disease: patterns of worldwide occurrence and the significance of familial and sporadic clustering. Ann Neurol 5:177–188, 1978

Masters CL, Gajdusek DC, Gibbs CJ Jr: Creutzfeldt-Jakob disease virus isolations from the Gerstmann-Straussler syndrome. Brain 104:559–588, 1981

Medori R, Montagna P, Tritschler HJ, et al: Fatal familial insomnia: a second kindred with mutation of prion protein gene at codon 178. Neurology 42: 669–670, 1992a

Medori R, Tritschler H-J, LeBlanc A, et al: Fatal familial insomnia, a prion disease with a mutation at codon 178 of the prion protein gene. N Engl J Med 326: 444–449, 1992b

Meggendorfer F: Klinische und genealogische Beobachtungen bei einem Fall von spastischer Pseudosklerose Jakobs. Zeitschrift für die Gesamte Neurologie und Psychiatrie 128:337–341, 1930

Mullan M, Houlden H, Windelspecht M, et al: A locus for familial early-onset Alzheimer's disease on the long arm of chromosome 14, proximal to the α1-antichymotrypsin gene. Nat Genet 2:340–342, 1992

Palmer MS, Dryden AJ, Hughes JT, et al: Homozygous prion protein genotype predisposes to sporadic Creutzfeldt-Jakob disease. Nature 352:340–342, 1991

Pan K-M, Baldwin M, Nguyen J, et al: Conversion of αhelices into β-sheets features in the formation of the scrapie prion proteins. Proc Natl Acad Sci U S A 90:10962–10966, 1993

Parry HB: Scrapie: a transmissible and hereditary disease of sheep. Heredity 17: 75–105, 1962

Parry HB: Scrapie Disease in Sheep. Edited by Oppenheimer DR. New York, Academic Press, 1983

Pattison IH, Millson GC: Scrapie produced experimentally in goats with special reference to the clinical syndrome. J Comp Pathol 71:101–108, 1961

Prusiner SB: Novel proteinaceous infectious particles cause scrapie. Science 216:136–144, 1982

Prusiner SB: The biology of prion transmission and replication, in Prions—Novel Infectious Pathogens Causing Scrapie and Creutzfeldt-Jakob Disease. Edited by Prusiner SB, McKinley MP. Orlando, FL, Academic Press, 1987, pp 83–112

Prusiner SB: Scrapie prions. Annu Rev Microbiol 43:345–374, 1989

Prusiner SB: Molecular biology of prion diseases. Science 252:1515–1522, 1991

Prusiner SB: Molecular biology and genetics of neurodegenerative diseases caused by prions. Adv Virus Res 41:241–280, 1992

Prusiner SB: Inherited prion diseases. Proc Natl Acad Sci U S A 91:4611–4614, 1994

Prusiner SB, McKinley MP, Bowman KA, et al: Scrapie prions aggregate to form amyloid-like birefringent rods. Cell 35:349–358, 1983

Prusiner SB, Scott M, Foster D, et al: Transgenetic studies implicate interactions between homologous PrP isoforms in scrapie prion replication. Cell 63: 673–686, 1990

Prusiner SB, Groth D, Serban A, et al: Ablation of the prion protein (PrP) gene in mice prevents scrapie and facilitates production of anti-PrP antibodies. Proc Natl Acad Sci U S A 90:10608–10612, 1993a

Prusiner SB, Groth D, Serban A, et al: Attempts to restore scrapie prion infectivity after exposure to protein denaturants. Proc Natl Acad Sci U S A 90: 2793–2797, 1993b

Race RE, Graham K, Ernst D, et al: Analysis of linkage between scrapie incubation period and the prion protein gene in mice. J Gen Virol 71:493–497, 1990

Riesner D, Kellings K, Meyer N, et al: Nucleic acids and scrapie prions, in Prion Diseases of Humans and Animals. Edited by Prusiner SB, Collinge J, Powell J, et al. London, Ellis Horwood, 1992, pp 341–358

Rogers M, Serban D, Gyuris T, et al: Epitope mapping of the Syrian hamster prion protein utilizing chimeric and mutant genes in a vaccinia virus expression system. J Immunol 147:3568–3574, 1991

Rogers M, Yehiely F, Scott M, et al: Conversion of truncated and elongated prion proteins into the scrapie isoform in cultured cells. Proc Natl Acad Sci U S A 90:3182–3186, 1993

Rosen DR, Siddique T, Patterson D, et al: Mutations in Cu/Zn superoxide dismutase gene are associated with familial amyotrophic lateral sclerosis. Nature 362:59–62, 1993

Safar J, Roller PP, Gajdusek DC, et al: Conformational transitions, dissociation, and unfolding of scrapie amyloid (prion) protein. J Biol Chem 268: 20276–20284, 1993

Schellenberg GD, Bird TD, Wijsman EM, et al: Genetic linkage evidence for a familial Alzheimer's disease locus on chromosome 14. Science 258:668–671, 1992

Scott M, Foster D, Mirenda C, et al: Transgenic mice expressing hamster prion protein produce species-specific scrapie infectivity and amyloid plaques. Cell 59:847–857, 1989

Scott MR, Kohler R, Foster D, et al: Chimeric prion protein expression in cultured cells and transgenic mice. Protein Sci 1:986–997, 1992

Scott M, Groth D, Foster D, et al: Propagation of prions with artificial properties in transgenic mice expressing chimeric PrP genes. Cell 73:979–988, 1993

Sigurdsson B: Rida, a chronic encephalitis of sheep with general remarks on infections which develop slowly and some of their special characteristics. Br Vet J 110:341–354, 1954

Sparkes RS, Simon M, Cohn VH, et al: Assignment of the human and mouse prion protein genes to homologous chromosomes. Proc Natl Acad Sci U S A 83:7358–7362, 1986

Stahl N, Borchelt DR, Hsiao K, et al: Scrapie prion protein contains a phosphatidylinositol glycolipid. Cell 51:229–240, 1987

Stahl N, Baldwin MA, Teplow DB, et al: Structural analysis of the scrapie prion protein using mass spectrometry and amino acid sequencing. Biochemistry 32:1991–2002, 1993

St. George-Hyslop P, Haines J, Rogaev E, et al: Genetic evidence for a novel familial Alzheimer's disease locus on chromosome 14. Nat Genet 2:330–334, 1992

Taraboulos A, Jendroska K, Serban D, et al: Regional mapping of prion proteins in brains. Proc Natl Acad Sci U S A 89:7620–7624, 1992

Tateishi J, Kitamoto T: Inherited prion diseases and transmission to rodents. Brain Pathol 5:53–59, 1995

Tateishi J, Sato Y, Ohta M: Creutzfeldt-Jakob disease in humans and laboratory animals, in Progress in Neuropathology, Vol 5. Edited by Zimmerman HM. New York, Raven, 1983, pp 195–221

Tateishi J, Doh-ura K, Kitamoto T, et al: Prion protein gene analysis and transmission studies of Creutzfeldt-Jakob disease, in Prion Diseases of Humans and Animals. Edited by Prusiner SB, Collinge J, Powell J, et al. London, Ellis Horwood, 1992, pp 129–134

Telling GC, Scott M, Hsiao KK, et al: Transmission of Creutzfeldt-Jakob disease from humans to transgenic mice expressing chimeric human-mouse prion protein. Proc Natl Acad Sci U S A 91:9936–9940, 1994

Telling GC, Scott M, Mastrianni J, et al: Prion propagation in mice expressing human and chimeric PrP transgenes implicates the interaction of cellular PrP with another protein. Cell 83:79–90, 1995

Van Broeckhoven C, Haan J, Bakker E, et al: Amyloid β protein precursor gene and hereditary cerebral hemorrhage with amyloidosis (in Dutch). Science 248:1120–1122, 1990

Van Broeckhoven C, Backhovens H, Cruts M, et al: Mapping of a gene predisposing to early-onset Alzheimer's disease to chromosome 14q24.3. Nat Genet 2:335–339, 1992

Westaway D, Goodman PA, Mirenda CA, et al: Distinct prion proteins in short and long scrapie incubation period mice. Cell 51:651–662, 1987

Westaway D, Mirenda CA, Foster D, et al: Paradoxical shortening of scrapie incubation times by expression of prion protein transgenes derived from long incubation period mice. Neuron 7:59–68, 1991

Westaway D, Cooper C, Turner S, et al: Structure and polymorphism of the mouse prion protein gene. Proc Natl Acad Sci U S A 91:6418–6422, 1994a

Westaway D, DeArmond SJ, Cayetano-Canlas J, et al: Degeneration of skeletal muscle, peripheral nerves, and the central nervous system in transgenic mice overexpressing wild-type prion proteins. Cell 76:117–129, 1994b

Whittington MA, Sidle KCL, Gowland I, et al: Rescue of neurophysiological phenotype seen in PrP null mice by transgene encoding human prion protein. Nat Genet 9:197–201, 1995

Wickner RB: [URE3] as an altered URE2 protein: evidence for a prion analog in Saccharomyces cerevisiae. Science 264:566–569, 1994

Wilesmith JW, Ryan JBM, Hueston WD, et al: Bovine spongiform encephalopathy: epidemiological features 1985 to 1990. Vet Rec 130:90–94, 1992

Ziegler DR: Genetic Maps—Locus Maps of Complex Genomes, 6th Edition. Edited by O'Brien SJ. Cold Spring Harbor, NY, Cold Spring Harbor Laboratory Press, 1993, pp 4.42–4.45

Chapter 6

Clinical, Pathological, and Genetic Heterogeneity of Alzheimer's Disease

Marshal F. Folstein, M.D., and Susan E. Folstein, M.D.

———◆———

T he pace of research on Alzheimer's disease accelerated rapidly in the 1990s. Recent advances have been based on the application of a disease perspective. According to this view, Alzheimer's disease, similar to Huntington's disease (for example), is defined by a broken part of an organ such as the brain or genome. Investigators therefore may explain clinical and pathological manifestations (the phenotype) by identifying predisposing and precipitating factors (etiology); these factors produce neurochemical changes (pathogenesis), which lead to structural changes in an organ such as the brain (pathology)—which lead, in turn, to the presentation of particular symptoms: the cortical dementia syndrome.

In this chapter, we review advances in clinical, pathological, and genetic concepts related to Alzheimer's disease; we redefine the disorder as a family of diseases with similar pathologies but different etiologies. This process resembles the reclassification of anemia that differentiated sickle cell disease from hemolytic anemia and hemolytic anemia from anemia in general. In the case of Alzheimer's disease, genetic mutations on chromosomes 21, 14, and 19 are responsible for the majority of cases. These genetic defects lead to overproduction or faulty processing of amyloid preprotein to produce βA4 protein—and cell death.

Advances in Clinical Concepts

⌈Typically, Alzheimer's disease is a regularly progressive syndrome, usually beginning at about age 80 years with anosmia and amnesia, followed by aphasia, apraxia, and agnosia, and finally gait disorder and incontinence.⌉ These three clinical stages (Table 6–1) correspond roughly to the progression of neuropathological features from the limbic system to the parietal lobe and finally to the frontal cortex. Death occurs an average of 10 years after onset.

Researchers have identified several clinical subtypes of Alzheimer's disease, in addition to the typical syndrome and course. The designation of a subtype requires that the symptom pattern occurs with some regularity in a proportion of cases and that the subtype can be validated by a predictable prognosis, pathology, or etiology. Physicians currently recognize subtypes by age at onset, extrapyramidal symptoms, and noncognitive symptoms such as depression, delusions, and hallucinations (Table 6–2).

Onset occurs before age 65 years in half of all clinical cases; in community samples, however, the prevalence of cases with age at onset under 75 years is less than 2%, compared with a prevalence of 20%–40% with an age at onset of 85 years or older. A small proportion of early-onset cases involve seizures and myoclonus; these symptoms were present, for example, in a large family with chromosome 14 mutation (Campion et al.

Table 6–1. Syndrome progression

Limbic stage
Anosmia
Amnesia

Parietal stage
Aphasia
Apraxia
Agnosia

Frontal stage
Gait disorder
Incontinence

Table 6–2. Validation of clinical subtypes of the syndrome

Subtype	Validation
Early onset	Etiology: Down's, 14, 21
Late onset	Etiology: 19
Extrapyramidal	Pathology: Lewy bodies; prognosis: rapid decline
Depression	Pathology: locus coeruleus; prognosis: institutionalization, mortality
Delusions, hallucinations	Prognosis: rapid cognitive decline

1995; Kennedy et al. 1995). Early-onset cases probably are related to mutations on chromosome 21 or 14; late-onset cases probably are linked to chromosome 19.

Approximately 20% of all patients with Alzheimer's disease have comorbid depression, which researchers associate with severe locus coeruleus cell loss (Zweig et al. 1988), higher rates of institutionalization, and higher mortality within institutions (Sattell et al. 1993; Steele et al. 1990), and 20%–40% exhibit extrapyramidal syndrome, which investigators associate with Lewy bodies in the cortex and substantia nigra, neuroleptic sensitivity, and rapid progression of disease (Armstrong et al. 1991; Forstl et al. 1993; McKeith et al. 1992). Delusions and hallucinations, which occur in 40% of patients, also appear to be associated with rapid course of Alzheimer's disease (Folstein and Bylsma 1994; Stern et al. 1993).

Advances in Pathology

Cell loss, neurofibrillary tangles, and neuritic plaques characterize the typical pathology of Alzheimer's disease (Masliah et al. 1991). Loss of cortical cells and their synapses is closely related to cognitive decline. Cell loss in Alzheimer's disease does not involve diffuse or random cortical degeneration; rather, it entails systematic neuron-to-neuron progression, perhaps via cortical glutamatergic neurons. The pathology of the disorder mirrors the clinical stages of disease: changes occur first and most severely in the limbic system, followed by the parietal cortex.

The relation of cortical cell death to subcortical cell groups is unclear. In some cases, the nucleus basalis of Meynert, locus coeruleus, dorsal raphe, and substantia nigra may all be affected. Most investigators now assume that subcortical nuclei are affected secondarily. Because cholinergic stimulation decreases amyloid production in vitro, however, selective cholinergic cell death may lead to increased amyloid production in a positive feedback loop (Buxbaum et al. 1992; Felsenstein et al. 1994).

In addition to the typical pathology, several pathological variants relate to Lewy bodies, locus coeruleus, absent tangles, and prion stains. A significant proportion of cases involve Lewy bodies in the cortex and substantia nigra (St. Clair et al. 1994). The presence of these intracellular structures is associated with an extrapyramidal syndrome in 20% or more of cases (Zweig et al. 1988). Patients with greater locus coeruleus cell loss have more depression (Zweig et al. 1988). In a few cases, patients with clinical symptoms lack plaques and tangles (Kim et al. 1981; R. Terry, personal communication, May 1995). One family had plaques that stained with antibody to prion protein (DeArmond 1993).

The late changes of head trauma—especially in boxers—resemble Alzheimer's disease pathology; however, such cases have other signs of trauma, such as a patent septum pellucidum (Roberts et al. 1989). A minority of cases exhibit maximum pathology in frontal regions.

The structural neuropathological changes in Alzheimer's disease involve amyloid processing. Amyloid is produced by the aggregation of a protein B4; this protein is secreted in soluble form after processing from membrane preprotein *APP*, which is coded on chromosome 21. This process is regulated by cholinergic stimulation, estrogen, and interleukins (Buxbaum et al. 1992).

This theory of pathogenesis characterizes Alzheimer's disease as a form of cerebral amyloidosis: amyloid is first deposited as diffuse plaques; over many years, these diffuse plaques develop into neuritic plaques. Diffuse amyloid plaques appear before neurofibrillary tangles. The amyloid plaque is related to an overproduction of amyloid in Down's syndrome cases, in the amyloid preprotein mutation on chromosome 21, and in chromosome 14 cases (Brachova et al. 1993).

Theories of Cell Death in Alzheimer's Disease

Amyloid is central to the process.   *APP* is processed to $\beta A4$, which aggregates and forms amyloid plaques and neurofibrillary tangles and leads to cell death. Under this hypothesis, interventions should be designed to increase the soluble form or decrease the production of $\beta A4$ (Smith-Swintosky and Mattson 1994).

Soluble P3 ← amyloid precursor protein → βA4 → amyloid

Amyloid is an epiphenomenon.   An opposing view holds that the amyloid preprotein is an adhesive molecule that is secreted after cells are damaged and hence is a repair mechanism like inflammation. In this theory, cell death occurs from the production of hyperphosphorylated microtubule-associated protein tau or from the effects of naturally occurring excitotoxins on a defective cell membrane.

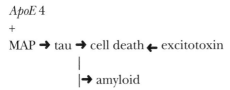

Research findings that apolipoprotein E *(ApoE)* 4 is an important risk factor for Alzheimer's disease and that *ApoE* 2 is protective are consistent with either theory (Chartier-Harlin et al. 1994). Consistent with the first theory, *ApoE* 4 enhances amyloid production in vitro (Castano et al. 1995); *ApoE* 4 also promotes the syntheses of tau from MAP, consistent with the second theory (Berr et al. 1994). Because Alzheimer's disease is etiologically heterogenous, both models could be correct for different proportions of cases (Hyman et al. 1995).

Differences in quantitative neuropathology suggest that the mechanism of plaque formation differs in Down's syndrome and chromosome 19 disease (Hyman et al. 1995). These neurochemical changes are triggered by environmental events or the accumulation of abnormal gene products over a lifetime.

Advances in Etiology

Scandinavian researchers in the 1950s and 1960s suggested that early- and late-onset Alzheimer's disease were genetic disorders (Larsson et al. 1963; Sjogren et al. 1952); most British and American investigators, however, were unconvinced by the evidence. Our own clinical work suggests that Alzheimer's disease, carefully defined, is an autosomal dominant disorder and that the genetic form is the most common dementia (Breitner and Folstein 1984a, 1984b; Folstein 1982, 1989; Folstein and Breitner 1981; Folstein and Powell 1989; Folstein and Warren 1991; Folstein et al. 1983,

1984; Powell and Folstein 1984). Our observations were based on the application of life-table methods to family data; after accounting for individuals who died from competing causes before passing through the age at risk, we estimated the proportion of affected members of families (Breitner et al. 1986; Chase et al. 1983).

In a study that involved tracing families through previous generations to an unaffected founder, we applied the appropriate statistics to account for maternal age and discovered advanced paternal age in the founder (Powell and Folstein 1981). This finding was consistent with other genetic disorders involving advanced paternal age, such as achondroplasia and Marfan's syndrome. Phenotypic analysis suggested that Alzheimer's disease would be genetically heterogeneous (Folstein 1989; Folstein et al. 1988). Subsequent studies have confirmed these early hypotheses.

Loci Linked to Alzheimer's Disease in Families

Alzheimer's disease is genetically heterogeneous because it is caused by mutations on chromosomes 19, 21, and 14. In 60% of cases, late-onset Alzheimer's disease is caused by a mutation on chromosome 19 close to the gene for *ApoE* 3,4 (Corder and Woodbury 1993; Farrer and Stice 1993; Pericak-Vance et al. 1991; Strittmatter et al. 1993). The absence of *ApoE* 2 appears to increase the risk for disease (Corder et al. 1994; Rubinsztein et al. 1994; Smith-Swintosky and Mattson 1994; Tamaoka 1994).

Early-onset Alzheimer's disease is caused by loci on chromosome 21 (Balbin et al. 1992; Goate et al. 1989, 1991; Heston et al. 1991) and chromosome 14 (Schellenberg et al. 1992; St. George-Hyslop et al. 1992; van Broeckhoven et al. 1992). Chromosome 21 trisomy and mutation account for fewer than 1% of cases and chromosome 14 fewer than 5% of cases. Researchers have found several families with a mutation in codon 670 of the *APP* gene on chromosome 21 (Axelman et al. 1994; Johnston et al. 1994; Lampe et al. 1994; Lannfelt et al. 1994; Mullan et al. 1992; Nagano et al. 1992; Peacock et al. 1994; Zeldenrust et al. 1993).

Overproduction of amyloid occurs in trisomy 21, the *APP* mutation on chromosome 21, and the locus on chromosome 14 (Querfurth et al. 1995). Researchers have not identified a gene or gene product for the chromosome 14 locus (Campion et al. 1995; Kennedy et al. 1995).

Researchers found a chromosome 20 locus mutation producing prion protein in a single family with Alzheimer's disease and the typical Alzheimer's disease pathology. In this case, however, the neuritic plaques stained with an antibody for prion protein. Other prion diseases, such as Creutzfeldt-Jakob disease and kuru, have amyloid plaques that stain for prion protein; these disorders do not exhibit significant numbers of neurofibrillary tangles. Volga Germans and others (Brown et al. 1993) have not been linked to any known locus, suggesting that another major locus is present but undiscovered (Bird et al. 1988).

Sporadic Alzheimer's Disease

Nonfamilial Alzheimer's disease is sometimes genetic: *ApoE* frequency is higher in sporadic cases than in control subjects (Dai et al. 1994) (Table 6–3), and new mutations associated with advanced paternal age may produce a sporadic case that will become familial in the next generation. Researchers do not know the mutation rate (Breitner et al. 1986; Chase et al. 1983; Powell and Folstein 1984).

Gene-Gene Interactions

Several investigations of mitochondrial genes are under way. The *CYP2D6B* gene, which is associated with Parkinson's disease, is more common in Alzheimer's disease patients with extrapyramidal symptoms (Chandrasekaran et al. 1994; Saitoh et al. 1995; Simonian and Hyman 1994).

Another gene interaction occurs in cases involving Alzheimer's disease and comorbid depression. These cases entail not only the pathological subtype described above but also a higher frequency of family members

Table 6–3.   ApoE 4 frequencies

Author	Date	% E4 in Alzheimer's disease patients	% E4 in control subjects
Forstl et al.	1994	58	24
Galasko et al.	1994	40	15
Hendrie et al.	1995	40	14
Kuusisto et al.	1994	39	17
Lehtimaki et al.	1995	55	20
Liddell et al.	1994	33	12
Poirier et al.	1993	38	12
Strittmatter et al.	1993	50	16
Yoshizawa et al.	1994	34	10
Yu et al.	1994	51	19

Note.   See Betard et al. (1994) for E4 frequency in various diseases; more E4 frequency (Brousseau 1994).

affected with depression apparently independent of Alzheimer's disease. This pattern suggests that the gene responsible for familial predisposition to depression in Alzheimer's disease modifies the expressions of the syndrome and pathology (Pearlson et al. 1988).

Gene-Environment Interactions

Environmental factors may be important modifiers of gene expression in Alzheimer's disease. For example, a history of head trauma increases the risk for Alzheimer's disease in individuals with the *ApoE* 4 allele (Mayeux et al. 1995). Aluminum and other metals affect amyloid deposition and protein phosphorylation (Shin et al. 1994); thus, they may be more potent risk factors in genetically vulnerable individuals.

Low levels of education, which are a risk factor for Alzheimer's disease, may implicate another intelligence-related gene that predisposes an individual to Alzheimer's disease (Katzman and Kawas 1994). Alternatively, early environmental deprivations may mediate the effect.

As with other genetic diseases, phenocopies—environmentally caused cases with characteristic phenotypes—are likely. To date, however, dementia following head trauma is the only known example. Protective factors include nicotine, estrogen (Paganini-Hill and Henderson 1994) and cholinergic stimulation, nonsteroidal anti-inflammatory agents (Breitner et al. 1994; Rich et al. 1994), and *ApoE* 2.

Conclusion

The foregoing developments suggest reclassifying Alzheimer's disease into five variants: the Duke variant, the Seattle variant, the London-Swedish variant, the Down's syndrome variant, and the idiopathic variant (Tables 6–4 and 6–5).

The Duke variant is caused by a mutation on chromosome 19 and is associated with *ApoE* 4. This variant usually entails late onset, although many early-onset cases occur. The Duke variant is familial or (apparently) sporadic; it accounts for 60%–70% of all cases of Alzheimer's disease.

The Seattle variant is caused by a mutation on chromosome 14 in an unidentified gene. This variant involves early onset—with some cases appearing in the forties and fifties—although a few cases entail later onset. The Seattle variant is familial; it accounts for the majority of early-onset cases and perhaps 5% of all cases of the disorder.

Table 6–4.   Seattle, London-Swedish, and Down's variants

Seattle variant

  2%–5% of cases
  Early onset
  Myoclonus and seizures
  Chromosome 14 linkage
  ?*C-FOS* candidate

London-Swedish variant

  1% of cases
  Early onset
  Amyloid overproduction
  Chromosome 21 linkage
  APP gene mutations

Down's variant

  50%–100% of cases
  Early onset
  Amyloid overproduction
  Trisomy 21

Table 6–5.   Classification of variants

Variant	% of all Alzheimer's disease	Onset	Amyloid production	Family history	Locus	Genes
Duke	50–80	Late	?	+ or −	19	*ApoE*
Seattle	5	Early	Increase	+	14	?*C-FOS*
London-Swedish	< 1	Early	Increase	+	21	*APP*
Down's syndrome	< 1	Early	Increase	−	21	*APP*
Idiopathic	20–50	?	?	+ or −	?	?

The London-Swedish variant is caused by a mutation on chromosome 21 in the amyloid precursor gene. Onset is early; this variant is familial but extremely rare. The gene product is βA4, which is produced in excess.

The Down's syndrome variant is caused by trisomy 21, which leads to an overproduction of amyloid. The idiopathic variant accounts for 10%–25% of cases, many of which are genetic (e.g., the Volga German families).

A number of factors may affect the clinical and pathological expression of these variants. These considerations include genes for depression and Parkinson's disease; environmental factors such as nicotine (van Duijn et al. 1994, 1995), nonsteroidal anti-inflammatory drugs, trauma, or aluminum and other metals; and early developmental factors that lead to low levels of education.

References

Armstrong TP, Hansen LA, Salmon DP, et al: Rapidly progressive dementia in a patient with the Lewy body variant of Alzheimer's disease. Neurology 41: 1178–1180, 1991

Axelman K, Basun H, Winblad B, et al: A large Swedish family with Alzheimer's disease with a codon 670/671 amyloid precursor protein mutation: a clinical and genealogical investigation. Arch Neurol 51:1193–1197, 1994

Balbin M, Abrahamson M, Gustafson L, et al: A novel mutation in the beta-protein coding region of the amyloid beta-protein precursor (APP) gene. Hum Genet 89:580–582, 1992

Berr C, Haus JJ, Delaere P, et al: Apolipoprotein E allele epsilon 4 is linked to increased deposition of the amyloid beta-peptide (A-beta) in cases with or without Alzheimer's disease. Neurosci Lett 178:221–224, 1994

Betard C, Robitaille V, Gee M, et al: Apo E allele frequencies in Alzheimer's disease, Lewy body dementia, Alzheimer's disease with cerebrovascular disease and vascular dementia. Neuroreport 5:1893–1896, 1994

Bird TD, Lampe TH, Nemens EJ, et al: Familial Alzheimer's disease in descendants of Volga Germans: probable genetic founder effect. Ann Neurol 23:25–31, 1988

Brachova L, Lue F, Schultz J, et al: Association cortex, cerebellum, and serum concentrations of C1q and factor B in Alzheimer's disease. Brain Res Mol Brain Res 18:329–334, 1993

Breitner JC, Folstein MF: Familial Alzheimer dementia: a prevalent disorder with specific clinical features. Psychol Med 14:63–80, 1984a

Breitner JC, Folstein MF: Familial nature of Alzheimer's disease (letter). N Engl J Med 311:192, 1984b

Breitner JC, Murphy EA, Folstein MF: Familial aggregation in Alzheimer dementia, II: clinical genetic implications of age-dependent onset [published erratum appears in J Psychiatr Res 21:331, 1987]. J Psychiatr Res 20:45–55, 1986

Breitner JC, Gau BA, Welsh KA, et al: Inverse association of anti-inflammatory treatments and Alzheimer's disease: initial results of a co-twin control study. Neurology 44:227–232, 1994

Brousseau T: Confirmation of the epsilon 4 allele of the apolipoprotein E gene as a risk factor for late-onset Alzheimer's disease. Neurology 44:342–344, 1994

Brown J, Gydesen S, Sorensen SA, et al: Genetic characterization of a familial non-specific dementia originating in Jutland, Denmark. J Neurol Sci 114: 138–143, 1993

Buxbaum JD, Oishi M, Chen HI, et al: Cholinergic agonists and interleukiregulate processing and secretion of the Alzheimer beta/A4 amyloid protein precursor. Proc Natl Acad Sci U S A 89:10075–10078, 1992

Campion D, Brice A, Hannequin D, et al: A large pedigree with early-onset Alzheimer's disease: clinical, neuropathologic, and genetic characterization. Neurology 45:80–85, 1995

Castano EM, Perelli F, Wisniewski T, et al: Fibrillogenesis in Alzheimer's disease of amyloid beta peptides and apolipoprotein E. Biochem J 306:599–604, 1995

Chandrasekaran K, Giordano T, Brady DR, et al: Impairment in mitochondrial cytochrome oxidase gene expression in Alzheimer's disease. Brain Res Mol Brain Res 24:336–340, 1994

Chartier-Harlin MC, Parfitt H, Legrain S, et al: Apolipoprotein E, epsilon 4 allele as a major risk factor for sporadic early and late-onset forms of Alzheimer's disease: analysis of the 19q13.2 chromosomal region. Hum Mol Genet 3: 569–574, 1994

Chase GA, et al: The use of life tables and survival analysis in testing genetic hypotheses, with an application to Alzheimer's disease. Am J Epidemiol 117: 590–597, 1983

Corder EH, Woodbury MA: Genetic heterogeneity in Alzheimer's disease: a grade of membership analysis. Genet Epidemiol 10:495–499, 1993

Corder EH, Saunders AM, Risch NJ, et al: Protective effect of apolipoprotein E type 2 allele for late onset Alzheimer's disease. Nat Genet 7:180–184, 1994

Dai XY, et al: Association of apolipoprotein E4 with sporadic Alzheimer's disease is more pronounced in early onset type. Neurosci Lett 175:74–76, 1994

DeArmond SJ: Alzheimer's disease and Creutzfeldt-Jakob disease: overlap of pathogenic mechanisms. Curr Opin Neurol 6:872–881, 1993

Farrer LA, Stice L: Susceptibility genes for familial Alzheimer's disease on chromosomes 19 and 21: a reality check. Genet Epidemiol 10:425–430, 1993

Felsenstein KM, Ingalls KM, Hunihan LW, et al: Reversal of the Swedish familial Alzheimer's disease mutant phenotype in cultured cells treated with phorbol 12,13-dibutyrate. Neurosci Lett 174:173–176, 1994

Folstein M: Inheritability of Alzheimer's disease. Am Fam Physician 26:56–57, 1982

Folstein M, Bylsma F: Noncognitive symptoms of Alzheimer's disease, in Alzheimer's Disease. Edited by Terry R, Katzman R, Bick K. New York, Raven, 1994, pp 27–41

Folstein MF: Heterogeneity in Alzheimer's disease. Neurobiol Aging 10:434–435, 1989

Folstein MF, Breitner JC: Language disorder predicts familial Alzheimer's disease. Johns Hopkins Med J 149:145–147, 1981

Folstein MF, Powell D: In search of the Alzheimer's disease gene, in Familial Alzheimer's Disease: Molecular Genetics and Clinical Perspectives. Edited by Miner GD, Richter RW, Blass JP, et al. New York, Marcel Dekker, 1989, pp 3–13

Folstein MF, Warren A: Genetics of Alzheimer's disease. Res Publ Assoc Res Nerv Ment Dis 69:129–136, 1991

Folstein MF, Powell D, Breitner JC: The cognitive pattern of familial Alzheimer's disease (FAD), in Banbury Report 15: Biological Aspects of Alzheimer's Disease. New York, Banbury Center, Cold Spring Harbor Laboratory, 1983, pp 337–349

Folstein M, Breitner JCS, Powell D: Familial Alzheimer's disease, in Biology and Treatment of Dementia in the Elderly. Edited by Shamoian CA. Washington, DC, American Psychiatric Press, 1984, pp 40–47

Folstein MF, Warren A, McHugh PR: Heterogeneity in Alzheimer's disease: an exercise in the resolution of a phenotype, in Molecular Genetic Mechanism in Neurological Disorders: Genetic Mechanism in Alzheimer's Disease and Down's Syndrome, Vol 3. Edited by Brown P, Bolis L, Gajdusek DC. Geneva, Switzerland, FESN, 1988, pp 85–89

Forstl H, et al: Lewy body variant of Alzheimer's disease: clinical and pathological findings. Br J Psychiatry 163:692, 694–695, 1993

Forstl H, Czech C, Sattell H, et al: Apolipoprotein E and Alzheimer dementia: personal results and brief literature review (in German). Nervenarzt 65: 780–786, 1994

Galasko D, Saitoh T, Xia Y, et al: The apolipoprotein E allele epsilon 4 is overrepresented in patients with the Lewy body variant of Alzheimer's disease. Neurology 44:1950–1951, 1994

Goate A, Owen MJ, James LA, et al: Predisposing locus for Alzheimer's disease on chr 21. Lancet 1:352–355, 1989

Goate A, Chartier, Harlin MC, Mullan M, et al: Segregation of a missense mutation in the amyloid precursor protein gene. Nature 349:704–706, 1991

Hendrie HC, Hall HS, Hui S, et al: Apolipoprotein E genotypes and Alzheimer's disease in a community study of elderly African Americans. Ann Neurol 37: 118–120, 1995

Heston LL, Orr HT, Rich SS, et al: Linkage of Alzheimer disease susceptibility locus to markers on chr 21. Am J Med Genet 40:449–453, 1991

Hyman BT, West HL, Rebeck GU, et al: Quantitative analysis of senile plaques in Alzheimer's disease: observation of log-normal size distribution and molecular epidemiology of differences associated with apolipoprotein E genotype and trisomy 21 (Down syndrome). Proc Natl Acad Sci U S A 92: 3586–3590, 1995

Johnston JA, Cowburn RF, Norgren S, et al: Increased beta-amyloid release and levels of amyloid precursor protein (APP) in fibroblast cell lines from family members with the Swedish Alzheimer's disease APP670/671 mutation. FEBS Lett 354:274–278, 1994

Katzman R, Kawas C: Alzheimer disease: senile dementia and related disorders, in Alzheimer's Disease. Edited by Terry R, Katzman R, Blick KL. New York, Raven, 1994, pp 105–123

Kennedy AM, Newman SK, Frackowiak RS, et al: Chromosome 14 linked familial Alzheimer's disease: a clinico-pathological study of single pedigree. Brain 118:185–205, 1995

Kim R, et al: Familial dementia of adult onset with pathological findings of a nonspecific nature. Brain 104:61–78, 1981

Kuusisto J, Koivisto K, Kervinen K, et al: Association of apolipoprotein E phenotypes with late onset Alzheimer's disease: population based study. BMJ 309(6955):636–638, 1994

Lampe TH, Bird TD, Mochlin D, et al: Phenotype of chromosome 14-linked familial Alzheimer's disease in a large kindred. Ann Neurol 36:368–378, 1994

Lannfelt L, Bogdanovic N, Appelgren H, et al: Amyloid precursor protein mutation causes Alzheimer's disease in a Swedish family (letter). Neurosci Lett 168:254–256, 1994

Larsson T, Sjogren T, Jacobson G: Senile dementia. Acta Psychiatr Scand 39(suppl 167):1–259, 1963

Lehtimaki T, Pirttila T, Mehta PD, et al: Apolipoprotein E (APOE) polymorphism and its influence on APOE concentrations in the cerebrospinal fluid in Finnish patients with Alzheimer's disease. Hum Genet 95:39–42, 1995

Liddell M, Williams J, Boyer A, et al: Confirmation of association between the ε4 allele of apolipoprotein E and Alzheimer's disease. J Med Genet 31:197–200, 1994

Masliah E, Terry RD, Alford M, et al: Cortical and subcortical patterns of synaptophysin immunoreactivity in Alzheimer's disease. Am J Pathol 138: 235–246, 1991

Mayeux R, Ottman R, Maestre G, et al: Synergistic effects of traumatic head injury and apolipoprotein-epsilon 4 in patients with Alzheimer's disease. Neurology 45:555–557, 1995

McKeith IG, Perry RH, Fairbairn AF, et al: Operational criteria for senile dementia of the Lewy body type. Psychol Med 22:911–922, 1992

Mullan M, Crawford F, Axelman K, et al: A pathogenic mutation for probable Alzheimer's disease in the APP gene at the N-terminus of beta-amyloid. Nat Genet 1:345–347, 1992

Nagano K, Miki T, Yoshioka K, et al: Two kindreds with familial Alzheimer's disease—analysis of the APP717 mutation and the mutated genes for the prion protein (in Japanese). Nippon Ronen Igakkai Zasshi 29:509–514, 1992

Paganini-Hill A, Henderson VW: Estrogen deficiency and risk of Alzheimer's disease in women. Am J Epidemiol 140:256–261, 1994

Peacock ML, Murman DL, Sima AA, et al: Novel amyloid precursor protein gene mutation (codon 665Asp) in a patient with late-onset Alzheimer's disease. Ann Neurol 35:432–438, 1994

Pearlson GD, Ross CA, Lohr WD, et al: Association between family history of affective disorder and the depressive syndrome of Alzheimer's disease. Am J Psychiatry 147:452–456, 1988

Pericak-Vance M, et al: Linkage studies in familial Alzheimer's disease—evidence for chromosome 19 linkage. Am J Hum Genet 48:1034–1050, 1991

Poirier J, Davignon J, Bouthillier D, et al: Apolipoprotein E polymorphism and Alzheimer's disease. Lancet 342(8873):697–699, 1993

Powell D, Folstein MF: Pedigree study of familial Alzheimer's disease. J Neurogenet 1:189–197, 1984

Querfurth HW, Wijsman Em, St. George-Hyslop PH, et al: Beta APP mRNA transcription is increased in cultured fibroblasts from the familial Alzheimer's disease—1 family. Brain Res Mol Brain Res 28:319–337, 1995

Rich JB, Rasmusson DX, Folstein MF, et al: Nonsteroidal anti-inflammatory drugs in Alzheimer's disease. Neurology 45:51–54, 1994

Roberts GW, Allsop D, Burton C: The occult aftermath of boxing. Neuropathol Appl Neurobiol 15:273–274, 1989

Rubinsztein DC, Hanlon DC, Irving RM, et al: Apo E genotypes in multiple sclerosis, Parkinson's disease, schwannomas and late-onset Alzheimer's disease. Mol Cell Probes 8:519–525, 1994

Saitoh T, Xia Y, Chen X, et al: The CYP2D6B mutant allele is overrepresented in the Lewy body variant of Alzheimer's disease. Ann Neurol 37:110–112, 1995

Sattell H, Geiger-Kabisch C, Schreiter-Gasser U, et al: Incidence and importance of non-cognitive symptoms in dementia of the Alzheimer type: productive psychotic symptoms, depressive disorders and behavioral disorders. Zeitschrift fur Gerontologie 26:275–279, 1993

Schellenberg GD, Bird TD, Wijsman EM, et al: Genetic linkage evidence for a familial Alzheimer's disease locus on chromosome 14. Science 258(5082): 668–671, 1992

Shin RW, Lee VM, Trojanowski JQ: Aluminum modifies the properties of Alzheimer's disease. J Neurosci 14:7221–7233, 1994

Simonian NA, Hyman BT: Functional alterations in Alzheimer's disease: selective loss of mitochondrial-encoded cytochrome oxidase mRNA in the hippocampal formation. J Neuropathol Exp Neurol 53:508–512, 1994

Sjogren T, Sjogren H, Lindgren AGH, et al: A genetic study of morbus Alzheimer and morbus Pick. Acta Psychiatr Scand 9(suppl 82):1–152, 1952

Smith-Swintosky VL, Mattson MP: Glutamate, beta-amyloid precursor proteins, and calcium mediated neurofibrillary degeneration. J Neural Transm Suppl 44:29–45, 1994

St. Clair D, Rennie M, Storach E, et al: Apolipoprotein E epsilon 4 allele frequency in patients with Lewy body dementia, Alzheimer's disease and age-matched controls. Neurosci Lett 176:45–46, 1994

St. George-Hyslop PS, Haines J, Rogaev E, et al: Genetic evidence for a novel familial Alzheimer's disease gene on chromosome 14. Nat Genet 2:330–334, 1992

Steele C, Rovner B, Chase GA, et al: Psychiatric symptoms and nursing home placement of patients with Alzheimer's disease. Am J Psychiatry 147:1049–1051, 1990

Stern Y, Folstein M, Albert M, et al: Multicenter study of predictors of disease course in Alzheimer's disease (the predictors study), I: Study design, cohort description, and intersite comparisons. Alzheimer Dis Assoc Disord 7:3–21, 1993

Strittmatter WJ, Saunders AM, Schmechel D, et al: Apolipoprotein E: high-avidity binding to beta-amyloid and increased frequency of type 4 allele in late-onset familial Alzheimer's disease. Proc Natl Acad Sci U S A 90:1977–1981, 1993

Tamaoka A: Apolipoprotein E4 and late-onset Alzheimer's disease (in Japanese). Nippon Rinsho 52:3257–3265, 1994

van Broeckhoven C, Backhovens H, Cruts M, et al: Mapping of a gene predisposing to early-onset Alzheimer's disease to chromosome 14q24.3. Nat Genet 2:335–339, 1992

van Duijn CM, Clarton DG, Chandra V, et al: Interaction between genetic and environmental risk factors for Alzheimer's disease: a reanalysis of case-control studies. EURODEM Risk Factors Research Group. Genet Epidemiol 11: 539–551, 1994

van Duijn CM, Havekes LM, van Broeckhoven C, et al: Apolipoprotein E genotype and association between smoking and early onset Alzheimer's disease. BMJ 310(6980):627–631, 1995

Yoshizawa T, Yamakawa-Kobayashi K, Komatsuzaki, Y, et al: Dose-dependent association of apolipoprotein E allele epsilon 4 with late-onset, sporadic Alzheimer's disease. Ann Neurol 36:656–659, 1994

Yu CE, Payami H, Olson JM, et al: The apolipoprotein E/CI/CII gene cluster and late-onset Alzheimer disease. Am J Hum Genet 54:631–642, 1994

Zeldenrust SR, Murrell J, Farlow M, et al: RFLP analysis for APP 717 mutations associated with Alzheimer's disease. J Med Genet 30:476–478, 1993

Zweig RM, Ross, CA, Hedreen JC, et al: The neuropathology of aminergic nuclei in Alzheimer's disease. Ann Neurol 24:233–242, 1988

Chapter 7

Unstable Triplet Repeats in Neurological Disease

Spinocerebellar Ataxia Type 1

Harry T. Orr, Ph.D., and
Huda Y. Zoghbi, M.D.

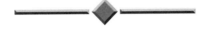

H uman geneticists have recently identified a new form of DNA alteration—unstable trinucleotide repeats—that seems to occur only in humans and causes specific neuropsychiatric disorders. This alteration involves repeated units of three nucleotides in human DNA that (when expanded in size) cause certain diseases that primarily affect the central nervous system. These diseases are characterized by *anticipation,* an unusual genetic feature in which the severity of the disease increases and the age at onset decreases in successive generations.

In fragile X syndrome and myotonic dystrophy, the unstable trinucleotide repeat is located within the transcribed region of the respective genes but outside the coding region. Five other disorders—Huntington's disease,

We thank the members of the SCA1 families, without whose participation this work would not have been possible. This work was supported by grants from the National Institutes of Health, the National Ataxia Foundation, and the Muscular Dystrophy Association.

spinal and bulbar muscular atrophy (SBMA or Kennedy's disease), spino-cerebellar ataxia type 1 (SCA1), dentarubro-pallidoluysian atrophy (DRPLA) and the related Haw-River syndrome, and Machado-Joseph disease (MJD, or SCA3)—are caused by an unstable CAG triplet located within the coding region of the affected gene. The CAG repeats in these genes all direct the synthesis of tracts repeating glutamine amino acids.

Over the past several years, researchers have found evidence suggesting that certain idiopathic neuropsychiatric disorders have genetic features that are consistent with anticipation and thus might be caused by unstable trinucleotide repeats. In this chapter, we describe the strategy that geneticists used to isolate the SCA1 gene. We hope that this discussion will benefit investigators interested in the characterization of genes associated with neuropsychiatric disorders that involve genetic anticipation.

Spinocerebellar Ataxia Type I: Clinical Features

Autosomal dominantly inherited ataxias, or spinocerebellar ataxias (SCAs), are a complex group of disorders with variable degrees of neurodegeneration that cause dysfunction of the cerebellum, spinal tracts, and brain stem (Greenfield 1954). Clinical presentation among various forms of SCA exhibits considerable overlap; as a result, the development of a clinical classification scheme has been difficult and controversial. The recent advent of molecular genetic approaches to disease classification has resulted in gradual formation of a genetic classification scheme for SCAs.

Spinocerebellar ataxia type 1 (SCA1) is one form of SCA that has been classified for several years. Geneticists have classified this disease based on its genetic or chromosomal localization in the short arm of chromosome 6 within band 6p22.1–23 (Jackson et al. 1977). Clinical features of early-stage SCA1 include gait ataxia, dysarthria, and nystagmus. As the disease worsens, ataxia progresses and other cerebellar signs develop, including dysmetria and hypotonia. In later stages of SCA1, muscle atrophy, decreased deep tendon reflexes, and loss of proprioception and vibration sense become common. For the most part, cognitive functions remain unimpaired, although Kish et al. (1994) reported some loss of cognitive function in SCA1 patients at later stages of the disease. The final stage of SCA1 is characterized by facial weakness and loss of bulbar signs, including severe dysarthria and dysphagia, which lead to frequent choking and coughing spells, poor cough reflex, food aspiration, and recurrent pneumonia; these symptoms usually result in death.

SCA1 is characterized as a late-onset disease: onset typically occurs in the third or fourth decade. In a few instances, researchers have reported juvenile onset of SCA1 (Schut 1950; Zoghbi et al. 1988). Interestingly, these juvenile cases of SCA1 were the result of disease transmissions from an affected father to his offspring. In most cases, the disease progresses over a period of 10–15 years; in juvenile cases, however, disease progression is much more rapid (Currier et al. 1982; Zoghbi et al. 1988).

Neuropathological studies at autopsy reveal considerable loss in the cerebellar cortex, with severe degeneration of Purkinje cells and dentate nuclei neurons. Pathological analysis also reveals neuronal degeneration within inferior olive and cranial nerve nuclei III, IV, IX, X, and XII, as well as demyelination of spinocerebellar tracts and dorsal columns.

Genetic and Physical Characterization of the SCA1 Locus

Researchers initially determined that the SCA1 gene was located on the short arm of chromosome 6 through linkage to the human leukocyte antigen (HLA) complex (Yakura et al. 1974). Further investigation placed the SCA1 locus distal to the HLA complex on chromosome 6p (Rich et al. 1987). Subsequent research refined the genetic position of the SCA1 gene by demonstrating very close linkage to a polymorphic DNA marker, D6S89. This marker maps distal to the HLA complex in chromosomal band 6p22–p23 (Kwiatkowski et al. 1993; Ranum et al. 1991; Zoghbi et al. 1991).

Combined analysis of approximately 120 affected individuals using D6S89 revealed a single individual in whom a chromosomal recombination event had occurred between SCA1 and the marker D6S89 (Kwiatowski et al. 1993). This finding indicated that D6S89 is located very close to the SCA1 gene—at a genetic distance of less than 1 centimorgan (cM) distal or telomeric to the SCA1 gene.

The next step in the genetic definition of the SCA1 locus involved the identification of marker D6S274 as lying proximal or on the centromeric side of the SCA1 gene. Again, researchers found a single individual with a recombination between SCA1 and D6S274 in a large population of SCA1-affected individuals (Kwiatkowski et al. 1993).

Importantly, researchers determined that the genetic distance between the markers flanking the SCA1 gene, D6S89 and D6S274, was less than 2.0 cm (Kwiatkowski et al. 1993). This genetic distance roughly corresponds to a physical distance of less than 2.0 megabases (mb) of DNA—an amount of DNA that can be fairly readily cloned in overlapping yeast artificial chromosomes (YACs). Thus, geneticists isolated the SCA1 region from D6S274 to D6S89 in a series of overlapping YAC clones that formed a contig of 1.2 mb. For the isolation of the SCA1 gene itself, investigators subsequently converted these YAC clones into cosmid clones, which are easier to handle and manipulate than YACs.

Molecular Basis of SCA1

Geneticists have identified unstable trinucleotide repeats as the underlying cause of three disorders that display anticipation: fragile X syndrome, myotonic dystrophy, and, most recently, Huntington's disease. Based on the observation of anticipation in families with SCA, researchers hypothesized that the mutational mechanism causing SCA1 could be an unstable trinucleotide repeat. To test this hypothesis, we examined cosmid clones from the SCA1 candidate region with a probe containing oligonucleotides representing all of the permutations of trinucleotide repeats (10 in all) (Orr et al. 1993).

Investigators had found that Huntington's disease was caused by the expansion of an unstable CAG triplet repeat; because the degree of anticipation SCA1 (as in Huntington's) was very subtle, we initiated our analysis with the oligonucleotide probe containing CAG. We found 23 cosmids from the SCA1 critical region that hybridized this CAG probe and had in common a 3.2-kb EcoRI fragment. Sequence analysis of this fragment revealed that it contained a CAG repeat with a configuration of $(CAG)_{12}CATCAGCAT(CAG)_{15}$. We used this 3.2-kb EcoRI fragment to examine Southern blots of DNA prepared from members of families with a juvenile case of SCA1. This analysis revealed an enlarged fragment in DNA from the juvenile patients (Figure 7–1).

Further Southern analyses indicated that an enlarged restriction fragment was present in the DNA of all SCA1-affected patients but in none of the DNA from unaffected individuals. We sequenced the 3.2-kb fragment further and synthesized oligonucleotide primers immediately flanking the CAG repeat to develop a polymerase chain reaction (PCR)-based test

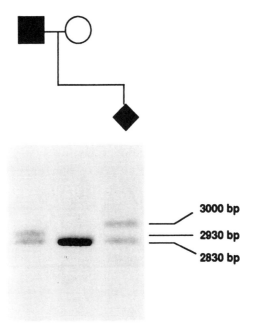

Figure 7–1. Demonstration of expanded SCA1 allele in a juvenile patient by Southern analysis. Genomic DNA from members of a family affected with SCA1 was digested with *Taq*I, blotted onto a nylon membrane, and probed with a radio-labeled 3.2-kb *Eco*RI fragment containing the CAG triplet repeat. Affected individuals are indicated by solid symbols. The father was affected with SCA1 at age 35; his child was diagnosed at age 4.   *Source.*   Reprinted with permission from Orr H, Chung M-y, Banfi S, et al: "Expansion of an Unstable Trinucleotide (CAG) Repeat in Spino-cerebellar Ataxia Type 1." *Nature Genetics* 4:221–226, 1993.

of repeat expansion. This test revealed that unaffected individuals carried two SCA1 alleles, each with a repeat size ranging from 6 to 39 CAGs. In contrast, individuals with SCA1 had one allele with a repeat number within the unaffected range and a second allele of the SCA1 gene with 40–81 CAG triplet repeats (Table 7–1).

The analysis of every family known to have SCA1 by linkage analysis revealed an expanded allele in each of the affected individuals examined. These data indicated that CAG triplet expansion to a size of 40 or greater is the mutational cause of SCA1 and that other types of mutations are less likely to have occurred within the SCA1 gene.

With regard to the relationship between the CAG repeat and the development of disease, the number of triplet units correlated inversely with age at onset and disease severity (Ranum et al. 1994). We evaluated the relationships between age at onset and number of CAG repeats on unaffected and SCA1 chromosomes in 113 individuals (Ranum et al. 1994). We found a correlation coefficient of – 0.815 for age at onset, compared with the number of SCA1 CAG repeats on expanded alleles in affected individuals (Figure 7–2); this finding indicated that the size of the CAG repeat accounts for 66% of the variability in age at onset. We also found a correlation (– 0.58) between CAG triplet number and disease severity, as measured by age at death minus age at onset—suggesting that 43% of the variation in disease duration is a result of the number of CAG triplets on an expanded allele. We found no correlation with any feature of disease between the number of SCA1 CAG repeats on the unexpanded allele in patients. Other investigators reported similar data on the correlation between SCA1 CAG repeat number and age at onset (Dubourg et al. 1995; Jodice et al. 1994).

Researchers have examined the intergenerational stability of the CAG repeat size at SCA1 for unaffected and expanded affected alleles. In more than 1,000 examples of parent-to-offspring transmission, investigators have reported no instances of instability for the CAG repeat on unaffected alleles. However, the CAG repeat number on affected alleles of SCA1 are unstable on transmission from affected parent to offspring. Researchers have noted decreases and increases in the number of CAG repeats in transmissions from an affected parent (Ranum et al. 1994).

Interestingly, Chung et al. (1993) found a significant difference in the type and size of repeat number change in maternal versus paternal transmission of an affected allele: 63% of the 16 paternal transmissions they examined resulted in an increase in the number of SCA1 CAG triplets, with an average increase of 3.3 repeats; in contrast, in 28 cases of maternal

Table 7–1. SCA1 CAG triplet repeat numbers on unaffected and affected chromosomes

Unaffected chromosomes		Affected chromosomes		
$(CAG)_n$	# of chromosomes studied	$(CAG)_n$	# of chromosomes studied	Reference
19–36	304	40–81	114	Ranum et al. 1994
6–39	68	41–57	10	Matilla et al. 1993
26–37	365	46–66	64	Jodice et al. 1994
27–36	116	42–67	61	Dubourg et al. 1995

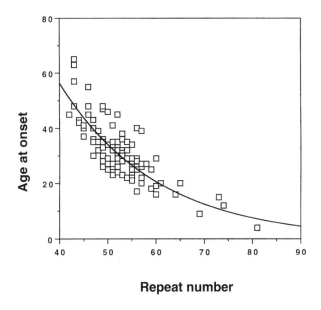

Figure 7–2.   Correlation between number of CAG triplet repeats in expanded allele of SCA1 gene and age at onset of disease for 113 patients. *Source.*   Reprinted with permission from Ranum LPW, Chung M-y, Banfi S, et al: "Molecular and Clinical Correlations in Spinocerebellar Ataxia Type 1 (SCA1): Evidence for Familial Effects on the Age of Onset." *American Journal of Human Genetics* 55:244–252, 1994. © University of Chicago Press, 1994.

transmission of an affected allele, 69% of the transmissions resulted in no change or a decrease in the number of CAG triplets, with an average change of − 0.4 triplets. The difference in the intergenerational stability of the CAG repeat between maternal and paternal transmissions is statistically significant ($P<.005$). This finding explains the fact that all juvenile cases of SCA1 reported to date have been the result of transmission of an affected allele from father to offspring. Moreover, the most dramatic intergenerational increase in SCA1 CAG repeat number—an increase of 28 CAG triplets—involved paternal transmission (Orr et al. 1993).

   Other investigators have described the effects of paternal origin on the stability and size of repeat expansion for SCA1 alleles. Matilla et al. (1993), for example, found that the majority of the larger intergenerational increases in CAG repeat number occurred in paternal transmissions. Jodice et al. (1994) observed that all transmissions of repeat numbers 54 and greater were from affected fathers, whereas alleles with repeat sizes between 46 and 54 were transmitted equally by fathers and mothers.

The presence of CAT trinucleotides interposed between two tracts of CAG triplet repeats on an unaffected SCA1 allele suggests that this interruption may have a role in the stability of the CAG repeat. To test this idea, Chung et al. (1993) examined the sequence configuration of the CAG repeat on unaffected and affected SCA1 alleles using a combination of direct sequence analysis and digestion of PCR products with the restriction enzyme $SfaNI$, which cleaves $GCATC(N)_5$—thereby allowing a determination of the presence of at least one CAT interruption within the CAG repeat. Analysis of 126 chromosomes with an unaffected allele of SCA1 revealed an interrupted repeat configuration with one, two, or three CAT triplets in 123 of 126 chromosomes studied. The three chromosomes with an unaffected allele without a CAT interruption were the two smallest unaffected alleles: one had 19 CAG triplets, and two had 21 CAG repeats. Thus, 98% of the unaffected and stable alleles of SCA1 had a CAG repeat configuration containing at least one CAT trinucleotide interruption within the CAG repeat tract. In contrast, of 30 affected SCA1 chromosomes, every one had a perfect, uninterrupted tract of CAG triplet repeats. Seven unrelated kindreds with at least four different haplotypes at D6S288 and D6S274 had perfect CAG repeat tracts on all affected chromosomes.

Jodice et al. (1994) also reported perfect repeats for all of the affected SCA1 alleles in 19 other SCA1 families. These data indicate that the loss of the CAT interruption in alleles of 21 or more repeats renders the CAG repeat unstable and susceptible to subsequent intergenerational expansion (Chung et al. 1993).

The SCA1 Gene and Protein

The transcript expressed from the SCA1 gene is 10,660 base pairs (bp) long and is found in a wide variety of cell and tissue types (Banfi et al. 1994; Orr et al. 1993). The coding region is 2,448 bp long and encodes a protein of 792–829 amino acids, depending on the number of CAG repeats that encode a polyglutamine tract within the protein. The SCA1-encoded protein, ataxin-1, is a novel protein without any detectable homologies to previously identified genes or proteins in the databases. The 5' untranslated and 3' untranslated regions of the SCA1 transcript are extremely long: 935 bp and 7,277 bp, respectively.

At the genomic level, the SCA1 gene spans about 450 kb of DNA and consists of nine exons (Banfi et al. 1994). The structure of the SCA1 gene exhibits an unusual feature: the 5' untranslated region is found in the first seven exons, whereas the region encoding the ataxin-1 protein is located within two large exons—eight and nine—of 2,079 bp and 7,805 bp, respectively.

Recently, researchers have generated polyclonal antibodies against the ataxin-1 protein (Servadio et al. 1995); they have used these antisera to determine that the ataxin-1 protein also is found in a wide variety of cell and tissue types. When investigators use these antibodies to probe Western blots of cellular extracts prepared from lymphoblastoid cells established from SCA1 patients with differing numbers of SCA1 CAG repeats, they detect two bands. One band, about 100 K in size, is identical in size to the band found in extracts prepared from unaffected individuals. The second ataxin-1 band in extracts from SCA1-affected individuals is larger, by an amount proportional to the number of CAG repeats found on the affected allele of SCA1. These results confirm that the CAG repeat is located within the coding region of the ataxin-1 protein and that an expansion of CAG repeat number leads to the production of an ataxin-1 protein with an increased number of amino acids.

A Model of Pathogenesis

The exact mechanism of pathogenesis in SCA1—or any of the diseases caused by the expansion of an unstable CAG triplet repeat—is unclear. Certain aspects of SCA1 and these other disorders favor, however, some models of pathogenesis over others. The mechanism of neurodegeneration probably has common aspects in all of the diseases caused by the expansion of an unstable CAG repeat that encodes a polyglutamine tract (i.e., SCA1, Huntington's disease, SBMA, DRPLA, and MJD).

The expansion of the polyglutamine tract in proteins encoded by genes affected in these disorders most likely leads to a gain in function mutation. Thus, deletions of the androgen receptor, the gene affected in SBMA and hemizygosity at the Huntington's disease locus, do not result in neurodegenerative disease. Moreover, expansion of the CAG repeat in the androgen receptor gene does not result in the same pattern of symptoms (e.g., testicular feminization) as deletion of the androgen receptor gene. Thus, expansions of the CAG repeat probably do not disrupt the normal functions of any of these genes. The most likely hypothesis is that the expansion of the polyglutamine tract in ataxin-1 causes it to interact with another cellular protein whose expression is cell-specific, which would explain the selective loss of neurons in SCA1.

Summary

By combining a positional cloning strategy with the directed identification of an unstable trinucleotide repeat, geneticists have isolated and characterized the novel gene affected in the neurodegenerative disorder SCA1. These results have important implications for families affected by this degenerative disease. On a broader level, the cloning of the SCA1 gene and the identification of an unstable CAG repeat as the molecular basis of disease indicate that the approach used to isolate SCA1 can be effective even for disorders in which the degree of genetic anticipation is extremely subtle. A strategy directed at identifying an unstable trinucleotide repeat might be extremely valuable for investigators working toward the isolation of a gene affected by a disease in which there is evidence for anticipation.

References

Banfi S, Servadio A, Chung M-y, et al: Identification and characterization of the gene causing type I spinocerebellar ataxia. Nat Genet 7:513–519, 1994

Chung M-y, Ranum LPW, Duvick L, et al: Analysis of the CAG repeat expansion in spinocerebellar ataxia type I: evidence for a possible mechanism predisposing to instability. Nat Genet 5:254–258, 1993

Currier RD, Jackson JF, Meydrech EF: Progression rate and age at onset are related in autosomal dominant neurologic diseases. Neurology 32:260–266, 1982

Dubourg O, Durr A, Cancel G, et al: Analysis of the SCA1 CAG repeat in a large number of families with dominant ataxia: clinical and molecular correlations. Ann Neurol 37:176–180, 1995

Greenfield JG: The Spino-Cerebellar Degenerations. Springfield, IL, Charles C Thomas, 1954

Jackson JF, Currier RD, Terasaki PI, et al: Spinocerebellar ataxia and HLA linkage: risk prediction by HLA typing. N Engl J Med 296:1138–1141, 1977

Jodice C, Malaspina P, Persichetti F, et al: Effect of trinucleotide repeat length and parental sex on phenotypic variation in spinocerebellar ataxia 1. Am J Hum Genet 54:959–965, 1994

Kish SJ, El-Awar M, Stuss D, et al: Neuropsychological test performance in patients with dominantly inherited spinocerebellar ataxia: relationship to ataxia severity. Neurology 44:1738–1746, 1994

Kwiatkowski TJ Jr, Orr HT, Banfi S, et al: The gene for autosomal dominant spinocerebellar ataxia (SCA1) maps centromeric to D6S89 and shows no recombination, in nine large kindreds, with a dinucleotide repeat at the AM10 locus. Am J Hum Genet 53:391–400, 1993

Matilla T, Volipini V, Genis D, et al: Presymptomatic analysis of spinocerebellar ataxia type 1 (SCA1) via the expansion of the SCA1 CAG-repeat in a large pedigree displaying anticipation and parental male bias. Hum Mol Genet 2:2123–2128, 1993

Orr H, Chung M-y, Banfi S, et al: Expansion of an unstable trinucleotide (CAG) repeat in spinocerebellar ataxia type 1. Nat Genet 4:221–226, 1993

Ranum LPW, Duvick LA, Rich SS, et al: Localization of the autosomal dominant, HLA-linked spinocerebellar ataxia (SCA1) locus in two kindreds within an 8cM subregion of chromosome 6p. Am J Hum Genet 49:31–41, 1991

Ranum LPW, Chung M-y, Banfi S, et al: Molecular and clinical correlations in spinocerebellar ataxia type 1 (SCA1): evidence for familial effects on the age of onset. Am J Hum Genet 55:244–252, 1994

Rich SS, Wilkie P, Schut L, et al: Spinocerebellar ataxia: localization of an autosomal dominant locus between two markers on human chromosome 6. Am J Hum Genet 41:524–531, 1987

Schut JW: Hereditary ataxia: clinical study through six generations. Archives of Neurology and Psychiatry 63:535–568, 1950

Servadio A, Koshy B, Armstrong D, et al: Expression analysis of the ataxin-1 protein in tissues from normal and spinocerebellar ataxia type 1 individuals. Nat Genet 10:94–98, 1995

Yakura H, Wakisaka A, Fujimoto S, et al: Hereditary ataxia and HLA genotypes. N Engl J Med 291:154–155, 1974

Zoghbi HY, Pollack MS, Lyons LA, et al: Spinocerebellar ataxia: variable age of onset and linkage to human leukocyte antigen in a large kindred. Ann Neurol 23:580–584, 1988

Zoghbi HY, Jodice C, Sandkuijl LA, et al: The gene for autosomal dominant spinocerebellar ataxia (SCA1) maps telomeric to HLA complex and is closely linked to the D6S89 locus in three large kindreds. Am J Hum Genet 49:23–30, 1991

Chapter 8

What a Dementing Illness Is Doing to My Family

Denise Heinrichs

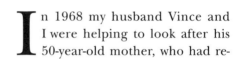

In 1968 my husband Vince and I were helping to look after his 50-year-old mother, who had received a diagnosis of hardening of the arteries. We were a young family, with three children, and Vince was planning to go to graduate school for 2 years for a Ph.D. in English literature. He had completed 2 years of classes, passed his comprehensive examinations, and started his dissertation.

As my mother-in-law's illness became progressively worse, our interest in her condition led to the discovery that three of her brothers and her mother had died at an early age in nursing homes or state mental hospitals. Vince's dissertation studies were no longer in English; they became a study in genetics. We tried to unlock the family secret that was hidden for many years: that people had died with their minds destroyed. This family secret was difficult to uncover because the healthy persons in each generation thought that their loved ones had died of a mental condition that was not to be discussed. Our search led us to a physician studying genetics, education about possible genetic diseases, and finally—

Our thanks go to Dr. Leonard Heston, our physician and friend; his colleague, June White, who searched through cemeteries to find our ancestors and collect data; all of the wonderful people who cared for Vince at NIH; the people who supported our family through the hard times; scientists to come who will find the cure for Alzheimer's disease; and Vince, who continues to give to us.

after 8 years—an autopsy of a first cousin and the discovery of genetic Alzheimer's disease in Vince's family.

Vince was 39 years old and a college teacher; by this time, we had six children. The physicians told us that because Vince's mother had died of familial Alzheimer's disease, he had a 50% risk of developing the same disease. He contacted all living members of his mother's family with the information about his mother, her brothers who had died before her, and their grandmother—all of whom probably had Alzheimer's disease. Over the next few years, we watched helplessly as three more cousins and Vince's brother received diagnoses in their early- to mid-forties of Alzheimer's disease. Some family members were angry with Vince for making them aware of what was happening: Vince had discovered that, in addition to his grandmother, four of her seven children and (as it turned out) seven of their 12 children had Alzheimer's disease.

I soon realized that the disease was starting to rob Vince of his memory. By the time he was 43 years old, he could no longer function in the class-room without assistance; his diagnosis was confirmed just after he turned 44 years old. Our oldest child was a senior in high school; the youngest was in kindergarten.

Coping with Alzheimer's disease led the branches of his family in different directions. Because Vince had done so much research, he and I knew what was ahead and tried to plan as best we could for the decisions to come. We became involved with the Alzheimer's Association and searched for more information about the disease and what we could do to prepare ourselves. For example, we learned about powers of attorney and making end-of-life decisions. By the time Vince's condition was diag-nosed, his brother was already in a nursing home and had a gastric feed-ing tube. We talked about the inappropriateness of that treatment, and Vince decided that nothing such as that should ever be done to him. In the early stages of the disease, we attended as many educational programs as possible, where we made plans for the later stages. At the same time, we were trying to prepare our children by providing them with genetic counseling, so they would understand that they also had a 50% risk of developing Alzheimer's disease.

For the first 3 years after Vince's condition was diagnosed, he did everything to maintain his independence. We both became part of Alzheimer's support groups; we took an active part in educational pro-grams and spoke to other people in our community who had possible Alzheimer's disease. In addition, Vince became a research patient at the National Institutes of Health, and we went to Bethesda, Maryland, every

6–8 months for tests to monitor the course of the disease. We knew nothing could be done to stop the progression of the disease for Vince, but he agreed to do whatever he could for research that might help our children and the millions of other people with Alzheimer's disease.

Because of Vince's background in academia, he did well as a research participant in the beginning. Little by little, however, these trips became more difficult; the last two trips required a great deal of convincing and coaxing to get him to cooperate. At the beginning of the study in 1983, Vince's IQ was 138, but by our last visit in 1987, it was less than 50.

As the disease progressed, our family roles changed. I became the head of the household, and the children helped out as caregivers. By the time our youngest child was 9 years old, for example, she could dress and change her father. The older children helped when Vince's mood swings and frustrations caused him to become violent.

Vince became depressed as he lost more and more of his abilities. He could no longer lace his shoes, tie a tie, or remember the proper order of getting dressed.

As with many Alzheimer's disease patients, giving up driving was one of the hardest things for Vince. As the disease progressed, he would get lost and lose the car. Eventually, he had an accident: he knew how to drive, knew he had to stop at a stop sign, but did not understand that he had to wait for the other cars to go by and drove into a car that had the right of way. We then got him a bicycle, and he maintained a sense of independence by riding his bike. Eventually, riding a bike became too much for him, and the fear of getting lost finally stopped him.

The greatest fear Vince had in the initial stage was that he might harm me or the children. He once described the disease as a slow drowning, which he could do nothing to stop. Indeed, because Alzheimer's disease is progressive, patients may not recognize when they can no longer care for themselves. Forgetfulness, lack of concentration, disorientation, and disruption of verbal skills slowly turn into mental impairment, personality change, wandering, loss of verbal skills, and eventually inability to communicate or recognize others.

Vince became extremely angry, frustrated, and argumentative with everyone. Noise upset him, as did any disruption in his routine. We could no longer be with a group of people because he was unable to understand conversations. He was anxious and paranoid. When he became frustrated and upset, he often would ride his bike to be alone and away from the confusion of the family. He fought hard to control himself, but as the impairment became more severe, he could no longer think of anyone else. More and more decisions had to be taken from him, which caused him even more frustration. He also began to have grand mal seizures. He took phenytoin to control the seizures, but the medication caused hallucinations. His condition changed dramatically, and he experienced a severe decline.

I had to continue to work. In the morning, I would take Vince with me to the school where I was a cook and give him small tasks to perform until our eldest son could pick him up and care for him. Our son had to pick him up before the children came in for lunch because Vince would not allow some of the children to come into the lunchroom.

We tried to place him in day care, but after one day at the program, he refused to go back because of his hallucinations. The day care center was decorated with Valentine hearts hanging from the ceiling; in Vince's confused state, he was terrified because he was sure blood was dripping from the ceiling. We found a woman who tried to care for him during the day, but he refused to stay with her and took off on his own and could not be coaxed back.

We soon learned that television also was too much stimulation. The people on television became real for him; even programs that he had liked in the past—such as *National Geographic*—became frightening because Vince thought, for example, that the lion on television actually was in our house.

As Vince's condition continued to decline, caring for him became more impractical for us. When Vince's violent outbursts began to endanger our children, I knew that nursing home placement was necessary, and we took him to the veterans hospital closest to us. From there, he was transferred to a Veterans Administration (VA) nursing home.

I was told that Vince would receive no more than 6 months of care from the VA at that facility; after that, the responsibility for paying the $85 per day would be up to me. Thus, I not only experienced the stress of watching him deteriorate but also the knowledge that soon I would have no money left for the care of the family.

Life in the nursing home was tragic for Vince. The only way to control his symptoms entailed large doses of thioridazine. Vince could no longer hold his head up, and he could barely walk. He became incontinent and could no longer feed himself. He lost almost all of his language skills and had a change in his visual perceptions. We would take him for walks, but he did not know how to go up and down stairs.

Little by little, however, he mellowed. We transferred him to a nursing home in our hometown that had a low-stimulus unit for extremely agitated Alzheimer's patients. After this transfer, he was slowly removed from medication. As the thioridazine wore off, he gradually became a little more alert. Unfortunately, his losses were permanent, and he required total care.

While Vince was in the nursing home, our family continued to take an active role in his caregiving. One of us would try to be available to feed him one meal a day or just to visit him briefly. There would be brief moments in his life of bewilderment when a window would seem to open and he might say one of our names, but most of the time he did not seem to know us and was unable to communicate. Life at the nursing home became routine for all of us, and we developed an extended family with all the patients and staff on his floor.

As we adjusted to the routine of the nursing home, my worries about how I would pay for his care became more stressful. Vince's salary as a teacher had not allowed us to save much money by the time he had to quit work at age 44 years. My job as director of a lunch program in a school brought in only enough money to care for the family at home and did not leave anything for the cost of nursing home care. The situation seemed impossible; the Department of Human Services advised me I would have to spend down all our assets, including the cash value of Vince's life insurance, until only $1,800 in assets were left to qualify for Medicaid. The system did not consider the possibility that paying for Vince's care and allowing me to continue to care for the rest of the family would make more sense than forcing me to ask for welfare.

Eventually, Vince developed pneumonia; I think it was his final attempt to care for his family. The children and I all agreed that we would stay with him and care for him as best we could, but we would not allow anything to be done to keep him alive. Difficult as it was, we chose not to treat the pneumonia with antibiotics but to administer "comfort only" measures. He died in less than 3 days. It was a beautiful death, with his family around him, telling him stories of our wonderful life together, the fun things he did with his children, and the love we all had for him.

We were fortunate. The physician at the nursing home knew that medical efforts could cure Vince's pneumonia but not his Alzheimer's disease. Vince's body had wasted from 235 pounds before he entered the nursing home to 124 pounds at the time of his death. Unlike his brother, however, Vince did not lie in a bed for years with a feeding tube and restraints, being treated three and four times a year for pneumonia. Our decision was right for us.

Perspectives From Our Experience

I now work as director of our local chapter of the Alzheimer's Association and help families find assistance through the long journey of this disease. We have learned a lot about the proper care of Alzheimer's patients and the need for specialized care. Supportive home care and early intervention with day care, for example, can help delay early placement in nursing homes and provide the necessary respite for caregivers to sustain their well-being. Specialized units within nursing homes with specially trained staff members can promote dignity for the patient—without chemical and physical restraints, in most cases. We now know that the patient's environment plays an important part in the course of the disease. Current research and theories of care suggest that special programming can provide most patients with a more normalized life.

Alzheimer's disease affects each patient differently, but the destruction ultimately is the same: it is complete. Each family has to find its own way to handle the emotional strain, to survive feelings of helplessness and loneliness, and to make some sense out of the hopelessness of the disease. Some members of a family may not accept the decline of their loved one; they may not take part in the caregiving process. In our family, for example, three of our children were comfortable going to the nursing home and interacting with Vince and the other patients, whereas the other three children were not as comfortable in that situation. These feelings did not mean they loved Vince less or cared less; we all had to accept our strengths and limitations.

Physicians and professional caregivers must acknowledge the path that families take in making this journey and offer support and understanding. Stress, depression, and loneliness can lead to physical as well as mental breakdowns among caregivers. Support groups can educate families and help them cope with the losses in Alzheimer's slow death. Ironically, caregivers often are better prepared to accept the death of their loved ones than are physicians or nursing home staff. Because Alzheimer's disease is terminal, families need a supportive hospice approach as life ends.

As a family, we now face the challenge of continuing to take part in research, being available for additional testing, and making decisions about how much information each person wants to discover about the future. Soon, for example, physicians will be able to test my adult children for the gene that will determine if they will develop Alzheimer's disease. As a parent, I wonder how much information is too much. The results of such testing could lead individuals to change their plans regarding family, job choices, and other significant aspects of their lives. However, people at risk for the disease may choose not to be tested or not to ask for the results, proceeding instead with a positive attitude and leading their lives as if they did not carry the gene.

My children are concerned for one another: they do not want the others to be afflicted, but they may not be ready to accept the possibility for themselves. They hope that researchers will find a cure or treatment soon enough for them—or at least for their children, if they should have families. They sometimes talk seriously about the possibility of getting Alzheimer's disease, but more often they make jokes about it as a release of their fears. My children are fiercely loyal to one another and also want to protect one another. One son has said that some days he feels that if anyone in the family has to have the disease he wants it to be himself; other times, however, he would give almost anything to avoid it. Another son has said that he has always felt that his life has a short ceiling and that he wants to accomplish as much as possible during the time he has, and leave behind something of himself that will be good.

As I watch my children choose marriage partners, I wonder if their spouses will be able to handle the pressures of caring for someone with Alzheimer's disease. I can only hope that we will all be available to help if the time comes—and that, with our increased knowledge, we will find a way to provide good care for the patient and the family.

My eldest daughter—who is now a nurse in the critical care unit at our local hospital—still likes to go back to our home and sit in her dad's office to be surrounded by "his" space, which is where he would go even after he was sick to be in his own space. This daughter talks about the fear the children had after Vince's diagnosis, thinking that their dad was going to die in a short time and realizing how important the time we had together became. Looking back, she remembers exhaustion, sadness, fear, anger, and triumph. She feels that the fact that Alzheimer's disease could happen to any of them has brought them closer and made them more special to one another. She regards Alzheimer's disease as an awful disease that makes no sense to her, but she also knows that she has become a better person, a more patient nurse, and a more appreciative daughter because of her experience with it.

My eldest son recalls using humor to get through the hard times. He notes how close our family has become and feels that we have become a more loving family, albeit at a great cost. He also is upset by the genetic counseling that was provided for the children when they were still teenagers: they were told not to have children of their own. He and his wife have talked at length about this issue; they have decided to have children. He feels that curing the disease by wiping out the gene pool is not the answer. He offers himself for testing to help cure the disease or improve his possibilities for a quality, memorable life.

Our family has always been committed to understanding as much as possible about Alzheimer's disease and helping with research to find the cure or effective treatment to delay the disease's onset or mitigate its effects. We understand that research into genetic Alzheimer's disease is so competitive, but we are not competitive—just frightened that it will not happen fast enough. We will go anywhere and do anything to make the answer come quickly.

Research into the cause and eventual cure of this disease is vital. There are now 4 million people in the United States with Alzheimer's disease; because Alzheimer's disease typically affects the elderly—the fastest growing segment of the population—researchers estimate that there will be 14 million people with Alzheimer's disease by the year 2050. Researchers now know that most Alzheimer's disease cases are sporadic, but families such as ours may constitute 10% of all cases.

In a way, Vince lives on; his brain and blood cells have been shared with research programs. These studies helped lead to the discovery that the genetic defect that causes the familial form of Alzheimer's disease is located on chromosome 14. I regard that finding as a small victory in the large war against this terrible disease. My plea is for support of research and understanding of patients and families. We also must maintain pressure on the government to support research and not allow these victories to lie dormant.

Congress would be shortsighted in cutting back research monies to balance the budget; in the long run, such a policy will cost so much more. Senator Tom Harkin of Iowa has addressed the need for continuing research—asserting that no amount of money appropriated for the care of the 4 million patients who now have the disease will help if we do not find the cure. Moreover, simply caring for 14 million patients by the year 2050 will bankrupt this country. Senator Harkin contends that we are only rearranging the deck chairs on the Titanic if we do not put money into finding the cure for Alzheimer's disease, AIDS, cancer, and other diseases that are costing this country so much in money and diminished value of life.

Chapter 9

Genetic Testing for Neuropsychiatric Disease

Experiences From 8 Years of Genetic Testing for Huntington's Disease

Richard H. Myers, Ph.D.,
Catherine A. Taylor, L.C.S.W., and
Judith A. Sinsheimer, L.I.C.S.W.

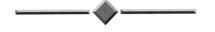

Researchers have identified genes responsible for inherited disorders such as Huntington's disease (Huntington's Disease Collaborative Research Group 1993), spinocerebellar ataxia type I, fragile X syndrome (Fisch et al. 1994; Warren and Nelson 1994), neurofibromatosis type I (Hofman and Boehm 1992), neurofibromatosis type II (MacCollin et al. 1993, 1994), dentatorubral pallidoluysian atrophy, myotonic dystrophy, and Machado-Joseph disease. In addition, geneticists now know that the apolipoprotein E gene is associated with increased risk for Alzheimer's disease.

These findings have generated a battery of genetic test opportunities. Such tests are now widely available to clinicians; they are offered as a clinical diagnostic service whereby a physician may send a blood specimen to one of about a dozen DNA diagnostic laboratories in the United States. At least one genetic diagnostic company has prematurely offered a test for

Alzheimer's disease on the basis of the apolipoprotein E (*ApoE*) gene. A host of genetic tests for familial forms of cancer also are under development.

Despite progress in DNA diagnostic methods, however, the poor prognosis for these diseases makes the emotional impact of testing a profound consideration in genetic testing. Testing has significant implications not only for the individual being tested but also for the spouse or other family members who may be faced with the prospect of losing the companionship of a loved one—as well as the burden of care—and for children who are newly identified as being at risk for disease. In addition, siblings and offspring, and possibly larger extended family, may be confronted with significant threats to their health, which influence prospects for marriage and family and have the potential for discrimination in employment and access to insurance coverage.

Genetic testing may involve one of two methods, depending on whether the mutation events responsible for disease expression have been identified. For a time in the 1980s, researchers had not identified most of the genes responsible for neuropsychiatric disease, although they did know the chromosomal locations of these genes. Even without identifying the gene, geneticists could characterize polymorphic markers genetically linked to the disease gene by studying affected relatives. These genetic "linkage" tests were cumbersome and expensive because they required the participation of affected living relatives to characterize the chromosome bearing the disease gene. Researchers have now cloned genes for virtually all of the major dominantly inherited neuropsychiatric diseases, however, and testing for the responsible mutation is possible by "direct" testing.

We have been supervising or involved in genetic testing for Huntington's disease at Massachusetts General Hospital and the Boston University Medical Center for the past 8 years. In this chapter, we share some of our observations from that experience, including our impressions of the extent to which our observations may be relevant to other diseases.

Cost and Accuracy

Medical professionals tout genetic testing as cost-efficient and diagnostically precise. Establishing an accurate diagnosis is a critical factor in the process of determining appropriate treatment and follow-up care; thus, the availability of genetic tests may enhance medicine's ability to diagnose and treat inherited illnesses.

A genetic diagnostic test may be an efficient and relatively inexpensive way to establish a diagnosis. In the past, for example, assessment of individuals with a suspected diagnosis of Huntington's disease might include a neurological evaluation, collection of an extensive family history, a neuropsychological test battery of cognitive function, brain imaging by magnetic resonance, and various blood studies. Such a workup could cost $1,500–$2,000; now, however, confirmation by DNA diagnostic methods costing about $250 to $300 dramatically reduces the expense of diagnosis.

Availability of Treatment

Recent identification of the breast cancer gene (*BRCA1*) (Futreal et al. 1994) and other oncogenes demonstrates the potential value of genetic testing for the identification of persons at risk for inherited diseases; such testing, for example, may enable physicians to closely monitor women for early detection of breast malignancies or to suggest prophylactic mastectomy. Although monitoring of high-risk oncogene carriers is still in its early stages, the potential benefits that such efforts offer for physicians to provide early treatment prior to metastatic complications may lead to enhanced survival for carriers of these oncogenes. Nevertheless, observers have raised concerns about testing, particularly for children (Garber and Diller 1993; Malkin and Friend 1994).

Similarly, testing for neurofibromatosis may offer opportunities for early detection of tumors and surgical intervention. In contrast, however, most inherited neuropsychiatric diseases have no available treatment; therefore, the availability of medical intervention is rarely a justification for testing.

Current Genetic Test Utilization

In spite of the power of genetic testing, it is not without risk. We review three main circumstances under which genetic testing may be considered: confirmation testing of persons with suspected symptoms of disease, presymptomatic testing of persons at risk for disease, and prenatal testing to determine the risk for a fetus.

Confirmation of Diagnosis

Physicians may consider genetic testing when a patient has had a provisional diagnosis of disease for some time and the advent of a new genetic test permits confirmation of the existing diagnosis. Such confirmation may be particularly helpful when there is no known family history because of adoption, suspected nonpaternity, or a possible new mutation. Under these circumstances, confirmation of existing disease is almost certainly helpful in establishing proper care of the individual and accurately determining genetic risk for relatives.

Consider, for example, confirmation of diagnosis in Huntington's disease for persons without a family history for this disorder. Individuals evaluated in neurological movement disorder clinics often present with symptoms that suggest Huntington's disease in the differential diagnosis despite the absence of family history of the disease. Because researchers have now established the presence of new mutations to Huntington's disease (Myers et al. 1993), genetic testing is appropriate in these cases.

Misdiagnosis of Huntington's disease is rare when an individual presents with a family history and characteristic symptoms and undergoes tests to rule out other illnesses. Nevertheless, clinicians occasionally misdiagnose familial forms of Alzheimer's disease or ataxia as Huntington's disease. Therefore, the genetic test is appropriate for persons suspected to have Huntington's disease, particularly if no relative has had an autopsy confirming the disorder.

A difficult diagnostic situation may arise when an individual at risk for Huntington's disease presents with symptoms of an uncertain neurological impairment. Indeed, indiscriminate use of genetic testing increases the possibility that physicians will miss non-Huntington's disease neurological disorders occurring among individuals at risk for Huntington's disease. One particular situation that came to our attention illustrates this point.

Staff members at a pediatric neurology clinic examined a 4-year-old boy with a seizure disorder of unknown etiology. A routine workup revealed that the mother was at risk for Huntington's disease. Although the mother had no symptoms of Huntington's disease, the clinic staff raised the possibility that the child had a juvenile onset of the illness. They requested a genetic linkage test for Huntington's disease and referred the family to us for the procedure.

For a variety of reasons, however, we did not perform the test. First, the mother did not wish to learn her carrier status. Moreover, juvenile

Huntington's disease is virtually never transmitted from mothers; therefore, the chance that this child's seizure disorder was a consequence of his being a gene carrier was essentially nil. However, we recognized the strong possibility that the mother and the child were both Huntington's disease gene carriers. Had we performed the test and found the child to be a carrier, we might have reached the obvious conclusion that the seizure disorder was caused by the gene. This inference, however, almost certainly would have been erroneous. In fact, the test would not have established the actual cause of the seizure disorder. Yet the child would have been labeled as a gene carrier; this labeling would have altered his access to health insurance and changed his life in ways difficult to predict.

A note of caution. The circumstances under which confirmation of diagnosis is appropriate constitute the most frequently misunderstood aspect of genetic testing. These factors are particularly evident when the individual has an unequivocal family history of the illness but equivocal symptoms.

Again, consider the example of Huntington's disease. Persons with a family history of Huntington's disease for whom a definite diagnosis of the disease cannot be made—with or without the presence of "soft signs"—are not appropriate candidates for testing under the rubric of confirmation of diagnosis. This point is critical. Any person presenting with a positive family history of Huntington's disease for whom a definite diagnosis of Huntington's disease cannot be made is considered "presymptomatic." A genetic test can only establish whether an individual is a carrier of the gene in question; it cannot confirm that equivocal signs of disease are a consequence of that gene. Physicians can establish the onset of Huntington's disease only through clinical neurological evaluation. Therefore, they should advise persons with "soft signs" about the limitations of genetic tests. Such individuals are appropriately tested under protocols for presymptomatic testing (described in the section on "Presymptomatic Testing of Persons at Risk").

Contraindications for genetic testing. For adult-onset diseases, genetic testing of children is rarely appropriate (Tyler et al. 1992). Fragile X syndrome and neurofibromatosis usually manifest in childhood, however, so these diseases are not constrained by some of the indications for adult-onset diseases. Several authors have addressed this topic (e.g., Ball and Harper 1992); many have questioned whether appropriate consent is possible for minors. Given the potential for discrimination and other adverse

personal and emotional consequences (which may be difficult to anticipate), testing minors for an untreatable disease probably is not in their
best interests. Many insightful persons who are at risk for neuropsychiatric
disease have carefully considered their options with regard to genetic testing and decided not to be tested. A minor who is tested is denied the opportunity to decline the test. We advise parents and clinicians seeking tests
for minors to give the child the opportunity when he or she reaches matu-
rity to decide for himself or herself whether to be tested.

The following prohibitions currently are the accepted standard for
Huntington's disease testing:

- Children should not be tested regardless of circumstances; this includes
  children with seizure disorders (with or without Huntington's disease
  family history), children with attention-deficit disorder (with or without Huntington's disease family history), children being placed for
  adoption (with or without Huntington's disease family history), and
  children of parents who request the test for their offspring.

- Adults should not be tested without providing informed consent or if
  they (or appropriate family members) cannot provide consent because
  of psychiatric, cognitive, or other impairment; they should never be
  tested against their wishes.

Hersch et al. (1994), Huntington's Disease Society of America (1994),
and World Federation of Neurology (1989/1990) address these issues further.

Presymptomatic Testing of Persons at Risk

When an individual has a family history of disease or a suspected family
history of disease and a neurological evaluation cannot establish a diagnosis (even in the presence of "soft signs"), the test is considered
presymptomatic. The main consideration in presymptomatic testing is
that the individual is making an informed choice concerning the risks,
benefits, and options surrounding genetic testing. In our program, we
deliver information in two counseling sessions; because of the emotional
impact of testing, we strongly encourage the individual to bring his or
her spouse or a friend to counseling sessions.

Most genetically at-risk people seeking testing want to learn their
genetic status so that they can plan for the future (marriage, family, career); many wish to reduce the uncertainty about their genetic risk
(Meissen et al. 1991). Many people want to be tested to minimize the

possible adverse consequences of Huntington's disease on family members by trying to prepare for the disease if they learn that they are probable gene carriers.

Risks associated with presymptomatic genetic testing.   Our experience with genetic testing for Huntington's disease between 1986 and 1994 highlighted some problematic issues. Although many people expressed an interest in being tested (several hundred people called our offices), the number of people who obtained a test result was relatively small (fewer than 100). The low rate of testing related in part to an awareness of possible negative consequences of testing. For example, a few individuals who learned that they were probable Huntington's disease gene carriers experienced significant depression; two people required psychiatric hospitalization.

Testing also raised significant concerns regarding continued access to health insurance. Because of the expense of the linkage test (often $3,000 or more), many people could not afford to pay for the testing themselves; they did not want to request third-party insurance payment because of concerns about confidentiality. These risks deterred many persons from obtaining the test.

The direct test is considerably cheaper (about $1,000), enabling persons to pay out of pocket and maintain a higher degree of confidentiality. In addition, the direct test can be used when all affected relatives are deceased and even when the family history of Huntington's disease is equivocal. Thus, we now use the direct test with greater frequency than the linkage test. We completed more than 30 tests between July 1994 and March 1995.

Circumstances of concern in presymptomatic testing.   Certain circumstances increase the risk for adverse reactions to genetic testing. Two types of individuals may be particularly vulnerable to such reactions: persons who have a great investment in learning that they are not gene carriers and persons who have learned of their risk for Huntington's disease only recently.

Occasionally, individuals request testing with unrealistic expectations of finding that they are non-gene carriers. For example, an at-risk individual who seeks testing after becoming engaged to be married—but who has not informed the prospective spouse about his or her risk status— may not fully acknowledge the possible adverse consequences if the test reveals the presence of the Huntington's disease gene. In these situations, persons who are influenced by, but not included in, the decision for testing (such as the fiancé) may experience negative reactions. Therefore, we encourage the inclusion of the fiancé in counseling about the decision for testing. Pretest counseling should involve all individuals directly influenced by the outcome.

Persons at risk for Huntington's disease who grow up with an awareness of their risk may develop emotional defense mechanisms to cope with the threat of the disease. Individuals who only learn of their Huntington's disease risk as adults, however, may find the sudden threat of a severely disabling, fatal illness unbearable. The prospect of the illness can be overwhelmingly frightening, and the desire to return to "the way things were" may compel some people to seek testing. Yet the possible adverse consequences of seeking testing before developing defense mechanisms to cope with a 50% risk of illness are apparent.

We consider a period of adjustment to be prudent; whenever possible, we encourage individuals who are newly aware of their risk to take a year to adjust to their 50% risk status before proceeding with a test that could reveal a 100% risk for the disease. Because there is no urgency for immediate medical intervention, such individuals can take time to adjust to and assimilate information in contemplating available testing options— including the option not to be tested.

Prenatal Testing

Prenatal testing follows a course similar to that for presymptomatic testing. Several factors complicate the situation, however.

Persons who already are pregnant when they seek genetic testing face a potentially difficult situation. Most often, individuals who are pregnant have not undergone presymptomatic testing themselves. Therefore, the pregnant individual will be inquiring about a presymptomatic test and a prenatal test simultaneously. In instances in which both the parent and the fetus are found to be Huntington's disease gene carriers, the emotional impact is dramatic. When an individual learns that he or she is a gene carrier and shortly thereafter learns that the unborn child is as well, profound despair and grieving can create an extraordinary challenge to the emotional stability of both members of the couple. A deep sense of loss and mourning may follow the delivery of test results: not only does the affected parent face the prospect of severely debilitating, fatal disease; the couple also must come to grips with the fact that their child faces the same prospect.

Unfortunately, couples have little time to prepare for the potential adversities that they may face. Consequently, prenatal testing may pose an increased risk to the well-being of the individual at risk and to the spouse. At-risk individuals seeking testing for family planning purposes and considering prenatal testing may wish to seek presymptomatic testing before attempting to become pregnant.

Persons who are uncertain about their views regarding the termination of a pregnancy face another dilemma. When a couple chooses not to terminate the pregnancy after learning that the fetus is a carrier, their decision may have significant implications for their child later in life concerning possible insurance or career discrimination; such implications may be difficult to anticipate. Couples who are uncertain about terminating a pregnancy may want to consider whether prenatal testing is useful; pretest counseling must address this issue.

Impact of the Nature of the Disease

The experience of affected family members has a dramatic impact on an at-risk individual's perception of the disease. Because many of the diseases for which genetic tests are available are autosomal dominant, most persons genetically at risk have (or had) a parent with the disease. These experiences influence expectations about how it will affect the individual seeking testing and the impact of a gene-positive test result.

Huntington's disease is an autosomal dominant, midlife-onset disorder. The primary features of the disease include involuntary "choreic" movement; cognitive impairment, particularly memory disturbance; and a change in personality, tending to depression and/or temper outbursts. The average age at onset is 40 years, but the range is large: 24% of cases manifest initial symptoms after age 50 and 7% before age 20. The duration of the disease averages 20 years. The illness is progressive, without periods of remission, and the terminal stages are highly debilitating. Huntington's disease is always fatal.

The offspring of persons with Huntington's disease have a 50% risk of inheriting the illness. These offspring usually have first-hand experience in caring for the affected parent and observing the profound effects of the disease. When the parent becomes disabled, the family unit may dissolve, and the children may face a chaotic living situation. As the disease progresses, the affected parent not only is no longer able to work or care effectively for children but also requires care himself or herself that drains the resources (emotional as well as financial) of the family.

Huntington's disease clearly is a profoundly disabling disease. Many of the other illnesses for which genetic testing is available have similar prognoses, although each disease has its own characteristic disabilities. Some involve little or no cognitive impairment (e.g., Machado-Joseph disease) but nevertheless cause significant physical disability; others (e.g., fragile X syndrome) may involve significant cognitive deficits. The unique features of each disease, the manner in which the disease is expressed in the family, and the impact of the disease on affected relatives influence family members' perceptions of what having the disease means and the emotional impact of a genetic test.

Genetic Test Protocols for Huntington's Disease

Testing protocols must include appropriate counseling so that at-risk individuals can make informed choices about testing. In our experience, individuals who are at risk for Huntington's disease only rarely express frustration with counseling visits; usually, they are relieved and grateful for an opportunity to discuss the implications of the test. Our experience in administering the Huntington's disease genetic test has reinforced our impression that these visits are valuable in minimizing possible adverse consequences of testing.

The goals of counseling are simple: to inform the individual about his or her options regarding testing or other alternatives, depending on personal circumstances; to ensure that the individual is aware of the risks and possible adverse consequences of testing; and to inform the individual of the limitations and accuracy of the procedure. During counseling, we do not try to discourage anyone from being tested; rather, we try to ensure that the individual is making an informed choice. Obviously, a test result cannot be taken back once it is delivered; thus, the person seeking testing must be knowledgeable before the delivery of a result.

Our protocol for Huntington's disease testing involves several steps. The protocol incorporates specific procedures for intake, counseling, neurological examination, and delivery of results.

Telephone Intake

Individuals seeking testing generally contact the testing program by telephone through referral from our affiliated neurology clinics, the

Huntington's Disease Society of America, or self-referral. Typically, one of our social workers informs persons requesting presymptomatic testing about the process. Our main goal throughout the process is to provide people with the best and most accurate information available to facilitate their decision to be tested.

We begin by making sure that the person knows what to expect during each step of the testing process. We inform them about the number of visits involved, who they will see at each visit, the length of time for each visit, and the purpose of each visit. We also discuss the cost of testing, as well as issues of confidentiality. We tell them that genetic testing information shared with health insurance companies may hinder their ability to acquire health insurance in the future; about 90% of the people who go through our testing program choose to pay out of pocket to avoid such discrimination.

The individual involved in the telephone intake must be thoroughly knowledgeable about the purposes of the testing protocol because individuals seeking testing may resist it; they may say, "I've already made the decision, I just want the test now." Persons seeking testing may be anxious to "get it over with" once they have made the difficult decision to be tested. A tendency to minimize the potential adverse emotional impact of the test may be one response to the threat of disease. This reaction may prevent the individual from acknowledging the magnitude of the threat and the significance of the test and produce a desire to avoid circumstances that necessitate attention to these issues. Nevertheless, the process of preparing for the test outcome requires that the individual consider the consequences of the choice to be tested.

We reassure the person seeking testing that the protocol is the same for everyone. We underscore this standardization because the Huntington's disease community is small; differential treatment of individuals within this community could create misunderstanding. Protocol consistency is comforting for the individual because it indicates that the program is a product of experience; it is not a casual process.

We emphasize that persons seeking testing may have different feelings when they are in the process of learning about their risk status and the impact of the test. For example, one man was adamant that because he was knowledgeable about Huntington's disease and had been in therapy for several years with his spouse he should be tested immediately. He reluctantly agreed to comply with the protocol, however; following counseling, he decided that he did not wish to be tested because the test would have no impact on any of the life decisions that he faced.

We also gather information about the person's family history to confirm the presence of Huntington's disease in the family and assess the person's risk status. We identify cases that warrant the inclusion of other family members in the testing process and discuss options for including those people.

Genetic tests may reveal risk information about other persons. Assessment is essential in certain circumstances:

- The genetic status of the parent may be unclear because the parent died before the appearance of symptoms or because the parent has not yet reached the age at disease onset. A positive result in this case would indicate that the parent also was a gene carrier, increasing the risk for all descendants of this parent. Therefore, these people should be involved in some way in the testing process and have a choice about what information they wish to receive.
- If an identical twin is seeking testing, implications for the co-twin must be considered. The co-twin must be counseled and involved in the decision to proceed with testing.

Finally, during the initial telephone interview we briefly explore the motivations for the person seeking testing. This inquiry often reveals that the genetic test may not be the best way to address the individual's concerns or that he or she is unclear about how the test may be beneficial. For example, the person may reveal that he or she is concerned primarily about lapses in memory; the individual may be afraid that he or she is showing signs of the disease. We emphasize that the genetic test will not reveal whether these are signs of disease onset and that only a neurological examination will answer this question. When possible symptoms are a concern, we recommend that the person delay testing and first see a neurologist who is knowledgeable about Huntington's disease.

A telephone inquiry for any other preexisting issues also is useful in obtaining preliminary information on family history, any apparent psychiatric difficulties, or substance abuse issues. Between the initial telephone contact and the first counseling visit, the individual can begin to identify psychological support mechanisms and document the family history of Huntington's disease.

First Counseling Visit

Most persons seeking genetic testing have had no prior genetic counseling for Huntington's disease. Therefore, about half of the first meeting addresses the basic genetics of Huntington's disease.

Genetic counseling. In this phase of the first visit (approximately 1 hour), counselors address the disease itself. Counselors undertake several steps:

- Collect family history.
- Explore basis for Huntington's disease diagnosis. (Have any confirming autopsies been performed?) Request medical records to assess whether relatives had Huntington's disease.
- Determine whether Huntington's disease has been confirmed in any other relative by the genetic test. If not, such testing is critical to ensure testing for the correct illness.
- Discuss genetic risk.
- Discuss specific questions about disease expression in parent and other relatives. Are there uncommon aspects of disease expression (e.g., psychiatric involvement, unusually early or late onset, predominantly one sex affected coincidentally) that may lead to misconceptions about the disease?
- Discuss the individual's specific concerns regarding the threat of the disease.

Test counseling. In this phase (approximately 1 hour), counselors discuss issues related to the testing process.

- Present manner in which test is performed (i.e., nature of the mutation, blood sample, associated visits).
- Explore motivations of individual seeking testing (e.g., implications for marriage, family/procreation, career).
- Explore options other than testing that may accommodate the specific desires of the individual (e.g., prenatal testing, nondisclosing linkage prenatal testing, artificial insemination, not being tested).
- Explore support network (i.e., family, friends, therapist).
- Discuss current and past emotional state of the individual (e.g., severe depressions, psychiatric treatment) and whether appropriate support resources are in place.
- Explore anticipated outcomes and implications of favorable and adverse test results. (Does the individual recognize and acknowledge potential for adverse outcome of test and its implications?)
- Discuss confidentiality risks (e.g., payment by insurance, future access to insurance).

We have found that when the individual is accompanied by someone with whom he or she can discuss the decision to be tested, this dramatically facilitates the counseling process; on the day the test result is delivered, furthermore, such a companion is not simply comforting but, in our view, essential. This person may be a spouse or a close friend; ideally, it would be someone who is not at risk for Huntington's disease. Some individuals seeking testing tell us that they have no one that they can ask to accompany them for this purpose; we consider such comments to be a strong indication that they may be emotionally isolated. In these instances, we try to assist the individual in finding an appropriate companion.

In our experience, 50% of persons who have come to a first visit seeking information about linkage testing never return for a second appointment, although the number of persons choosing to postpone or cancel testing has decreased with direct testing. We believe that the individual should leave the first visit without making a commitment to being tested and without making an appointment date for the second visit; instead, we ask the individual to take some time to think about the alternatives and call for a second appointment when he or she is ready to proceed.

Because many people do not make second appointments, a multiple-visit testing process is the only approach in which decision making is truly fluid. A few test programs have instituted a practice of collecting blood samples at the initial visit. Unfortunately, this protocol engenders an attitude of encouragement and commitment to proceeding with testing.

In some cases, the individual is clearly struggling with the emotional burden of the risk of Huntington's disease; such persons often are poorly prepared to proceed with the test at that time. Formal psychological evaluation may be appropriate in these situations. Alternatively, we may refer the individual for psychological counseling to address emotional concerns before proceeding with testing.

Most testing is performed through neurological and genetic clinics that do not provide psychological therapy. We therefore require that all individuals seeking testing identify a therapist (psychologist, psychiatrist, social worker, minister) following the first visit; that person serves as the primary post-test resource in addressing possible adverse emotional consequences of testing.

Neurological Examination

Virtually everyone who is at high risk for inheriting a serious illness has questions about his or her well-being. Occasionally, individuals may be convinced that they are symptomatic; these feelings may be a major factor in their decision to seek the test. As we have noted earlier—and as we emphasize throughout the process—the genetic test will not confirm that equivocal signs are caused by the disease gene. The appropriate method to assess whether an individual is exhibiting symptoms of the disease is a neurological examination. Thus, the neurological examination is a routine part of the testing process. The neurological examination usually follows the first counseling visit, although it may occasionally precede that initial visit.

In our experience, approximately 20% of persons who have requested predictive testing have been symptomatic at the time of the request. We believe that the best interests of the individual seeking testing require us to make the diagnosis, if we can do so unequivocally. We can then initiate appropriate treatment and address the impact of the onset of the illness on the individual and the family.

In addition, a normal neurological examination result can reassure an individual who suspects himself or herself to be symptomatic and later learns that he or she is a gene carrier. This approach is the only way to confirm that the illness is not yet manifest. Some people choose to postpone genetic testing when the neurological examination outcome is normal.

Second Counseling Visit

At the second counseling visit, individuals seeking testing should be accompanied by the person they expect to accompany them when they receive the result. We expect the individual to be better informed and better prepared at the second visit to address his or her test options, having had an opportunity to assimilate the information from the first visit.

At the second visit, we discuss in-depth the individual's specific motivations for testing and raise difficult issues as appropriate:

- What are the person's primary motivations for testing?
- Does the individual believe that he or she already is symptomatic for Huntington's disease?
- What emotional response is anticipated if the individual learns that he or she is a gene carrier? Specifically, inquiry about possible suicide risk is appropriate.
- What is the perceived impact of the different test outcomes?
- Does the individual believe that the test is likely to reveal that he or she is a gene carrier or a non-gene carrier?

Inquiry about the current and perceived emotional status of the individual is critical in Huntington's disease testing. Physical debilitation is so extensive in this disease that the risks for suicide are substantial in certain circumstances (Schoenfeld et al. 1984); the risks are particularly high at the time of disease onset. Every individual at risk for Huntington's disease will experience at some time or another events that lead him or her to question whether he or she is experiencing the initial signs of the disease. If an individual perceives himself or herself to be symptomatic—even though this perception may not be correct—and subsequently learns that he or she is a gene carrier, the effect will be to confirm the fear that the illness is beginning. That is why the neurological examination before testing is so critical and why inquiring about suicide intent around the time of onset is equally important.

Finally, at the second visit, we ask persons seeking testing to fill out brief self-report psychological inventories for depression, hopelessness, stress, and interpersonal resources. We then determine whether our clinical impressions match the self-report. Discrepancies between our impressions and the self-report may indicate that we need to meet again with the individual to sort out the differences.

We make it clear that we do not use these self-reports to "qualify" individuals for testing—because the decision to be tested rests fundamentally with the individual at risk—but rather to estimate the extent of psychological support necessary to ensure that the individual is well-grounded and equipped to deal with the test outcome. We do require persons who are at high risk for severe adverse emotional response to testing to establish rapport with a therapist for the post-test follow-up and prepare additional family or other support mechanisms before we proceed with testing.

Test counseling.   In the second visit, the counselor once again addresses issues related to the testing process.

- Answer new questions.
- Review information covered in first visit in greater depth.
- Ensure that the individual understands the potential for a result indicating the presence of the Huntington's disease gene and the implications of this outcome.
- Rehearse the manner in which the test result is to be delivered.

Assessment.   Virtually all of the established Huntington's disease testing facilities conduct structured interviews and brief assessments of emotional well-being (we conduct an interview and administer the Beck Depression Inventory, the Beck Hopelessness Scale, the Ways of Coping Scale, the SCL-90, and a few other brief self-report scales). At the end of the second counseling visit, the individual signs a consent form and provides a blood sample for the test.

Result Delivery

Rehearsal of the manner in which results are delivered, before result delivery, is crucial. We describe in detail the events that may happen on the result day, introduce the person who will greet the individual in the waiting room, and rehearse the delivery of the result. We also ensure that all details are prearranged. We confirm that a companion will be present on result day and discuss who the individual wants in the room when we deliver the results. We alert people that they may expect to spend some time with us in the office and that this period may be as long as they wish. We generally allocate 1 hour; although delivery of the gene-negative outcome averages about 20 minutes, delivery of the gene-positive result averages about 45 minutes.

We usually wait until the day before the visit to learn the actual test result; in two instances, individuals who have been tested have changed their minds about getting the results. We have found that knowing the result of the genetic test interferes with our ability to counsel these individuals in the future.

Without exception, we deliver test results in person. The intensity of result delivery cannot be overstated. Even the most stoic individuals are shaken by this experience. There is no appropriate scale to assess the magnitude of the emotional turmoil that people feel at the time of the delivery of the result.

The emotional response in the first few minutes is difficult to anticipate. Obviously, the gene-negative result prompts tremendous relief—and sometimes disbelief. These concerns are relatively easy to deal with, and these favorable outcomes are a joy to deliver.

The immediate impact of the gene-positive result varies dramatically. Some individuals acknowledge that this result is what they expected and appear calm; others are stunned, despairing, and grief-stricken. In one instance, we provided an individual with immediate acute psychiatric hospitalization after delivering the result. Appropriate care for such reactions must be available.

Impact of the Result

The most profound impact of genetic testing continues to be the emotional and personal implications of the result for the individual and the family. The emotional impact for a spouse is virtually equal to that for the individual who has been tested. Alerting the spouse to this impact ahead of time and advising him or her to identify a therapist or other resources before result delivery is prudent. Finding resources in the midst of emotional crisis is difficult, and assessing the clinical skills of a therapist often is impossible at this time. The testing staff must be able to provide emotional support to individuals who have no other resources.

The reactions of persons who receive genetic test results vary widely. In the following sections, we describe our observations regarding genetic testing for Huntington's disease.

Gene-Positive Outcome

We have learned that anticipating which individuals will be gene-positive for Huntington's disease is impossible. Although persons with existing "soft" neurological signals who have experienced significant depressive episodes may be slightly more likely to be gene-positive, such signs are poor prognostic indicators of gene status. In our program, some individuals with past suicide attempts have tested gene-negative; others with multiple graduate degrees and long-term, stable relationships and employment have tested gene-positive.

The gene-positive result invariably is more difficult to cope with than the individual and the family anticipate. Persons who say, "I have lived with this threat all my life; I have always assumed that I am a gene carrier, and therefore a [gene-positive] result will not be a surprise" find that the certainty of the genetic test is different from the at-risk state.

Immediately following delivery of the test result, the individual may struggle to get through each day. We call people within 2–3 days simply to say "hello" and arrange for a time to see them again. People react in different ways to follow-up. Most are not eager to discuss the profound sense of despair that they are experiencing. Many individuals present a composed demeanor that thinly veils tremendous emotional turmoil. For some, the sense of despair and grieving is so powerful that it is too painful to acknowledge. Gene-positive individuals often have a difficult time returning to the same office for future visits because the environment conjures up the image of the delivery of the result.

The period between 1 and 2 months post-test often is the most difficult. Sharing the result with family and friends causes pain and grieving among loved ones, making the outcome increasingly real and difficult to face. Frequently, family members do not respond supportively. In-laws may appear resentful or blaming; an unaffected parent may seem heavily burdened by guilt and be unable to provide hoped-for nurturing. A sibling who is still at risk may behave as though nothing has happened and disregard the significance of the result.

Gene-positive individuals commonly complain that within a few days or weeks—when they are only beginning to grapple with the impact of the test outcome—friends no longer seem comfortable talking about the result (or do not know what to say). Persons who were counting on friends and family as their primary sources of support may find that, after what seems to be a short time, these people act as if the test never happened and seem to pull away. Professional therapeutic resources become particularly important at this time.

The impact of a gene-positive result on marriage can be significant. Some gene-positive individuals push for divorce, with the intent of sparing their spouse the pain of the disease. Although none of the spouses of persons tested in our program has indicated a desire for divorce, when both members of the couple are in pain, sometimes neither can provide support for the other. Some couples report a sense that the union was destined not to succeed—as if the outcome were determined by fate. Nevertheless, only one couple in our program has divorced in the posttest period, yet one gene-positive individual got married.

Some of the people tested in our program several years ago have gained some insight into the impact of the test on their lives. One gene-positive individual has noticed that many events that cause persons around him to become upset do not bother him. His reaction is that "these events are small potatoes"; such things are of little concern to him. This individual describes a sense of remarkable tranquility. Many others have noted that they cherish even more the life events that they previously valued.

Although some gene-positive individuals have achieved a sense of greater intensity in living and appreciation of their existing health, others have not. Some persons (a minority, however) have not returned to working at their pretest level, even after several years. They seem to be paralyzed by foreboding and a dread of the future that prevents them from enjoying the present.

Gene-Negative Outcome

Although individuals undergoing testing usually cannot imagine any possible negative consequence to learning that they are not gene carriers, health care professionals should not assume that a gene-negative outcome will have no adverse repercussions. In the few hours and days following delivery of the result, gene-negative individuals may experience a sense of disappointment. Some expect that a favorable result would produce exhilaration or profound sense of relief; such reactions, however, are rare. Most people are emotionally exhausted by the time they receive the result; the relief of a favorable outcome may enable them to relax, and they may feel completely drained.

Individuals with favorable outcomes commonly report a period of depression that persists for a few days or even a few weeks. This depression most commonly relates to a realization that Huntington's disease may not be out of their lives forever, particularly if they have siblings.

Gene-negative individuals with siblings who are symptomatic, or even several asymptomatic siblings—where the likelihood that all of them will escape the disease is low—often find that they feel responsible for caring for or assisting those siblings. However, many feel an opposite urge: to move on from the cloud of Huntington's disease and move away from those who are threatened. Some gene-negative individuals report that relationships with siblings have changed and grown more distant. One individual, for example, expressed the feeling that she was "no longer part of the family" and that the siblings who were still at risk shared a closeness that she was no longer part of.

For many people, the risk of Huntington's disease has masked other significant difficulties in their lives. One individual, for example, attributed his chronic alcoholism to the stress that the risk for Huntington's disease had created; this individual experienced a severe relapse shortly after receiving a favorable test result. Health care workers must recognize the possibility of "scapegoating," whereby individuals may blame difficult or uncomfortable life circumstances on their Huntington's disease risk status. Many of these individuals expect these problems, which may have their roots only partly (if at all) in their Huntington's disease risk, to disappear with a favorable outcome; they find, however, that they still must address these issues.

In some cases, individuals who are at risk for Huntington's disease may use that knowledge as a way to "manage" the threat of death. One woman, for example, remarked that knowing how she most likely would die was somewhat "comforting." Individuals who have received gene-negative results, however, have reported amazement at the speed with which other threats to their lives replaced the threat of Huntington's disease. Accordingly, some have expressed sudden new concerns about other possibilities, such as cancer or a horrible accident.

Most gene-negative individuals are shocked to discover how much Huntington's disease was part of their identity. Many realize only after receiving a negative result that the threat of developing Huntington's disease factored into most, if not all, of their major life decisions. This awareness can be overwhelming; it can lead to emotional turmoil over whether they made the best decisions for themselves. Such persons, for example, may have chosen not to spend time in school, not to pursue a certain career path, or not to start a family given the threat of Huntington's disease. Such lost opportunities can produce remorse.

Some gene-negative individuals who had been active in the lay organization or very public in presenting the plight of Huntington's disease families have found that their mission in life seemed less focused and less clear. One individual, for example, expressed the concern that he now needed to plan for his retirement; he could no longer live in the present to the extent he had become accustomed. Some of these individuals seem to have a letdown that involves feeling that "I'm just like everyone else now; I'm not special any more." This letdown seems to be related to a sense of intensity that some people at risk for Huntington's disease achieve in their lives; such intensity is harder to maintain with a favorable result.

Insurance, Risks, and Benefits

The potential that the insurance industry will use genetic test information to deny coverage is a reality. We recently counseled an asymptomatic woman at risk for Huntington's disease who was denied health insurance on 13 applications and remains without health insurance coverage. The overwhelming majority of persons who currently are undergoing genetic testing for Huntington's disease are paying out of pocket to preserve their confidentiality. In addition, some individuals have used pseudonyms to disguise their identities in testing clinics.

Although the primary concern for these individuals is maintaining their access to health insurance, some have readily acknowledged that they will seek high levels of life and disability insurance if they find that they are gene carriers. Thus, the Huntington's disease test (which costs about $1,000) enables some individuals to gain information relevant to risk that permits "adverse selection" in insurance coverage.

Some states have enacted laws that explicitly limit the use of genetic tests by insurers. In Wisconsin, for example, insurers are prohibited from requesting or requiring genetic test information for health coverage, though not for life insurance coverage (Capron 1993). The distinction between health and life or disability insurance coverages is critical in the establishment of insurance guidelines. Unfortunately, most states currently have no legal safeguards to prohibit insurance companies from denying coverage for persons undergoing genetic testing.

Relevance to Other Diseases and Conclusion

In this chapter, we have focused heavily on our experiences in genetic testing for Huntington's disease. Nevertheless, our observations are relevant to other midlife-onset diseases for which medical interventions are unavailable. Clearly, a different approach to testing would be indicated if a medical intervention to postpone onset or slow the course of the disease were available.

Researchers have cloned genes for most of the major common inherited diseases; this process facilitates direct detection of mutation events that are responsible for these diseases. The major psychiatric diseases remain elusive, however, which may be an indication of their etiological complexity. Investigators recently found that the *ApoE* 4 allele is a significant risk factor for Alzheimer's disease. Unfortunately, at least one DNA diagnostic company has prematurely offered testing for the *ApoE* 4 allele as a "genetic test" for the disease. Investigation of the *ApoE* 4 allele in a randomly ascertained elderly population in the Framingham Heart Study, however, revealed that the majority of *ApoE* 4 gene carriers do not develop Alzheimer's disease and that only approximately half of Alzheimer's disease is associated with *ApoE* 4 (Myers et al. 1995). Thus, a positive test result for the *ApoE* 4 allele does not ensure development of the disease, and a negative result does not ensure absence of the disease. Genetic testing must include a process of evaluation of the specificity of the outcome before such procedures are implemented.

We were cautious in applying this new technology in Huntington's disease—in part because we had few precedents to follow. Health care professionals now know a great deal, however, about the risks associated with testing of this kind. Practitioners undertaking testing for diseases such as spinocerebellar ataxia type I, Machado-Joseph disease, and neurofibromatosis should consider the lessons from Huntington's disease in developing similar protocols for testing.

References

Ball DM, Harper PS: Presymptomatic testing for late-onset genetic disorders: lessons from Huntington's disease. FASEB J 6:2818–2819, 1992

Capron AM: Hedging their bets. Hastings Cent Rep 23 (May/June):30–31, 1993

Fisch GS, Nelson DL, Snow K, et al: Reliability of diagnostic assessment of normal and premutation status in the fragile X syndrome using DNA testing. Am J Med Genet 51:339–345, 1994

Futreal PA, Liu Q, Shattuck-Eidens D, et al: *BRCA1* mutations in primary breast and ovarian carcinomas. Science 266:120–122, 1994

Garber JE, Diller L: Screening children at genetic risk of cancer. Curr Opin Pediatr 5:712–715, 1993

Hersch SM, Jones R, Koroshetz WJ, et al: The neurogenetics genie: testing for the Huntington's disease mutation. Neurology 44:1369–1373, 1994

Hofman KJ, Boehm CD: Familial neurofibromatosis type 1: clinical experience with DNA testing. J Pediatr 120:394–398, 1992

Huntington's Disease Collaborative Research Group: A novel gene containing a trinucleotide repeat that is expanded and unstable on Huntington's disease chromosomes. Cell 72:971–983, 1993

Huntington's Disease Society of America: Guidelines for Genetic Testing for Huntington's Disease. New York, Huntington's Disease Society of America, 1994

MacCollin M, Mohny T, Trofatter J, et al: DNA diagnosis of neurofibromatosis 2: altered coding sequence of the merlin tumor suppressor in an extended pedigree. JAMA 270:2316–2320, 1993

MacCollin M, Ramesh V, Jacoby LB, et al: Mutational analysis of patients with neurofibromatosis 2. Am J Hum Genet 55:314–320, 1994

Malkin D, Friend SH: Screening for cancer susceptibility in children. Curr Opin Pediatr 6:46–51, 1994

Meissen GJ, Mastromauro CA, Kiely DK, et al: Understanding the decision to take the predictive test for Huntington disease. Am J Med Genet 39:404–410, 1991

Myers RH, MacDonald ME, Koroshetz WJ, et al: De novo expansion of a (CAG)n repeat in sporadic Huntington's disease. Nat Genet 5:168–173, 1993

Myers RH, Schaefer EJ, Wilson PWF, et al: Apolipoprotein E allele 4 is associated with dementia in the Framingham study, in Research Advances in Alzheimer's Disease and Related Disorders. Edited by Iqbal K, Mortimer J, Winblad B, et al. Chichester, England, John Wiley & Sons, 1995

Schoenfeld M, Berkman B, Myers RH, et al: Increased rate of suicide among patients with Huntington's disease. J Neurol Neurosurg Psychiatry 47:1283–1287, 1984

Tyler A, Morris M, Lazarou L, et al: Presymptomatic testing for Huntington's disease in Wales 1987–1990. Br J Psychiatry 161:481–488, 1992

Warren ST, Nelson DL: Advances in molecular analysis of fragile X syndrome. JAMA 271:536–542, 1994

World Federation of Neurology, Research Committee Group on Huntington's Disease: Ethical Issues Policy Statement on Huntington's Disease Molecular Genetics Predictive Test. J Neurol Sci 94:327–332, 1989, and J Med Genet 27: 34–38, 1990

Chapter 10

Depression in Alzheimer's Dementia

Benoit H. Mulsant, M.D.,
Bruce G. Pollock, M.D., Ph.D.,
Robert D. Nebes, Ph.D.,
Carolyn C. Hoch, Ph.D., and
Charles F. Reynolds III, M.D.

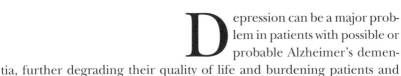

D epression can be a major problem in patients with possible or
probable Alzheimer's demen-
tia, further degrading their quality of life and burdening patients and
their caregivers with excess disability. In this chapter, we review current
knowledge on depression in Alzheimer's disease; we focus on epidemiology, diagnostic issues, neurological correlates, treatment issues, and impact on functioning.

This work was supported in part by grants from the National Institute of Mental
Health (MH49786, MH0140, MH0029, and MH52247) and a grant (AG05133)
from the National Institute of Aging.

Clinical Epidemiology

Clinically significant depression and depressive symptoms are common among patients with Alzheimer's disease; these symptoms are an important source of excess functional disability in Alzheimer's disease (Fitz and Teri 1994). Data from clinically referred samples indicate that depressed mood is present in 30%–50% of cognitively impaired patients, and a full depressive syndrome is present in 10%–20% (Knesevich et al. 1983; Lazarus et al. 1987; Reifler et al. 1982; Vida et al. 1994; Wragg and Jeste 1989; Zubenko et al. 1992). However, the prevalence of syndromal major depression in community-based samples of patients with Alzheimer's disease seems to be far lower—with estimates as low as 1.5% in the Dallas series and a 2-year incidence of 1.3% in the Consortium to Establish a Registry for Alzheimer's Disease (CERAD) series (Weiner et al. 1994).

Researchers have reported that the prevalence of syndromal major depression in institutionalized elderly persons—the population with the highest prevalence of dementia (Tariot et al. 1993)—is more than six times higher than in community-dwelling elderly individuals (Myers et al. 1984; Parmelee et al. 1989). Thus, differences in settings and population may explain, at least partially, differences in the reported prevalence of depression in Alzheimer's disease patients. Problematic case identification and diagnosis also may explain some of the reported differences in prevalence.

Diagnostic Issues

Several epidemiological studies reported an unexpected finding: the prevalence of major depression in community-dwelling individuals without dementia decreased with age (Blazer 1994; Myers et al. 1984; Snowdon 1990). Among the factors the investigators invoked to explain this controversial finding (Blazer 1994), several are particularly relevant to the diagnosis of depression in Alzheimer's disease. For example, cognitive problems may lead to underreporting of depressive symptoms; comorbid somatic disorders may cause undue "discounting" or misattribution of depressive symptoms; and current diagnostic criteria for syndromal major depression may be inadequate to accommodate clinically significant depressive symptoms in late life.

Elderly individuals with dementia are less likely to report depressive symptoms than are family members or other caregivers or informants (Logsdon and Teri 1995). Thus, using structured instruments specially developed for patients with dementia, Mackenzie et al. (1989) found a 4% prevalence of DSM-III-R (American Psychiatric Association 1987) major depressive episodes in interviews of Alzheimer's disease outpatients referred to a specialized dementia clinic, whereas information from their families yielded a 31% prevalence. Congruent with this study, Ott and Fogel (1992) reported that observer-rated and self-rated depression scales showed good agreement in outpatients with dementia (most with Alzheimer's disease) who presented with relatively preserved cognition and insight regarding their cognitive deficits; in patients with more severe dementia or loss of insight, however, observer-rated and self-rated scales showed divergent results. These findings justifiably raise questions about the results of studies that attempt to determine the presence and severity of depression in Alzheimer's disease patients without using explicit procedures to gather and integrate information from caregivers as well as from patients (Alexopoulos et al. 1988; Mulsant et al. 1994; Sunderland et al. 1988a).

Misattribution of depressive symptoms also may contribute to diagnostic errors in Alzheimer's disease patients with depression. Older persons often attribute their depressive symptoms to physical illness; this attribution—rather than lower endorsement of depressive symptoms—accounts for findings of decreased prevalence of major depression associated with increased age in some epidemiological studies that used structured interviews (Knauper and Wittchen 1994). Furthermore, attribution bias was independent of the physical status of older respondents, although it was related to their working-memory capacity and the verbal complexity of probe questions (Knauper and Wittchen 1994). These results support the use of an inclusive approach that considers all depressive symptoms—regardless of their possible etiology—in the diagnosis of depression in patients with dementia (Cohen-Cole and Stoudemire 1987; Vida et al. 1994).

Using this strategy, we distinguished Alzheimer's disease patients with major depressive syndromes from Alzheimer's disease patients with other behavioral disturbances; in addition, we validated this distinction *ex juvantibus* by demonstrating specific alleviation of depressive symptoms with antidepressant treatment in the group with depression (Mulsant et al. 1994; Zubenko et al. 1992). Regardless of the diagnostic approach used, however, elderly patients with and without dementia who have clinically significant depressive symptoms that warrant recognition and treatment nevertheless may not meet criteria for syndromal major depression (Blazer 1994; Blazer et al. 1987; Meyers 1994).

Further complicating the diagnosis of depression in Alzheimer's disease patients, the expression of various depressive syndromes may change as dementing illnesses progress (Forsell et al. 1993; Lazarus et al. 1987). Ultimately, the validation of depression diagnoses in patients with Alzheimer's disease will require correlations with external parameters such as personal and family history, course of illness, biological correlates, and response to treatment (Kathol et al. 1990). Research data suggest, for example, that Alzheimer's disease patients presenting with major depressive syndromes are more likely than Alzheimer's disease patients without depression to have a personal history of major depressive disorder (Zubenko et al., in press) or a family history of major depressive disorder (Rabins et al. 1984).

The presence of depression may relate to the course of the illness. Several studies have demonstrated that a depressive episode—particularly if it induces significant cognitive impairment—may constitute the earliest clinical manifestation of degenerative dementia (Alexopoulos et al. 1993; Emery and Oxman 1992).

Neurophysiological, Neurochemical, and Neuroanatomical Correlates of Depression in Alzheimer's Disease

Characteristic changes in sleep architecture demonstrated by sleep electroencephalography (EEG) constitute some of the most robust and reproducible biological correlates of major depression. These changes include short rapid eye movement (REM) sleep latency; prolonged first REM sleep period, with enhanced density of REM; shifting of EEG delta wave activity from the first to the second non-REM sleep period; and early morning awakening (Nemeroff et al. 1993). These abnormalities appear in patients with depression throughout the life cycle; older patients, however, show more pronounced changes than midlife patients, including more sleep continuity disturbances (particularly early morning awakening), shorter REM sleep latencies, and a more pronounced shift of REM sleep toward sleep onset.

In Alzheimer's disease patients without depression, sleep deteriorates as the dementia progresses. These patients develop an arrhythmic, polyphasic sleep pattern; they experience gradual loss of all phasic activity (decreased spindles and K-complexes in stage 2, decreased eye movements in REM), normal or prolonged REM sleep latency, and a decreased percentage of REM sleep (Prinz et al. 1982; Reynolds et al. 1988). These physiological differences allow researchers to discriminate, with 80%–90% accuracy, elderly patients with dementia and depression (Buysse et al. 1988; Reynolds et al. 1988). Moreover, sleep physiological changes (e.g., measures of sleep-disordered breathing and REM sleep generation) in Alzheimer's disease patients with depression provide a sensitive indicator of brain failure (i.e., they correlate with progressive cognitive decline) and a reliable correlate of mortality by 2-year follow-up (Hoch et al. 1989). Control of sleep disturbance may not only improve the quality of life for Alzheimer's disease patients and their caregivers, but it also may prolong community tenure because disruptive nocturnal behavior often leads to placement in long-term care (Pollak and Perlick 1987).

Clinical, pharmacological, and physiological studies have implicated the catecholaminergic and serotonergic systems in the pathophysiology of depression. Furthermore, dementia often is associated with degeneration of the locus coeruleus and the substantia nigra—the nuclei that contain the majority of the noradrenergic and dopaminergic neurons, respectively (Boller et al. 1980; Huber et al. 1986; Mayeux et al. 1981; Perry et al. 1993). Several studies have found that the occurrence of depression in patients with primary dementia was specifically associated with the degeneration of these nuclei (e.g., Mulsant and Zubenko 1994). Zweig et al. (1988) reported that brain autopsies of Alzheimer's disease patients with depression demonstrated a specific reduction in the numbers of neurons in raphe nuclei and in pigmented neurons in the locus coeruleus or ventral tegmental area.

In a series of brain autopsy studies, Zubenko (1992), Zubenko and Moossy (1988), and Zubenko et al. (1990, 1991) compared the morphological and neurochemical features of elderly control subjects without dementia, dementia patients with major depression, and dementia patients without depression. Depression was associated with significantly more severe neuropathological changes in the locus coeruleus and the substantia nigra but not in the cortex. The investigators determined concentrations of norepinephrine, dopamine (and its metabolite homovanillic acid), and serotonin (and its metabolite 5-hydroxyindoleacetic acid) in seven specific brain areas. Dementia patients with depression demonstrated a 10- to 20-fold reduction in norepinephrine in the neocortex and hippocampus and a trend in the same direction in other brain regions, compared with dementia patients without depression. Patients with depression also exhibited a trend toward reduction in serotonin in all brain areas, as well as a nonsignificant reduction in its metabolite.

The results of these and other studies suggest that patients with primary dementia who meet diagnostic criteria for major depression exhibit distinct neuropathological and neurochemical changes. Furthermore, these changes are consistent with existing neurochemical hypotheses of "functional" major depression that implicate the noradrenergic and serotonergic systems (Mulsant and Zubenko 1994). However, these studies do not address the question of whether patients with primary dementia who develop major depression constitute a distinct pathogenic subgroup or represent merely an extreme in terms of degeneration of their aminergic nuclei. Nevertheless, the neuropathological and neurochemical profile of major depression in the context of primary dementia suggests that effective therapies for "functional" depression also should be effective for the treatment of this syndrome.

The durability of antidepressant efficacy in Alzheimer's disease patients is an important but largely unaddressed issue. Because neurodegenerative changes in Alzheimer's disease are progressive, antidepressant response may be "brittle," or less durable, in patients with Alzheimer's disease than in elderly patients without concomitant dementia. This issue must be addressed in a controlled clinical trial of long-term efficacy.

Treatment Issues

Miller (1980) observed that even when psychiatrists recognized depression occurring in the context of dementia, they often undertreated the syndrome. Miller attributed this therapeutic nihilism to the fact that psychiatrists did not consider depression "a potentially treatable complication of dementia" (Miller 1980, p. 112).

Several subsequent studies suggested that depression in Alzheimer's disease may be responsive to acute therapy with cyclic antidepressants such as imipramine (Reifler et al. 1989) and nortriptyline (Mulsant et al. 1994; Reynolds et al. 1987; Stoudemire et al. 1991; Zubenko et al. 1992); selective serotonin reuptake inhibitors (SSRIs) such as citalopram (Nyth and Gottfries 1990; Nyth et al. 1992) or sertraline (Volicer et al. 1994);

and electroconvulsive therapy (Mulsant et al. 1991; Stoudemire et al. 1991). The imipramine and citalopram studies were double-blind, placebo-controlled, randomized clinical trials, whereas the other studies were open-label or naturalistic.

Reifler et al. (1989) showed that Alzheimer's disease patients who met criteria for a major depressive episode of moderate severity improved significantly when treated with either low-dose imipramine or placebo for 8 weeks. Over this brief period of time, however, patients receiving imipramine experienced a significant cognitive decline on the Mattis Dementia Rating Scale, whereas patients receiving placebo did not.

Nyth and Gottfries (1990) demonstrated a superior effect of citalopram, compared with placebo, not only on depressed mood but also on a broad range of behavioral dysfunctions, such as "emotional bluntness, confusion, irritability, anxiety, fear/panic, . . . and restlessness" (p. 894) among patients with Alzheimer's disease (but not in patients with vascular dementia). Nyth et al. (1992) subsequently conducted a 6-week, double-blind trial of citalopram versus placebo in elderly patients with depression who also had somatic disorders or "senile dementia." Even though few patients met criteria for major depression, cognitive and emotional functions improved significantly more in patients treated with citalopram than in patients receiving placebo. For example, citalopram-treated patients with concomitant dementia and depression showed more improvement than placebo-treated patients in measures of orientation to time, recent memory, ability to increase tempo, and frequency of fear/panic reactions. By 6 weeks, 60% of citalopram-treated patients were rated as much improved on the Clinical Global Impression Scale, versus only 24% in the placebo group ($P < .001$). There were no differences in side-effect global ratings between the two groups.

Data from acute open-trial treatment with nortriptyline, comparing the response of elderly patients with depression with and without Alzheimer's disease, showed good resolution of depressive symptoms in both groups (Buysse et al. 1988; Reynolds et al. 1987). Hamilton depression ratings dropped, but Folstein cognitive scores remained unchanged, after resolution of depressive symptoms on nortriptyline at doses associated with therapeutic plasma levels of 50–150 ng/mL for 6–8 weeks. Moreover, improvement in Hamilton depression ratings correlated with improvement in functional status as measured by the Blessed Dementia Rating Scale ($r = .65$, $n = 16$, $P < .01$). Improvement in functional status was particularly evident on Blessed items measuring regard for the feelings of others, reengagement in hobbies, and improved initiative; improvement on Hamilton items was most apparent in mood, early morning awakening, anxiety, and appetite. We also followed up Alzheimer's disease patients with depression maintained on nortriptyline up to 2 years (Buysse et al. 1988). The results from this open-maintenance trial suggested continuing antidepressant effects over 2 years despite worsening of cognitive and functional impairment over the same period.

Given the recognized sensitivity of Alzheimer's disease patients to the cognitive effects of anticholinergic agents (Sunderland et al. 1988b), these data raise the question of whether the added atropinic burden of nortriptyline may affect cognition—thus altering the risk-to-benefit ratio of long-term therapy. This noncontrolled study did not determine whether active medication affected the rate of cognitive decline positively or adversely. In the following section, we review the complex relationship between cognitive impairment, depression, and antidepressant treatment in Alzheimer's disease patients.

Effects of Depression on Cognitive Performance in Alzheimer's Disease Patients

Although the occurrence of depression in Alzheimer's disease contributes to excess functional disability (Teri and Wagner 1992), investigators have not determined conclusively whether it also worsens cognitive impairment. Cross-sectional studies comparing Alzheimer's disease patients with and without depression have produced inconsistent results. Some studies have suggested that depression does not increase the cognitive impairment of Alzheimer's disease (Fischer et al. 1990; Rubin et al. 1991; Teri and Wagner 1992), but others have found that performance on various psychometric instruments was lower in dementia patients with depression than in dementia patients without depression (Breen et al. 1984; Rovner et al. 1989). Fitz and Teri (1994) reported that Alzheimer's disease patients with moderate dementia showed increased cognitive impairment if they also had depression; this was not true of Alzheimer's disease patients with mild dementia.

These contradictory results may be caused by selection bias: depression may be more frequently diagnosed or more prevalent in Alzheimer's disease patients early in the course of the disease, when their dementia is less severe (Burns et al. 1990; Fischer et al. 1990; Mulsant and Zubenko

1994; Teri and Wagner 1992). Thus, cross-sectional studies may not be able to demonstrate any excess cognitive disability resulting from depression because they often compare Alzheimer's disease patients with depression with Alzheimer's disease patients without depression who are further advanced in the disease.

Another approach to determining the cognitive effects of depression in Alzheimer's disease involves examining whether cognitive performance improves when depression resolves (Mulsant et al. 1991; Stoudemire et al. 1991). If depression causes excess cognitive impairment in Alzheimer's disease patients, successful acute treatment of depression should be associated with cognitive improvement. The results of such studies are mixed, however. Greenwald et al. (1989) found that Alzheimer's disease patients with depression performed more poorly on cognitive tasks than Alzheimer's disease patients without depression; following treatment, performance by patients with depression improved, whereas performance by patients without depression did not. In contrast, however, Reifler et al. (1986) and Reynolds et al. (1987) found no evidence of cognitive improvement associated with treatment of Alzheimer's disease patients with depression.

As we noted earlier, these results may have been confounded by the anticholinergicity of the drugs used (Sunderland et al. 1988b). In the placebo-controlled study of imipramine by Reifler et al. (1989), the cognitive performance of Alzheimer's disease patients with and without depression treated with imipramine was worse than in patients receiving placebo, suggesting that imipramine impaired rather than improved cognitive functioning in Alzheimer's disease patients. However, Teri et al. (1991) reported that imipramine produced a decrease in cognitive performance in Alzheimer's disease patients without depression but not in Alzheimer's disease patients with depression.

These treatment studies had numerous limitations; these limitations complicate interpretation of the results. For example, patients in these studies were treated with tricyclic antidepressants, which by themselves can produce significant cognitive impairment in elderly individuals (Marcopulos and Graves 1990; Meyers et al. 1991; Moskowitz and Burns 1986). Alzheimer's disease patients are especially sensitive to the anticholinergic side effects of medications. Thus, the cognitive side effects of antidepressant treatment may mask improvement in cognitive function produced by remission of depression (Branconnier et al. 1982; Teri et al. 1991).

A second limitation involved the nature of cognitive tasks that the studies used. In most cases, investigators assessed cognitive performance either by screening tests—such as the Mini-Mental State Exam (Folstein et al. 1975) or the Dementia Rating Scale (Mattis 1976)—or by clinical neuropsychological tasks—such as the Wechsler Memory Scale, Block Design (Wechsler 1987)—that were not designed to examine the specific information processing operations known to be impaired in depression. For instance, deficiencies in allocation and maintenance of attention in complex tasks (Nebes et al. 1992; Poon 1992; Schwartz et al. 1989) are critical components of cognitive impairment in older persons with depression: these individuals perform poorly on tasks that require large amounts of sustained attentional capacity but normally on tasks that are performed automatically (Hartlage et al. 1993; Weingartner 1986).

The presence of major depression should exacerbate the severe impairment that Alzheimer's disease patients show on tasks that require them to divide their attention (Baddeley et al. 1991; Nebes and Brady 1989; Nestor et al. 1991); this excess decrement should diminish, at least acutely, as Alzheimer's disease patients recover from their depression. Similarly, Alzheimer's disease patients with depression should demonstrate excess impairment in cognitive tasks involving vigilance (Frith et al. 1983; Nebes and Brady 1993), psychomotor speed (Nebes et al. 1992), or differential recognition memory for concepts with negative or positive emotional tones (Dunbar and Lishman 1984). This excess cognitive disability should resolve with acute recovery from depression.

Conclusion

Research advances in the epidemiology and diagnosis of depression in Alzheimer's disease in the past decade suggest that a greater focus on treatment is warranted. The identification of specific biological correlates of major depression in the context of Alzheimer's disease suggests that such depression may respond to the same somatic treatments that are effective in the treatment of "functional" major depression in patients without dementia. Yet scant published data support the efficacy of antidepressant medications in the treatment of depression in Alzheimer's disease. Moreover, these data suggest that although tricyclic antidepressants and SSRIs may be effective in treating depression in Alzheimer's disease, tricyclic antidepressants may worsen cognition.

Research comparing the efficacy and toxicity of a tricyclic antidepressant and an SSRI under double-blind conditions is warranted. Such studies should assess not only acute response to treatment but also whether continued antidepressant medication maintains recovery from depression after acute and continuation therapy. In addition, investigators should determine whether depression produces reversible excess cognitive impairment in Alzheimer's disease patients. Comparison of cognitive performance after treatment with an antidepressant with minimal anticholinergic effects (such as an SSRI) and a tricyclic antidepressant would be particularly informative. Such research would have definite implications for treating depression in patients who are already cognitively impaired.

References

Alexopoulos GS, Abrams RC, Young RC, et al: Cornell scale for depression in dementia. Biol Psychiatry 23:271–284, 1988

Alexopoulos GS, Meyers BS, Young RC, et al: The course of geriatric depression with "reversible dementia": a controlled study. Am J Psychiatry 150:1693–1699, 1993

American Psychiatric Association: Diagnostic and Statistical Manual of Mental Disorders, 3rd Edition, Revised. Washington, DC, American Psychiatric Association, 1987

Baddeley AD, Bressi S, Della Sala S, et al: The decline of working memory in Alzheimer's disease. Brain 114:2521–2542, 1991

Blazer DG: Is depression more frequent in late life? An honest look at the evidence. American Journal of Geriatric Psychiatry 2:193–199, 1994

Blazer DG, Hughes DC, George LK: The epidemiology of depression in an elderly community population. Gerontologist 27:281–287, 1987

Boller F, Mizutani T, Roessmann U, et al: Parkinson disease, dementia, and Alzheimer's disease: clinicopathological correlations. Ann Neurol 1:329–335, 1980

Branconnier RJ, Cole JO, Ghazvinian S, et al: Treating the depressed elderly patient: the comparative behavioral pharmacology of mianserin and amitriptyline. Adv Biochem Psychopharmacol 32:195–212, 1982

Breen AR, Larson EB, Reifler BV, et al: Cognitive performance and functional competence in coexisting dementia and depression. J Am Geriatr Soc 32:132–137, 1984

Burns A, Jacoby R, Levy R: Psychiatric phenomena in Alzheimer's disease, III: disorders of mood. Br J Psychiatry 157:81–86, 1990

Buysse DJ, Reynolds CF, Kupfer DJ, et al: EEG sleep in depressive pseudodementia. Arch Gen Psychiatry 45:568–575, 1988

Cohen-Cole SA, Stoudemire A: Major depression and physical illness. Psychiatr Clin North Am 10:1–17, 1987

Dunbar GC, Lishman WA: Depression, recognition-memory, hedonic tone: a signal detection analysis. Br J Psychiatry 144:376–382, 1984

Emery VO, Oxman TE: Update on the dementia spectrum of depression. Am J Psychiatry 149:305–317, 1992

Fischer P, Simanyi M, Danielczyk W: Depression in dementia of the Alzheimer type and in multi-infarct dementia. Am J Psychiatry 147:1484–1487, 1990

Fitz AG, Teri L: Depression, cognition and functional ability in patients with Alzheimer's disease. J Am Geriatr Soc 42:186–191, 1994

Folstein MF, Folstein SE, McHugh PR: Mini-mental state: a practical method for grading the cognitive state of patients for the clinician. J Psychiatr Res 12: 189–198, 1975

Forsell Y, Jorm AF, Fratiglioni L, et al: Application of DSM-III-R criteria for major depressive episode to elderly subjects with and without dementia. Am J Psychiatry 150:1199–1202, 1993

Frith CD, Stevens M, Johnstone EC, et al: Effects of ECT and depression on various aspects of memory. Br J Psychiatry 142:610–617, 1983

Greenwald BS, Kramer-Ginsberg E, Marin DB, et al: Dementia with coexistent major depression. Am J Psychiatry 146:1472–1478, 1989

Hartlage S, Alloy LB, Vazquez C, et al: Automatic and effortful processing in depression. Psychol Bull 113:247–278, 1993

Hoch CC, Reynolds CF, Houck PR, et al: Predicting mortality in mixed depression and dementia using EEG sleep variables. J Neuropsychiatry Clin Neurosci 1:366–371, 1989

Huber SJ, Shuttleworth EC, Paulson GW: Dementia in Parkinson's disease. Arch Neurol 43:987–995, 1986

Kathol RG, Mutgi A, Williams J, et al: Diagnosis of major depression in cancer patients according to four sets of criteria. Am J Psychiatry 147:1021–1024, 1990

Knauper B, Wittchen HU: Diagnosing major depression in the elderly: evidence for response bias in standardized diagnostic interviews? J Psychiatr Res 28: 147–164, 1994

Knesevich JW, Martin RL, Berg L, et al: Preliminary report on affective symptoms in the early stages of senile dementia of the Alzheimer type. Am J Psychiatry 140:233–235, 1983

Lazarus LW, Newton N, Cohler B, et al: Frequency and presentation of depressive symptoms in patients with primary degenerative dementia. Am J Psychiatry 144:41–45, 1987

Logsdon RG, Teri L: Depression in Alzheimer's disease patients: caregivers as surrogate reporters. J Am Geriatr Soc 43:150–155, 1995

Mackenzie TB, Robiner WN, Knopman DS: Differences between patient and family assessments of depression in Alzheimer's disease. Am J Psychiatry 146: 1174–1178, 1989

Marcopulos BA, Graves RE: Antidepressant effect on memory in depressed older persons. J Clin Exp Neuropsychol 12:655–663, 1990

Mattis S: Mental status examination for organic mental syndromes in the elderly patient, in Geriatric Psychiatry: A Handbook for Psychiatrists and Primary Care Physicians. Edited by Bellak L, Karasu TB. New York, Grune & Stratton, 1976

Mayeux R, Stern Y, Rosen J, et al: Depression, intellectual impairment, and Parkinson's disease. Neurology 31:645–650, 1981

Meyers BS: Epidemiology and clinical meaning of "significant" depressive symptoms in later life: the question of subsyndromal depression. American Journal of Geriatric Psychiatry 2:188–191, 1994

Meyers BS, Mattis S, Gabriele BS, et al: Effects of nortriptyline on memory self-assessment and performance in recovered elderly depressives. Psychopharmacol Bull 27:295–299, 1991

Miller NE: The measurement of mood in senile brain disease: examiner ratings and self-reports, in Psychopathology in the Aged. Edited by Cole JO, Barrett JE. New York, Raven, 1980, pp 97–122

Moskowitz H, Burns MM: Cognitive performance in geriatric subjects after acute treatment with antidepressants. Neuropsychobiology 15(suppl 1):38–43, 1986

Mulsant BH, Zubenko GS: Clinical, neuropathological, and neurochemical correlates of depression and psychosis in primary dementia, in Dementia: Presentations, Differential Diagnosis, and Nosology. Edited by Emery VOB, Oxman TE. Baltimore, MD, Johns Hopkins University Press, 1994, pp 336–352

Mulsant BH, Rosen J, Thornton JE, et al: A prospective naturalistic study of electroconvulsive therapy in late-life depression. J Geriatr Psychiatry Neurol 4:3–13, 1991

Mulsant BH, Sweet RA, Rifai AH, et al: The use of the Hamilton rating scale for depression in elderly patients with cognitive impairment and physical illness. American Journal of Geriatric Psychiatry 2:220–229, 1994

Myers JK, Weissman MM, Tischler GL, et al: Six-month prevalence of psychiatric disorders in three communities. Arch Gen Psychiatry 41:959–967, 1984

Nebes RD, Brady CB: Focused and divided attention in Alzheimer's disease. Cortex 25:305–315, 1989

Nebes RD, Brady CB: Focused, divided attention in Alzheimer's disease. Cortex 29:77–90, 1993

Nebes RD, Brady CB, Reynolds CF: Cognitive slowing in Alzheimer's disease and geriatric depression. J Gerontol 47:331–336, 1992

Nemeroff CB, Escalona PR, Krishnan KRR, et al: The biology of late-life depression, in Biology of Depressive Disorders, Part B: Subtypes of Depression and Comorbid Disorders. Edited by Mann JJ, Kupfer DJ. New York, Plenum, 1993, pp 59–73

Nestor PG, Parasuraman R, Haxby JV: Speed of information processing and attention in early Alzheimer's dementia. Developmental Neuropsychology 7:243–256, 1991

Nyth AL, Gottfries CG: The clinical efficacy of citalopram in treatment of emotional disturbances in dementia disorders. Br J Psychiatry 157:894–901, 1990

Nyth AL, Gottfries CG, Lyby K, et al: A controlled multicenter clinical study of citalopram and placebo in elderly depressed patients with and without concomitant dementia. Acta Psychiatr Scand 86:138–145, 1992

Ott BR, Fogel BS: Measurement of depression in dementia: self vs. clinician rating. International Journal of Geriatric Psychiatry 7:899–904, 1992

Parmelee PA, Katz IR, Lawton MP: Depression among institutionalized aging: assessment and prevalence estimation. J Gerontol 44:M22–M29, 1989

Perry EK, Irving D, Kerwin JM, et al: Cholinergic transmitter and neurotrophic activities in Lewy body dementia: similarity to Parkinson's and distinction from Alzheimer disease. Alzheimer Dis Assoc Disord 7:69–79, 1993

Pollak CP, Perlick D: Sleep problems, institutionalization of the elderly. Sleep Research 16:407–412, 1987

Poon LW: Toward an understanding of cognitive functioning in geriatric depression. Int Psychogeriatr 4(suppl 2):241–266, 1992

Prinz PN, Peskind ER, Vitaliano PP, et al: Changes in the sleep and waking EEGs of nondemented and demented elderly subjects. J Am Geriatr Soc 30:86–93, 1982

Rabins PV, Merchant A, Nestadt G: Criteria for diagnosing reversible dementia caused by depression: validation by 2-year follow-up. Br J Psychiatry 144: 488–492, 1984

Reifler BV, Larson E, Hanley R: Co-existence of depression and cognitive impairment in geriatric outpatients. Am J Psychiatry 139:623–626, 1982

Reifler BV, Larson E, Teri L, et al: Dementia of the Alzheimer's type and depression. J Am Geriatr Soc 34:855–859, 1986

Reifler BV, Teri L, Raskin M, et al: Double-blind trial of imipramine in Alzheimer's disease patients with, without depression. Am J Psychiatry 146:45–49, 1989

Reynolds CF, Perel JM, Kupfer DJ, et al: Open-trial response to antidepressant treatment in elderly patients with mixed depression and cognitive impairment. Psychiatry Res 21:111–122, 1987

Reynolds CF, Hoch CC, Kupfer DJ, et al: Bedside differentiation of depressive pseudodementia from dementia. Am J Psychiatry 145:1099–1103, 1988

Rovner BW, Broadhead J, Spencer M, et al: Depression and Alzheimer's disease. Am J Psychiatry 146:350–353, 1989

Rubin EH, Kinscherf DA, Grant EA, et al: The influence of major depression on clinical and psychometric assessment of senile dementia of the Alzheimer type. Am J Psychiatry 148:1164–1171, 1991

Schwartz F, Carr AC, Munich RL, et al: Reaction time impairment in schizophrenia and affective illness: the role of attention. Biol Psychiatry 25:540–548, 1989

Snowdon J: The prevalence of depression in old age. International Journal of Geriatric Psychiatry 5:141–144, 1990

Stoudemire A, Hill CD, Morris R, et al: Cognitive outcome following tricyclic and electroconvulsive treatment of major depression in the elderly. Am J Psychiatry 148:1336–1340, 1991

Sunderland T, Alterman IS, Yount D, et al: A new scale for the assessment of depressed mood in demented patients. Am J Psychiatry 145:955–959, 1988a

Sunderland T, Tariot PH, Newhouse PA: Differential responsivity of mood, behavior and cognition to cholinergic agents in elderly neuropsychiatric populations. Brain Res 13:371–389, 1988b

Tariot PN, Podgorski CA, Blazina L, et al: Mental disorders in the nursing home: another perspective. Am J Psychiatry 150:1063–1069, 1993

Teri L, Wagner A: Alzheimer's disease and depression. J Consult Clin Psychol 60:379–391, 1992

Teri L, Reifler BV, Veith RC, et al: Imipramine in the treatment of depressed Alzheimer's patients: impact on cognition. J Gerontol 46:372–377, 1991

Vida S, Des Rosiers P, Carrier L, et al: Prevalence of depression in Alzheimer's disease and validity of research diagnostic criteria. J Geriatr Psychiatry Neurol 7:238–244, 1994

Volicer L, Rheaume Y, Cyr D: Treatment of depression in advanced Alzheimer's disease using sertraline. J Geriatr Psychiatry Neurol 7:227–229, 1994

Wechsler D: Wechsler Memory Scale—Revised. San Antonio, TX, Psychological Corporation, 1987

Weiner MF, Edland SD, Luszczynska H: prevalence and incidence of major depression in Alzheimer's disease. Am J Psychiatry 151:1006–1009, 1994

Weingartner H: Automatic, effort-demanding cognitive processes in depression, in Handbook for Clinical Memory Assessment of Older Adults. Edited by Poon LW. Washington, DC, American Psychological Association, 1986, pp 218–225

Wragg RE, Jeste DV: Overview of depression and psychosis in Alzheimer's disease. Am J Psychiatry 146:577–587, 1989

Zubenko GS: Biological correlates of clinical heterogeneity in primary dementia. Neuropsychopharmacology 6:77–93, 1992

Zubenko GS, Moossy J: Major depression in primary dementia: clinical and neuropathologic correlates. Arch Neurol 45:1182–1186, 1988

Zubenko GS, Moossy J, Kopp U: Neurochemical correlates of major depression in primary dementia. Arch Neurol 47:209–214, 1990

Zubenko GS, Moossy J, Martinez AJ, et al: Neuropathologic and neurochemical correlates of psychosis in primary dementia. Arch Neurol 48:619–624, 1991

Zubenko GS, Rosen J, Sweet RA, et al: Impact of psychiatric hospitalization on behavioral complications of Alzheimer's disease. Am J Psychiatry 149:1484–1491, 1992

Zubenko GS, Rifai AH, Mulsant BH, et al: Association of premorbid history of major depression with the depressive syndrome of Alzheimer's disease. American Journal of Geriatric Psychiatry (in press)

Zweig RM, Ross CA, Hedreen JC, et al: The neuropathology of aminergic nuclei in Alzheimer's disease. Ann Neurol 24:233–242, 1988

Chapter 11
Presidential Address

The Future Is Now (Provided We Recognize It)

Leonard L. Heston, M.D.

———————◆———————

Over the past couple of decades, researchers have wrought massive changes in our understanding of molecular biology and its causal role in illness. No one could have anticipated (except in the most general terms) the nature and extent of these changes, and no one immediately understood their significance because the implications are only beginning to emerge as the devils—and, perchance, the angels—in the details become known.

A few landmarks lend perspective to the pace of change. Scientists correctly established the number of human chromosomes less than 30 years ago; in roughly that same period, researchers worked out the basic rules governing DNA replication and the DNA-to-RNA-to-protein pathway. Investigators discovered restriction enzymes, those critical tools of molecular biology, in 1970; cloned the first gene in 1972; and detected exons and introns—central features of DNA structure—in 1977. Repeat DNA segments, which provide the most useful genomic landmarks—and which are causally associated with a whole new class of diseases (including fragile X syndrome and Huntington's disease)—date from the late 1980s. So does another critical tool, the polymerase chain reaction (PCR), whose acronym has entered the popular vocabulary.

177

Clearly, such developments in biological science introduce enormous complexities to our professional lives as we seek to understand illness and help patients. Yet we are well positioned to incorporate these findings and use their power to greatly speed the unraveling of errant mechanisms of psychopathology.

In this chapter, I present a few principles that have emerged to focus my thinking about our new world. This discussion is a personal view; I draw heavily on my experience with Alzheimer's disease to illustrate these principles.

Principle 1

Entities that we have regarded as single diseases most often are caused by several distinct genetic mechanisms. Heterogeneity is extremely widespread.

Twenty years ago, Alzheimer's disease seemed to provide a most enticing resource for genetic studies of brain disease. Unlike nearly all other psychopathological conditions, Alzheimer's disease involved a delimiting tissue pathology. Plaques and tangles in brain tissue ensured secure diagnosis—an Archemedian fixed point from which we might manipulate and study the firmament of the brain. The erosion of that innocent notion is instructive.

In fact, even 20 years ago researchers knew that the delimitation of a unique disease by plaques and tangles was imperfect. Other conditions also featured plaques and tangles. Yet the most important of these exceptions, Down's syndrome, provided insights that paradoxically strengthened the argument for Alzheimer's disease as unique and unitary. Down's syndrome was associated with excess DNA from chromosome 21. Down's DNA was normal DNA; there was simply too much of it. This finding implied that excessive amounts of one or more normal products from chromosome 21 produced the Down's phenotype. This phenotype included plaques and tangles in the brain, coupled—in most if not all cases—with Alzheimer's-like mental decline. Thus, Alzheimer's disease seemed to be a feature of the Down's phenotype. At long last, an exception seemed to prove a rule (even for those of us who had never quite grasped the logic of that aphorism).

Early studies found that the transmission of Alzheimer's disease within families resembled the transmission of other psychopathological entities. Close relatives of individuals with Alzheimer's disease had a greater risk for the disorder than more distant relatives or the general population.

Some families exhibited an autosomal-dominant pattern; in most, however, transmission was highly irregular and not recognizably Mendelian. Moreover, many cases were isolated, apparently sporadic. Thus, Alzheimer's disease presented a confusing and unsatisfying picture that—except for a later age at onset—could have fit schizophrenia or affective illness equally well.

The theory that Alzheimer's disease might be the outcome of a (small) number of separate causal pathways remained in the background. Evidence to support heterogeneity was inconclusive, however, until the separation of Alzheimer's disease from Gerstmann-Sträussler-Schenker disease. This rare degenerative disease is associated with a mutation in the prion protein gene on chromosome 20p (see Chapter 5). Brain tissue affected by this disease also may exhibit typical Alzheimer's plaques and tangles, however, and its clinical course often resembles that of an Alzheimer-type progressive dementia—albeit an unusually severe one.

Indeed, I once published a description of a large family affected by a dementing syndrome associated with plaques and tangles (Heston et al. 1966). My collaborating pathologists unanimously diagnosed Alzheimer's disease. I continued to follow the family, however, and 15 years later other groups demonstrated unequivocal prion disease—thus changing the diagnosis to Gerstmann-Sträussler-Schenker disease.

Thus far, I have described two non-Alzheimer pathways to Alzheimer's pathology: Down's syndrome and Gerstmann-Sträussler-Schenker disease. Of course, the latter is rare and so, perhaps, hardly seems worth mentioning. We tend to seek big-picture generalizations. Yet we must extinguish that reflex thought pattern because the great majority of diseases may well be rare at the molecular level, although we also will have to decide at what level we will apply the term *disease*. At any rate, the "splitters" won the first rounds: heterogeneity began eroding what had seemed to be a single secure base for psychopathology.

The next molecular genetic breakthrough came from a candidate gene study. In a study of one high-risk family, Chartier-Harlin et al. (1991) found a mutation in the gene that codes for amyloid, the peptide present in Alzheimer plaques; so far, the mutation has been present in family members who develop the disease and absent in those who do not—in proportions that strongly support the mutation's causal role. Researchers subsequently screened other families and found several other mutations in the same gene, all clustered tightly together in two codons. Perhaps 1% or 2% of Alzheimer cases can be attributed to these mutations in the amyloid gene.

Access to high-risk Alzheimer families also led to searches for genetic linkage. Essentially, linkage studies attempt to discover associations between DNA markers and diseases within families. If a DNA marker (a DNA segment whose location is known) and a disease tend to be nonrandomly transmitted together, the disease's causal gene probably is located close to the marker. Unfortunately, major problems—perhaps especially heterogeneity—made detecting linkage so unlikely that, in retrospect, we might wonder how any successful searches were mounted. The current availability of DNA markers closely spaced throughout the genome, as well as extensive automation in laboratories, now make linkage searches practical. Despite the primitive technology of the early 1990s, however, researchers did find linkages between certain markers and Alzheimer's disease.

The first positive reports described linkage between Alzheimer's disease and chromosome 21. This area was a natural place to search because of the Down's syndrome connection. The statistical probabilities were weak, however, and some of the positive results may have reflected the amyloid gene mutations described earlier. Thus, the question is not yet settled; chromosome 21 may yet turn out to have causal genes other than amyloid.

Researchers have discovered two additional undoubted linkages between Alzheimer's disease and DNA markers. Schellenberg et al. (1993) demonstrated linkage to chromosome 14 in several large high-risk families who also were distinguished by early onset of illness. The chromosome 14 linkage is secure: a family member possessing a defined marker is almost certain to develop Alzheimer's disease. Chromosome 19 also is linked to Alzheimer's disease, though here the evidence leads in a new direction.

Thus, researchers have identified at least five different gene-related pathways to Alzheimer's disease: Down's syndrome, Gerstmann-Sträussler-Schenker, amyloid mutations on chromosome 21, a chromosome 14 locus, and a chromosome 19 locus. We can, perhaps, dismiss Gerstmann-Sträussler-Schenker because its chemical pathology now separates it from Alzheimer's disease. The Down's phenotype is much broader than Alzheimer's disease, so it strains taxonomic sense to consider them together. Nevertheless, Down's syndrome patients do develop what must be called Alzheimer's disease; moreover, the Down's–Alzheimer's relationship continues to demand attention.

Those quibbles aside, researchers have found three definite linkages. These three linkages are independent; investigators have sought but not found cross-linkages. The evidence implies different disease mechanisms—quite possibly with different pathological mechanisms, including different environmental co-contributors; different prognoses; and, ultimately, different treatments.

These known genetic loci only scratch the surface, however. The chromosome 14 and 21 mechanisms together account for only a small fraction of Alzheimer's disease—generously, 5%—leaving the great bulk unknown; some large number of causal genes presumably remain to be discovered.

The implications of the model developed for major psychiatric diseases such as schizophrenia or bipolar illness for progress in Alzheimer's disease are humbling. Research in Alzheimer's disease, quite unlike research in schizophrenia or anxiety disorder, began with pathology comparable in specificity with any in medicine. Yet heterogeneity has turned out to be a critical confounding factor in Alzheimer's disease—as it has in nearly all other conditions known at the molecular level.

The chromosome 19 gene is more strongly associated with Alzheimer's disease, but it is predisposing only: it is neither a sufficient nor a necessary cause (Strittmatter et al. 1993). That conclusion leads to a second principle.

Principle 2

Genetic contributions to disease generally operate in surprising ways, through extremely intricate mechanisms.

The causal gene on chromosome 19 probably codes for apolipoprotein. In other words, although researchers have not absolutely ruled out another closely linked locus, the evidence strongly implicates the apolipoprotein gene cluster. This gene involves a "normal" variant: there is no pathogenic mutation.

Any two of three normal alleles—E2, E3, and E4—code for apolipoprotein. One of these alleles, E4, predisposes to Alzheimer's disease in older-onset cases. The relationship is imperfect, however: many family members with the predisposing allele do not develop Alzheimer's disease; many without it do.

In a series of studies of families in Minnesota, Oregon, and Washington, Chang-En et al. (1994) found that at least one E4 allele was present in 83% of older-onset ($\geq$ 65) cases, compared with 59% of control subjects. Among late-onset families, 35 (66%) of 53 affected cases had at least one E4 allele; 13 families had cases with and without E4; and in 5 families (10%), all cases lacked E4. Of 137 total cases, 113 (82%) had at least one E4. This allele is a much weaker factor in sporadic cases (26% versus 19%). The attributable risk in familial cases, however, approaches 65%—high enough to make E4 an important predisposing allele.

Moreover, researchers have found evidence for the effect of gene dosage, as well as hints of a complex sex effect. Persons with two E4 alleles, for example, have a risk eight times higher than persons with only E2 or E3 and no E4; for men, the risk is about twice that for E4 heterozygotes. Overall, the risk of Alzheimer's disease increases by 2.84% at each step as the number of E4 alleles increases from 0 to 1 to 2. Payami et al. (1994) found that women with only one E4 have a risk equal to men with two E4s. Thus, women appear to be more susceptible. Population surveys among older persons show an excess of healthy E4 homozygotes—implying some protective function.

Obviously, the complexities are far from unraveled. Researchers have studied apolipoprotein extensively because it is related to coronary artery disease. E4 homozygotes have an increased risk for coronary artery disease. The protein's major function relates to lipid transfer across cell membranes, but it also is involved in other capacities, including damage control in brain tissue. The mechanism of its effect in Alzheimer's disease is unknown. This example, however, brings us closer to a framework applicable to diseases such as schizophrenia. The variants of apolipoprotein are normal ones, widespread in the population. They do not themselves produce disease; instead, they act in conjunction with other factors—genes, combinations of genes, or environmental triggers—to promote disease.

Down's syndrome also illustrates complexity. For example, mothers of children with Down's syndrome who were age 35 years or younger when the affected child was born had a fivefold higher relative risk than control subjects for developing an Alzheimer-type dementia; there was no increased risk of dementia for older mothers or for fathers of children with Down's syndrome (Schupf et al. 1994). Most cases of Down's syndrome are caused by nondisjunction in maternal gametogenesis; the evidence is compatible with a shared susceptibility between Down's syndrome and Alzheimer's disease involving accelerated aging. This evolving story appears to illuminate a fascinating, though extremely complex, pathobiology.

Principle 3

A single gene may have several mutant forms. If a mutation is associated with a disease, the gene generally will exhibit several other causal mutations. Some of these mutations probably will be associated with clinical variation in the disease; others will be associated with distinctly different diseases. Most, however, will simply be normal variants, not associated with any disease.

The gene coding for amyloid illustrates this principle, in part. There are several distinct mutations tightly bunched in two codons of the precursor protein's DNA. In Alzheimer's disease, the different mutations apparently produce approximately the same clinical picture, although researchers have studied too few affected persons to be certain. Better known diseases, however, warn us to prepare for extensive clinical variation based on allelic variation. Neurofibromatosis, for example, is protean in its clinical manifestations; much of this variability is associated with different mutant sites affecting the same protein. Marfan's syndrome, which is associated with defects in the chromosome 15 gene coding for fibrillin, has clinical manifestations ranging from unnoticeable to death in early infancy. Indeed, most diseases defined by the nomenclature of a decade ago arguably are distinct disorders that may share some features but are now known to have different prognoses and likely will respond to different treatments.

The amyloid precursor gene illustrates other facets of allelic variation. A mutation at a different point in the gene is associated with the Dutch form of hereditary cerebral hemorrhage. This disease features massive amyloid deposits in cerebral arteries, leading to strokes and early death. The presence of amyloid implies some commonality between this disease and Alzheimer's disease, although otherwise the phenotypes are quite distinct. However, other mutations in the gene produce diseases that have nothing in common with either Alzheimer's disease or hereditary cerebral hemorrhage.

The prion protein also exemplifies this aspect of allelic variation. Completely different clinical entities may be related to different mutations in the prion gene. Diseases associated with this molecule may be based on a genomic mutation, or they may be environmentally acquired (see Chapter 5).

A final practical point about allelic variation: ethnic groups exhibit significant differences in the frequencies of mutant genes—both innocent and disease-producing. Researchers have learned that control groups must be carefully matched for ethnicity.

Principle 4

Predicting disease phenotype from knowledge of a gene's function or indicating a specific gene as causal from knowledge of a disease—though sometimes embarrassingly self-evident—generally is impossible.

Because researchers knew that amyloid was central to the pathology of Alzheimer's disease, DNA coding for amyloid would seem—at least in retrospect—to be a likely target for study. Such examples are rare, however. Investigators had no a priori basis, for example, to suspect that the lipoprotein gene complex had anything to do with Alzheimer's disease. Researchers also had no basis to predict either motor neuron death in androgen receptor deficiency or absence of the vas deferens as part of the cystic fibrosis phenotype.

Lesch-Nyhan syndrome provides another telling example. The pathway from the defective enzyme hypoxanthine guanosine phosphoribosyltransferase (HPRT) to the disorder's profound central nervous system dysfunction, compulsive self-injurious behavior, is completely unknown. Indeed, there is no compelling rationale to connect HPRT deficiency to brain function at all, which should remind us that the pathological bases of diseases that most concern us may not be in the brain at all. Schizophrenia might well be a liver disease.

Principle 5

First, a statement of faith. We are well on the way toward an understanding of molecular processes that surely will lead to effective diagnosis, prevention, and treatment of diseases that concern us. Nevertheless, we must acknowledge one unambiguous principle: getting there will not be easy.

Many observers have remarked ruefully that progress toward the sort of understanding of disease that would facilitate definitive corrective treatments has been slow. Perhaps our expectations were unrealistically optimistic. We naively thought that demonstration of linkages between DNA markers and disease should make rapid identification of causal genes possible. Not so: the linkage of Alzheimer's disease to chromosome 14, for example, placed the gene within a length of DNA that includes 10 million nucleic acids. Scores of genes, mostly unknown, could be incorporated within those bounds. Isolating one of these genes is technically feasible (see Chapter 7); it simply takes time and hard, slogging work: following the demonstration of linkage, researchers took more than a decade to identify the Huntington's defect.

We also thought that when researchers identified a pathogenic gene, we could quickly devise corrective treatments: wrong, of course. Much of this early optimism was based on a rigid string-of-beads view of DNA and the "one gene, one enzyme" doctrine. A more sophisticated understanding of DNA structure has developed over little more than a decade. This perspective entails several important features:

- Scientists generally accept that the human genome includes 100,000 genes. This estimate remains rough, however.
- Only 3%–4% of DNA codes for proteins. Some of the remainder is involved in regulating the amount of protein produced; some has no known function.
- The coding DNA of most genes is interrupted by noncoding segments known as introns. Introns are cut out of the RNA chain that is transcribed from DNA, and the ends of the coding segments are then spliced together to make up a new chain that codes for the final protein product. One length of DNA, however, may code for more than one protein product, through alternative sites for cutting and splicing. This mechanism is especially prominent in the human central nervous system.
- Some genes code for more than one protein; these proteins usually are produced at different times in different tissues. For example, a protease—an enzyme that degrades protein—is contained within the amyloid gene. Obviously, the production or function of this enzyme might be a factor in the pathogenesis of some Alzheimer's disease.

- Genes in a specific metabolic pathway generally are scattered throughout the genome: inconvenient but true.

Despite the all-too-evident problems, the ability to define mechanisms by which genes contribute to disease is well within researchers' grasp. The genome project is on schedule: this endeavor will produce a map of the human genome that will decisively facilitate the identification of pathological genes. Marvels of biotechnology—such as PCR, yeast artificial chromosomes, and transgenic animals—ensure this outcome.

The more difficult technical problem entails gaining an understanding of the gene-to-phenotype pathway and how to manipulate it to provide treatment. Skeptics point out that even after the identification of a pathological gene and its product, progress toward treatment has been disappointing. Researchers have known the defective protein structure underlying horrible diseases such as Lesch-Nyhan for years. Yet they have not developed treatments for such diseases for which the molecular bases are known.

This impasse is unlikely to persist, however. Gene products are proteins, so definitive treatments probably will involve modifying the structure of genes or correcting metabolic errors caused by defective proteins. Both approaches are technically feasible; indeed, investigators are actively exploring the possibilities. Optimism requires substantial faith, but history surely warrants such faith.

Does progress mean that the clinicians among us will become automatons? Will we deal with what we now call schizophrenia by ordering a test that will tell us precisely which among 500 varieties of illness we are dealing with and then prescribe for it a protocol called up on our computer screen? Perhaps, but human diversity surely will ensure that instances of disease will not fall neatly into compartments.

At the same time, serious ethical problems certainly will emerge as we begin to apply emerging technology. By and large, we cannot anticipate the forms such dilemmas will take. Each affected person and family brings unforeseen and unique problems to genetic clinics. Thus, we cannot prescribe general solutions on the basis of armchair theorizing. Ethical principles evolve out of humane practice, not the reverse.

On a societal level, a number of ethical conundrums glimmer on the horizon. Although we professionals must be prepared to give advice of the highest quality, we will not be decision makers in this context. There will be many questions we cannot address: What is the place of bipolar illness in human ecology? Does the energy and optimism of hypomania balance the detrimental effects of mania and depression, as sickle cell disease and malaria are balanced? What might be the societal consequences of gene replacement therapy? Is obsessional behavior by individuals sufficiently beneficial to society that we should not risk eradication of contributing genes? Although these questions may appear to embody visionary and impractical concerns, we must be sensitive to such concerns.

When the University of Washington developed the first kidney dialysis program in the early 1960s, its resources were limited; decisions had to be made regarding who would be treated and who would not: who would live and who would die. An independent committee with lay and professional membership—nicknamed the God Squad—was formed to deal with this question. These events marked the birth of high-technology medicine and the beginnings of formalized medical ethics.

The God Squad was unprepared for the political ramifications of its decisions, and the U.S. Congress soon superseded its functions by forming the federal end-stage renal disease program. No one could design a more well-intentioned program—or one more ineptly bureaucratic, more likely to produce silly and wasteful unintended consequences. A case study of this program would be one way to help us prepare ourselves for the future. Prepare we must, for our future is now.

References

Chang-En Y, Payami H, Olson JM, et al: The apolipoprotein E/CI/CII gene cluster and late-onset Alzheimer disease. Am J Hum Genet 54:631–642, 1994

Chartier-Harlin MC, Crawford F, Houlden H, et al: Early-onset Alzheimer's disease caused by mutations at codon 717 of the beta-amyloid precursor protein gene. Nature 353:844–846, 1991

Heston LL, Lowther DLW, Leventhal CM: Alzheimer's disease: a family study. Arch Neurol 15:225–233, 1966

Payami H, Montee KR, Kaye JA, et al: Sex difference in apolipoprotein E-associated risk for Alzheimer's disease: a genetic clue to the higher prevalence of Alzheimer's disease in women. JAMA 271:1316–1317, 1994

Schellenberg GD, Bird TD, Wijsman EM, et al: Genetic linkage evidence for a familial Alzheimer disease locus on chromosome 14. Science 258:668–671, 1993

Schupf N, Kapell D, Lee JH, et al: Increased risk of Alzheimer's disease in mothers of adults with Down's syndrome. Lancet 344:353–356, 1994

Strittmatter WJ, Saunders AM, Schmechel D, et al: Apolipoprotein E: high-avidity binding to β-amyloid and increased frequency of type 4 allele in late-onset familial Alzheimer disease. Proceedings of the National Academy of Sciences 90:1977–1981, 1993

Chapter 12

Onset of Alzheimer's Disease

Influence of Genes and Environmental Factors, Including Anti-Inflammatory Drugs

John C. S. Breitner, M.D., M.P.H.

R esearchers now know that most instances of Alzheimer's disease are associated with predisposing genes that act in Mendelian fashion (Roses 1994). There are several such genes; fortunately, most are rare. These genetic factors include a number of mutations in the protein precursor (APP) of the Aβ amyloid peptide, an anonymous locus on chromosome 14, and an uncharacterized Mendelizing trait in families of Volga German ancestry.

Although these factors are interesting for their implications regarding the pathogenesis of Alzheimer's disease, their scarcity limits their public health implications. In contrast, *ApoE*—the polymorphic genetic locus that encodes apolipoprotein E—has 3 common alleles, including allele ε4; the ε4 allele predisposes strongly to Alzheimer's disease. The allele frequency of ε4 is about 15% in most populations (Davignon et al. 1988). Thus, about 2% (0.15^2) of such populations are homozygous for this allele, and another 25% (2 x 0.15 x 0.86) are heterozygous. At least one other common gene is widely suspected; this gene is likely to hold comparable implications for risk at the population level.

Recent evidence suggests that each predisposing genotype is associated with its own distribution of onset ages. Although the onset of Alzheimer's disease occurs over a wide range of ages (from the forties to the nineties and beyond), the distribution of onset within any one genotype tends to be much narrower. Figure 12–1 illustrates data from the Duke neurogenetics laboratory, demonstrating that the disease-free survival characteristics of individuals in high-risk families vary dramatically with the subjects' genotype at *ApoE* (Roses et al. 1994). Subtracting the ordinate of these survival curves from 1 yields the respective cumulative distributions of Alzheimer's disease onset in these individuals.

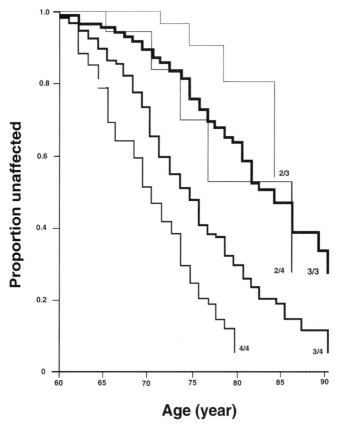

Figure 12–1.   Probability of disease-free survival for persons at high risk for Alzheimer's disease given the indicated apolipoprotein genotypes.

The cumulative curves may be differentiated in turn to yield what statisticians term the *onset probability density distributions* (Figure 12–2). The latter curves (which can be drawn only as crude estimates) represent the probability that a member of the group will experience onset of Alzheimer's disease at the age specified on the abscissa. Figure 12–2 raises several points:

- The means of the various distributions differ substantially. ε3/ε4 heterozygotes experience onset near age 80 years; unselected populations may experience onset somewhat later—perhaps around age 85 years. By contrast, ε4 homozygotes experience onset mainly in their sixties.
- Each distribution is (relatively) symmetrical. Thus, the probability of onset increases with age up to a point (the distribution node), after which it declines.
- Although these curves are drawn with equal amplitude (i.e., as true distributions), they apply to portions of the population that vary greatly in size. At the aforementioned allele frequency (and assuming Hardy Weinberg equilibrium), ε4 heterozygotes will be at least 12 times as common in the population as homozygotes.
- Although data are sparse, researchers widely believe that incidence and prevalence of Alzheimer's disease increase after age 85 years.

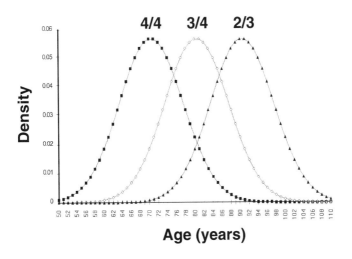

Figure 12–2. Probability of disease for population depicted in Figure 12–1.

Such increases are unlikely to result from the effects of ε4 because the probability of symptom onset[1] with this allele appears to decline shortly after age 80 years.

Inheritance does not necessarily equal fate. Whereas most inherited traits are expressed in "all or none" fashion, often from birth, the genes that predispose to Alzheimer's disease clearly act quite differently. These genes appear to control the rate of progression of a neurodegenerative process that may be ubiquitous. Some years ago, in fact, Allen Roses suggested that we all might develop Alzheimer's disease if we lived long enough; for many of us, however, that would mean living to age 120 years or older.

If the genes do act this way, the possibility remains that environmental influences might modify the expression of the process, which otherwise is conditioned by the genotype. Figure 12–3 presents a model for the effects of head injury—a probable risk factor for Alzheimer's disease. Figure 12–3 suggests that head injury may move the onset time of dementia symptoms forward by several years. Thus, the incidence of Alzheimer's disease at relatively youthful ages (when most people are still living) would increase, and epidemiologists would observe a relative risk (or odds ratio) of greater than 1. Head injury acts precipitously; other environmental influences (e.g., toxic exposures), however, may exert a cumulative effect.

On a more encouraging note, some environmental influences might retard the expression of the gene by slowing the neurodegenerative process (see Figure 12–4). Because the process is delayed, incidence is reduced at the ages at which Alzheimer's disease onset is common; however, it may increase later (i.e., delay implies deferral to a later time).

Researchers must seek environmental factors that accelerate the onset of Alzheimer's disease, as well as those that may delay it. Such understanding would allow at-risk individuals to avoid accelerating factors; alternatively, if their mechanism of action were understood, clinicians could prescribe treatments to diminish their effects. Similarly, identification of factors that delay onset would allow clinicians to prescribe them as a strategy for prevention.

The public health consequences of either strategy would be enormous, even if the effect on age at onset were slight. Alzheimer's disease

---

[1]Incidence actually is modeled by the hazard function, which divides the density by the fraction of the population remaining at risk (i.e., free of disease). However, because even ε3/ε4, the most common predisposing genotype, represents only about 25% of the population, the density function provides a reasonable approximation.

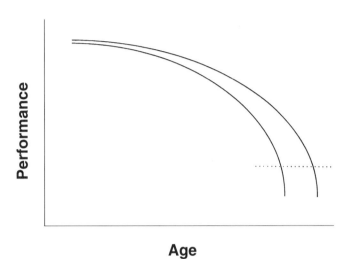

Figure 12–3.   Hypothetical effect of an environmental factor, head injury, lowering the age at onset.

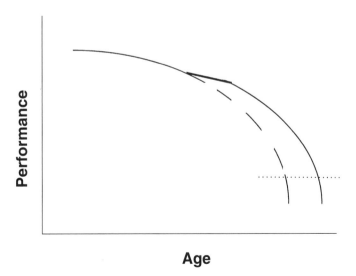

Figure 12–4.   Hypothetical effect of a beneficial environmental factor increasing the age at onset.

by its nature is a disease of old age; thus, many individuals who otherwise would develop the disorder die of other, unrelated causes before onset. Others may develop symptoms but experience an abbreviated course of progression before death intervenes. An average 5-year delay in onset would decrease the lifetime incidence of Alzheimer's disease by more than one-third (Breitner 1991). The prevalence of symptomatic cases would decrease even further—probably by about one-half—because prevalence depends on incidence and duration. Finally, because prevalent cases in the population would have shorter duration, affected individuals would experience less severe symptoms, further reducing the burden of the disease (defined as the product of prevalence and symptom severity).

How can researchers find the factors that are of such critical importance? Two complementary approaches are possible: reductionist/hypothetical or agnostic/empirical.

The reductionist/hypothetical approach is based on current thinking regarding etiology and pathogenesis; under this approach, researchers search for means of altering the mechanism of disease through the development of new drugs or similar interventions. The majority of research in Alzheimer's disease uses this approach—for example, through the study of amyloidogenesis, alterations in conformation of tau, and the actions of apolipoprotein E. The strengths of this approach are obvious in this day of high-resolution molecular science. The limitation, which researchers sometimes ignore, is that investigators cannot be sure that these factors are causes, rather than effects, of the underlying disease process in Alzheimer's disease.

The habitual (though rather inept) bank robber Willie Sutton, when asked why he persisted in robbing banks, replied, "that's where the money is." Researchers who adopt the reductionist/hypothetical approach hope they are acting analogously, although they also risk reenacting the story of the drunken sailor looking for his key in the dark: he invests great energy looking under the streetlamp because "that's where the light is."

Many investigators (including my own group) have chosen to pursue the agnostic/empirical method. In this approach, researchers seek environmental factors that are systematically associated with the occurrence of Alzheimer's disease.

My colleagues and I became intrigued with the idea that much of the modification in the risk of Alzheimer's disease must occur through alteration in the kinetics of disease expression. This led us to work with twin pairs whose members experienced the onset of Alzheimer's disease at different times (Breitner et al. 1993). We reasoned that, in theory, this approach would control genes (an obviously important determinant of Alzheimer's disease risk).

Although researchers have identified several important, easily detected genes, our approach continues to have merit because it controls genes that have not yet been identified, as well as those that have. Moreover, researchers now know that genes themselves act to influence the timing of disease expression; thus, epidemiological inquiries (e.g., case-control studies) clearly have limited value unless investigators can simultaneously control genotype as they seek other (probably less potent) factors that influence the timing of onset (Breitner 1994).

To pursue this inquiry, my colleagues and I began an ambitious study of Alzheimer's disease and other dementias in a population of 5,800 elderly residents of Cache County, Utah. This study involves the collection of buccal DNA from the entire elderly population and the use of genotype information (determined by polymerase chain reaction assays), as well as an extensive inventory of environmental exposures; we are seeking modifications in occurrence within specified genotypes for *ApoE* and (as they become available) other important loci. The data from the prevalence portion of this study will not be available until 1997, and the incidence-related data will not be available until 2000. In the meantime, however, we have used the co-twin control method and a similar approach of investigating environmental distinctions within siblings who differ in age at onset of Alzheimer's disease. We have reported two groups of findings.

In examining the distinctions within 50 sets of onset-discordant twin pairs (Breitner et al. 1994), we observed that the unaffected or late-affected member was four times more likely to have used glucocorticoids or nonsteroidal anti-inflammatory drugs (NSAIDs). Predictably, the effect was much stronger in monozygous (MZ) than in dizygous (DZ) pairs; the former achieve total, rather than partial, control of genotype.

The effect was not apparent, however, among pairs whose proband experienced onset of Alzheimer's disease before age 70 years. This finding puzzled us until we realized that most of the early-onset probands had developed Alzheimer's disease at an atypically early age. We now know that none of these probands had APP mutations, and only 4 (less than 10%) were homozygous for ε4. In the remainder, onset occurred at an unusually early age and therefore probably was provoked in large measure by environmental factors; there would be no reason, then, that environmental factors should account for the lack of disease in their co-twins. Exactly the opposite should hold for individuals with later (typical) onset whose co-twins escaped disease.

In an effort to replicate these findings, we studied 186 members of 45 late-onset familial Alzheimer's disease pedigrees containing sibships with multiple temporally distinct onsets, or those in which at least one sibling had survived for 3 or more years beyond onset in an index case (Breitner et al. 1995b). We found only limited exposure to glucocorticoids, but the odds ratio for sustained use of NSAIDs (daily for at least a month) was .22. The apparent protective effect was far more dramatic (odds ratio = .075) when the criterion for exposure required more than 1 year of continuous use. Again, the effect occurred almost exclusively among sibships in which Alzheimer's disease symptoms occurred after age 70 years, and it appeared mostly among individuals who lacked the ε4 allele.

Research that seeks environmental factors that increase the risk of Alzheimer's disease is logical among individuals with atypically early onset. Our twin studies produced an unexpected finding: 17 twin probands (almost 40%) from the population-based National Academy of Sciences–National Research Council (NAS-NRC) registry of World War II veteran twins (ages 62–73 years when screened for Alzheimer's disease) lacked an ε4 allele and (with one doubtful exception) a family history of Alzheimer's disease (Breitner et al. 1995a). In all instances, the co-twins were unaffected. Although none of these individuals had an APP mutation, 15 had experienced onset of Alzheimer's disease before age 65 years; their co-twins had all remained unaffected for at least 7 years (maximum 17, mean 11.3) after the proband's onset. We had complete exposure information on 10 of the latter pairs (6 MZ), which we used to conduct a co-twin control analysis (Breitner et al. 1994). We found six pairs in which the proband reported a history of chronic allergic conditions (e.g., hay fever, asthma) but the sibling did not (odds ratio = 6:0, exact P = .03, two-tailed). In 4 pairs, the proband reported an occupational history of machining, metal milling, welding, or sheetmetal working, whereas the sibling did not (D = .13, two-tailed).

Clearly, these data are preliminary, and the analyses do not consider the problem of multiple comparison. To our knowledge, however, this study is the first effort to seek environmental provocation in this unusual group, which would seem likely to have experienced environmental provocation.

In summary, the recent discovery of *ApoE* and other genes that modify the risk and timing of expression of Alzheimer's disease has important bearing on our understanding of the causes of this disease. We must not only continue to seek the mechanisms by which these genes exert their effect but also consider environmental influences that modify their expression. We cannot know which investigative approach will first yield the means of preventing this dreaded disease, but the two avenues in combination offer substantial hope that we may do so before the new millennium.

References

Breitner JCS: Clinical genetics and genetic counseling in Alzheimer's disease. Ann Intern Med 115:601–606, 1991

Breitner JCS: New epidemiologic strategies in Alzheimer's disease may provide clues to prevention and cause. Neurobiol Aging 15:S175–S177, 1994

Breitner JCS, Gatz M, Bergem ALM, et al: The use of twin cohorts for research in Alzheimer's disease. Neurology 43:261–267, 1993

Breitner JCS, Gau BA, Welsh KA, et al: Inverse association of anti-inflammatory treatments and Alzheimer's disease: initial results of a co-twin control study. Neurology 44:227–232, 1994

Breitner JCS, Welsh KA, Gau BA, et al: Alzheimer's disease in the NAS-NRC registry of aging twin veterans, III: detection of cases, longitudinal results, and twin concordance. Arch Neurol 52:763–771, 1995a

Breitner JCS, Welsh KA, Helms MJ, et al: Delayed onset of Alzheimer's disease with non-steroidal anti-inflammatory and histamine H2 blocking drugs. Neurobiol Aging 16:523–530, 1995b

Davignon J, Gregg RE, Sing CF: Apolipoprotein E polymorphism and atherosclerosis. Arteriosclerosis 8:1–21, 1988

Roses AD: The Alzheimer diseases, in Current Neurology, Vol 14. Edited by Appel SA. Chicago, IL, CV Mosby, 1994

Roses AD, Strittmatter WJ, Pericak-Vance MA, et al: Clinical application of apolipoprotein E genotyping to Alzheimer's disease. Lancet 343:1564–1565, 1994

Chapter 13

From Gene to Phenotype

A Transgenic Model of Alzheimer's Disease

Barbara Cordell, Ph.D., Linda S. Higgins, Ph.D., Jeffrey Higaki, Ph.D., Ziyang Zhong, Ph.D., Paula M. Moran, Ph.D., and Paul C. Moser, Ph.D.

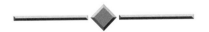

Transgenic technology allows researchers to evaluate the influence of a single gene in vivo. Investigators have applied this approach successfully to study Alzheimer's disease; our work has focused on the gene that encodes the human β-amyloid precursor protein (β-APP).

In this chapter, we describe the pathological influence of aberrant β-APP gene expression in transgenic mice. Characterization of these mice has revealed histological and behavioral features analogous to those in

We acknowledge Marion Merrell Dow Inc. for sponsoring the research described in this chapter.

early Alzheimer's disease. These features include extracellular diffuse deposits of β-amyloid derived from the exogenous gene and aberrancies in the neuronal cytoskeleton, as well as memory and learning impairments. These features are more pronounced in older transgenic animals. Although the typical transgenic mouse presents with an early Alzheimer's disease-like phenotype, occasionally some mice show advanced histopathology. Characteristics of more mature Alzheimer's disease-like pathology include large β-amyloid deposits associated with gliosis, vacuolization, and dystrophic neurites.

These findings indicate that the murine brain is capable of reproducing features of Alzheimer's disease. Moreover, the phenotype of this transgenic model indicates a central role for β-APP in the pathogenesis of Alzheimer's disease.

Experimental Strategy for Transgenic Model

Deposits of β-amyloid in the brain parenchyma and cerebrovasculature are unique histological hallmarks of Alzheimer's disease. Whether the formation of β-amyloid deposits is central to the pathology of Alzheimer's disease or an epiphenomenon, however, remains unclear. Our working hypothesis has been that β-amyloid formation and deposition is a critical component of the disease process. Therefore, our research has focused on elucidating the mechanisms of β-amyloid accumulation. Our experimental approach has been to generate and evaluate in vitro and in vivo models of this process.

β-amyloid is an approximately 4 kilodalton peptide produced by proteolytic processing of a larger precursor, β-APP (Kang et al. 1987). Investigators have described three major isoforms of β-APP, which arise by alternative splicing of a primary RNA transcript (Kang et al. 1987; Kitaguchi et al. 1988; Ponte et al. 1988; Tanzi et al. 1988). Two isoforms— β-APP751 and β-APP770—harbor a Kunitz proteinase inhibitor domain, whereas the third isoform, β-APP695, lacks this domain. In general, the β-APP695 isoform is expressed exclusively in neurons; the Kunitz inhibitor-containing isoforms are expressed ubiquitously (Neve et al. 1988; Ponte et al. 1988).

Researchers have shown that β-amyloid is produced by normal cellular metabolism and that this peptide is secreted from mammalian cells in culture (Haass et al. 1992; Shoji et al. 1992). We investigated the details of molecular and cellular events leading to β-amyloid peptide formation (Zhong et al. 1994). In these studies, we detected metabolically labeled β-amyloid peptide produced in vitro by immunoprecipitation with antibodies specific for the β-amyloid protein, followed by polyacrylamide gel electrophoresis and autoradiography. We also produced the β-amyloid peptide from genetically engineered mammalian cells that express wild-type β-APP695, β-APP751, or mutated derivatives of β-APP (Zhong et al. 1994).

Untreated cultured cells produced only small amounts of β-amyloid; after amplification of β-APP expression through recombinant introduction of β-APP isoforms into cells permitting overexpression of β-APP, however, β-amyloid levels increased significantly. Thus, increased β-APP expression appeared to promote increased β-amyloid formation (Zhong et al. 1994).

Modest amounts β-amyloid were formed when β-APP695 was expressed in its native neuronal cell background. By contrast, β-amyloid peptide levels were elevated when β-APP695 was expressed in a fibroblastic cell—a background not normally expressing this isoform. The converse situation obtained for β-APP751 expression: higher levels of β-amyloid peptide were present when β-APP751 was expressed in neuronal cells versus the fibroblastic cell background. These results suggest that an atypical host-cell background can lead to increased β-amyloid production. Furthermore, quantities of β-amyloid were 10 to 50 times larger when mutant β-APP—including mimics of naturally occurring mutations, as well as those produced artificially—was expressed than with wild-type β-APP. This significant increase in β-amyloid peptide formation by aberrant β-APP occurred despite equal synthesis of wild-type and mutant precursor proteins (Zhong et al. 1994).

These observations, in conjunction with other data, led us to propose that β-amyloid is derived by an intracellular degradative pathway used to discard aberrant nascent proteins (Zhong et al. 1994). Simply put, the β-amyloid peptide is a catabolic by-product of β-APP (Figure 13–1). A β-APP molecule might qualify as aberrant in a variety of ways, including mutations, misfolded structures, abnormal post-translational processing, excess amounts, or expression of an incorrect isoform in a cell.

Several observations on the molecular pathology of Alzheimer's disease support this model of β-amyloid formation. Naturally occurring, disease-specific examples include mutated β-APP, overexpression of β-APP, and expression of an incorrect β-APP isoform. One β-APP genetic mutation is especially relevant. This human β-APP mutation segregates with the disease phenotype (Mullan et al. 1992). Alzheimer's disease patients with this mutation have extensive β-amyloid deposition in their

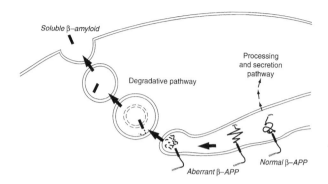

Figure 13–1. Hypothetical scheme of β-amyloid formation. Aberrant β-APP molecules are discarded by an intracellular editing process. On catabolism of the discarded β-APP, an 11-kilodalton amyloidogenic fragment is generated by proteolytic processing. This 11-kilodalton β-APP fragment bears an intact β-amyloid domain at its amino-terminus. Continued proteolytic processing of the 11-kilodalton fragment, which involves a cleavage producing the carboxyl-terminus of β-amyloid, results in the mature β-amyloid peptide. Degradative by-products of β-APP catabolism, including the β-amyloid peptide, are secreted from the cell.

brains, and skin fibroblasts cultured from these individuals secrete several times more β-amyloid peptide than age-matched control subjects (Citron et al. 1994). Furthermore, recombinant expression of this β-APP mutant in cultured cells leads to a five- to eightfold increase in β-amyloid production (Cai et al. 1993; Citron et al. 1992).

Down's syndrome, or trisomy 21, represents another example of abnormal β-APP expression with an associated increase in β-amyloid production. The gene encoding β-APP is located on chromosome 21, within the obligate Down's region (Tanzi et al. 1987). Individuals with Down's syndrome invariably develop Alzheimer's disease—and at a very early age (Burger and Vogel 1973; Wisniewski et al. 1985). In fact, individuals with Down's syndrome have a twofold increase in β-APP expression over age-matched control subjects (Rumble et al. 1989).

Furthermore, abnormalities in cell-specific β-APP isoform expression are selectively present in the brains of Alzheimer's disease patients (Golde et al. 1990; Johnson et al. 1990). Johnson et al. (1990) demonstrated that the Kunitz inhibitor-bearing isoforms of β-APP, which are not normally expressed at high levels in neurons, were increased in entorhinal, cortical, and hippocampal neurons in cases of sporadic Alzheimer's disease. In fact, Johnson et al. (1990) observed a direct linear relationship between increased expression of neuronal β-APP751/770 and amyloid plaque density.

Higaki et al. (1995) used a unique inhibitor of β-APP processing to generate additional data supporting the hypothesis that β-amyloid is a nonobligatory degradative by-product formed from the catabolism of discarded β-APP molecules. This inhibitor, MDL, prevents β-amyloid formation by inhibiting the enzyme that produces the carboxyl-terminus of the β-amyloid peptide. Higaki et al. (1995) found that application of MDL to cultured mammalian cells resulted in degradation of β-APP to non-amyloidogenic by-products through an alternative catabolic process. Moreover, biosynthesis of β-APP was unaltered in the presence of this inhibitor, lending additional support to the hypothesis. Figure 13–2 illustrates the effects of MDL on β-APP degradation and β-amyloid formation.

We used transgenic technology to test our hypothesis regarding β-amyloid formation at the in vivo level. This experiment also served as an

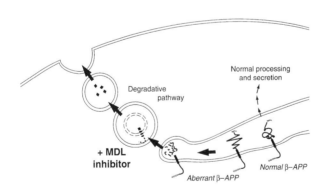

Figure 13–2. Inhibition of β-amyloid formation by inhibitor MDL. As in Figure 13–1, aberrant β-APP molecules are discarded from the biosynthetic pathway. The inhibitor blocks cleavage, yielding the carboxyl-terminus of the β-amyloid peptide. In the presence of MDL, the 11-kilodalton amyloidogenic fragment of β-APP is produced but not processed to a mature β-amyloid peptide. Instead, the 11-kilodalton fragment is degraded to nonamyloidogenic by-products. No β-amyloid peptide is formed.

approach toward developing a small-animal model of Alzheimer's disease. Our experimental strategy was to mimic the alterations in β-APP isoform expression that occur in Alzheimer's disease neurons. As noted earlier, β-APP751—a Kunitz proteinase inhibitor-containing isoform of β-APP—is not normally expressed at high levels in neurons, yet the mRNA for this β-APP isoform is elevated in neurons in Alzheimer's disease (Johnson et al. 1990). In vitro experiments with cultured neuronal cells also showed increased β-amyloid generation when expressing β-APP751, but not β-APP695 (Zhong et al. 1994).

Transgenic Mice Abnormally Expressing Beta-APP Have Beta-Amyloid Deposits in Their Brains

Quon et al. (1991) generated mice that were genetically programmed for increased neuronal expression of human β-APP751, as well as transgenic mice engineered for increased neuronal expression of human β-APP695. The β-APP695 isoform normally is expressed only in neurons (Neve et al. 1988; Ponte et al. 1988).

To genetically program the neurons of transgenic mice for increased expression of β-APP, we prepared an artificial gene, or transgene, using the rat neuronal-specific enolase promoter (NSE) linked to the human cDNA encoding either β-APP751 or β-APP695. We identified six NSE: β-APP751 and four NSE:β-APP695 founders as carrying their respective transgene. We bred these founders to yield homozygous pedigrees; each pedigree stably transmitted the transgene to all progeny. Furthermore, each pedigree was characterized and shown by molecular methods to express the transgene at both the RNA and the protein levels (Quon et al. 1991). Mice from these pedigrees, in addition to wild-type mice of the parental strain, constituted the set of animals used to characterize the pathological consequences of neuronal overexpression of human β-APP isoforms.

Using standard immunohistochemical methodology, we surveyed wild-type mice and multiple pedigrees of transgenic mice for production of β-amyloid immunoreactive deposits in their brains. We prepared and stained tissue sections with a collection of antibodies specific for β-amyloid—including a monoclonal antibody, 4.1 mAb, produced by our laboratory, as well as several polyclonal antisera used by other researchers. All of these antibodies were raised against human β-amyloid synthetic peptides, and all had been used in specific staining of plaques in Alzheimer's disease brain tissue.

Only mice of the NSE:β-APP751 pedigrees displayed β-amyloid immunoreactive deposits in their brains (Higgins et al. 1993, 1994; Quon et al. 1991). These deposits varied in size and morphology: the deposits were 5–50 mm in diameter; some were diffuse, others compact. In addition, we observed β-amyloid deposits most frequently in the cortex and hippocampus and occasionally in the thalamus; we did not find any such deposits in the cerebellum.

Immunoreactive deposits in NSE:β-APP751 brains were infrequent—generally only a few per tissue section. A large survey of animals spanning all NSE:β-APP751 pedigrees detected deposits in 67% of the animals in the study. Three tissue sections from 33 mice were examined; presumably, more positive mice would have been scored if a larger number of sections had been evaluated. Data from the NSE:β-APP751 animals in this study were subdivided by sex and transgene hemi- or homozygosity. The frequency of deposits was no different in male and female mice. Animals homozygous for the transgene, however, displayed twice the frequency that hemizygous animals exhibited.

One of the β-amyloid antibodies, 4.1 mAb, is specific for human, but not rodent, β-amyloid protein. Thus, the positive immunoreactivity of amyloid deposits with this monoclonal antibody indicates that deposits in the NSE:β-APP751 transgenic mouse brain were derived from protein encoded by the exogenous human transgene.

Histopathology in Beta-APP751 Transgenic Mice Resembles Early Alzheimer's Disease

To place our understanding of β-amyloid immunoreactive deposits in the brains of the NSE:β-APP751 transgenic mice into the context of human pathology, we compared these deposits with β-amyloid immunoreactive structures in the brain tissue of patients with Alzheimer's disease and Down's syndrome. Because individuals with Down's syndrome develop Alzheimer's disease by the fourth decade of life (Burger and Vogel 1973;

Wisniewski et al. 1985), the Down's brain offers a temporal glimpse of events in the progression of Alzheimer's disease pathology.

In young adult Down's brain, 4.1 mAb immunohistochemistry revealed only diffuse β-amyloid deposits; mature plaques were not yet present at this stage. This observation agreed with reports describing immature Alzheimer's disease pathology in Down's brain (Allsop et al. 1989; Giaccone et al. 1989; Mann and Esiri 1989). Although 4.1 mAb immunoreactivity in NSE:β-APP751 mouse brain was morphologically similar to the diffuse deposits in young Down's syndrome brain tissue, classic mature plaques were absent in the transgenic mouse brain. Thus, β-amyloid deposits in NSE:β-APP751 brain most closely resembled amyloid deposits in early Alzheimer's disease.

Studies using classic histological reagents—including methenamine silver, Bielschowsky silver, thioflavine S, and Congo red—provided further evidence that NSE:β-APP751 transgenic mice display early Alzheimer's disease β-amyloid pathology. Only reagents that exclusively stain diffuse amyloid deposits or preplaques (methenamine silver and thioflavine S, respectively) reacted with the structures in the transgenic mouse brain.

Other Histopathological Features in NSE: Beta-APP751 Transgenic Mice

A second major histological feature of Alzheimer's disease brain tissue is the presence of neurofibrillary tangles. Neurofibrillary tangles are composed primarily of the microtubule-associated protein, tau, in an aberrantly hyperphosphorylated state.

The β-APP751 transgenic mice were also characterized for abnormalities in tau protein. Aberrant tau was assessed immunohistologically with the Alz50 antibody. Extensive research has documented that in immunohistological staining of Alzheimer's disease tissue, the Alz50 antibody recognizes only the abnormal form of tau in neurofibrillary tangles (Wolozin et al. 1986). Our staining revealed Alz50-immunoreactive neuronal soma and processes in the brain tissue of NSE:β-APP751 mice (Higgins et al. 1995).

The aberrant subcellular localization of tau to neuronal soma in transgenic mice stained with Alz50 was identical to the abnormal subcellular distribution of tau in Alzheimer's disease. Stained neuronal soma in the NSE:β-APP751 mice were exclusively localized to the cerebral cortex, thalamus, and amygdala. Immunoreactive processes were frequently noted in these same brain regions and occasionally in the hippocampus. This Alz50 staining profile was unique to transgenic mice overexpressing β-APP751 in their neurons; no reactivity was seen in NSE:β-APP695 or in wild-type mice. As in the case of β-amyloid immunoreactivity, Alz50 staining of NSE:β-APP751 mouse brain was similar to the pathology present in young adult Down's brain (Mann and Esiri 1989).

Frequency of Beta-Amyloid and Alz50 Immunoreactivities in Transgenic Mice Increases With Age

As noted earlier, NSE:β-APP751 transgenic mice displayed two histopathological characteristics of early Alzheimer's disease: diffuse β-amyloid deposits and aberrant tau protein. These mice further paralleled the human condition in that the number of β-amyloid deposits and abnormal Alz50-immunoreactive structures increased with the age of the NSE:β-APP751 animal.

In a blinded study, β-amyloid deposition and aberrant tau-positive neurons were approximately twice as prevalent in brains from old (age 22 months) β-APP751 transgenic mice as in brains from young (ages 2–3 months) mice (Higgins et al. 1995). Specifically, 49% of the tissue sections scored positive for β-amyloid deposition in 22-month-old mice, compared with 29% in 2- to 3-month-old animals; 69% of the older mice had Alz50 reactive neuronal structures, in contrast to 33% of the younger group. Thirteen homozygous mice from a single pedigree were included in each age group, and three brain tissue sections were stained per animal.

Mature Histopathology in Transgenic Mice

The pathology observed in NSE:β-APP751 transgenic mice most frequently resembled an early, subtle stage of Alzheimer's disease. In rare instances, however, brains from these transgenic pedigrees contained features of a more mature disease state (Higgins et al. 1994). These histological features included extensive and dense β-amyloid deposition that co-localized with gliosis, vacuolization, and Alz50-immunoreactive structures morphologically identical to the swollen synaptic processes of dystrophic neurites.

These areas of extensive pathology also were stained by Bielschowsky silver staining method, again indicating a somewhat more mature Alzheimer's disease-like histopathology in the β-APP751 overexpressing transgenic mouse brain. None of these unique transgenic animals displayed congophilic deposits. We do not know why certain animals of the pedigree display a more advanced pathology. Although this pathology was rare—occurring in only 4% of the animals examined—these results indicate that the mouse brain is capable of recapitulating many of the histopathological features of advancing Alzheimer's disease. In addition, these findings have positive ramifications for the development of a faithful small-animal model of Alzheimer's disease.

Behavioral Abnormalities in Transgenic Mice

Moran et al. (1994) conducted an extensive behavioral comparison of β-APP751 transgenic and wild-type mice. This blinded study evaluated animals in areas of general neurological, general behavioral, and cognitive performance. Although transgenic mice did not display any gross neurological or behavioral impairments, they showed significant impairment in learning, compared with their wild-type counterparts. This impairment was evident in several learning models (e.g., Morris water maze paradigm of spatial navigation). Furthermore, the learning impairment of the β-APP751 transgenic mice was age-dependent: older animals (age 12 months) showed more pronounced impairment of learning acquisition than their younger (age 6 months) transgenic cohorts. Thus, the behavioral phenotype of NSE:β-APP751 mice also exhibited an early clinical manifestation of Alzheimer's disease: impairment in cognitive ability.

Conclusion

The age-dependent appearance of learning deficits, β-amyloid deposits, and aberrant tau structures in mice expressing human β-APP751 parallel cardinal features of Alzheimer's disease. Results obtained with this transgenic model indicate that a single genetic alteration produces a number of changes. These modulations suggest a cascade of events triggered by abnormal neuronal β-APP expression, which may mimic an analogous process in the human disorder.

These findings suggest a simple cause-and-effect linkage of some—though clearly not all—of the pathological events in Alzheimer's disease (Figure 13–3). Results obtained with β-APP751 transgenic mice lend additional support to our overall hypothesis that β-amyloid is a degradative by-product resulting from the elimination of aberrant β-APP expression. This conclusion implies that transgenic mice genetically engineered to express other aberrant β-APPs are likely to have pathological phenotypes.

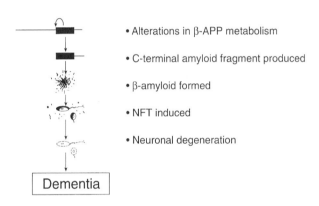

• Alterations in β-APP metabolism

• C-terminal amyloid fragment produced

• β-amyloid formed

• NFT induced

• Neuronal degeneration

Dementia

Figure 13–3. Proposed pathogenic cascade in Alzheimer's disease. This scheme represents some, but not all, of the events known to occur in the disease. The order of this pathogenic sequence of events is based on observation with transgenic mice abnormally expressing β-APP. These mice have a single perturbation in β-APP biosynthesis, yet the animals display aberrant tau structures in their brains and possess cognitive impairments. NFT designates neurofibrillary tangles.

References

Allsop D, Haga S-I, Haga C, et al: Early senile plaques in Down's syndrome brains show a close relationship with cell bodies and neurons. Neuropath Appl Neurobiol 15:531–542, 1989

Burger PC, Vogel FC: The development of the pathological changes in Alzheimer's disease and senile dementia in patients with Down's syndrome. Am J Pathol 73:457–476, 1973

Cai X-D, Golde TE, Younkin SG: Release of excess amyloid β protein from a mutant amyloid β precursor. Science 259:514–516, 1993

Citron M, Osltersdorf T, Haass C, et al: Mutation of the β-amyloid precursor protein in familial Alzheimer's disease increases β-protein production. Nature 360:672–674, 1992

Citron M, Vigo-Pelfrey C, Teplow DB, et al: Excessive production of amyloid β-protein by peripheral cells of symptomatic and presymptomatic patients carrying the Swedish familial Alzheimer's disease mutation. Proc Natl Acad Sci U S A 91:11993–11997, 1994

Giaccone G, Tagliavini F, Linoli G, et al: Down syndrome patients: extracellular preamyloid deposits precede neuritic degeneration and senile plaques. Neurosci Lett 97:232–238, 1989

Golde TE, Estus T, Usuk M, et al: Expression of β-amyloid protein precursor mRNAs: recognition of a novel alternatively spliced form and quantitation in Alzheimer's disease using PCR. Neuron 4:253–267, 1990

Haass C, Schlossmacher MG, Hung AY, et al: Amyloid β-peptide is produced by cultured cells during normal metabolism. Nature 359:322–325, 1992

Higaki J, Quon D, Zhong Z, et al: Inhibition of β-amyloid formation identifies proteolytic precursors and subcellular site of catabolism. Neuron 14:651–659, 1995

Higgins LS, Catalano R, Quon D, et al: Transgenic mice expressing human β-APP751, but not mice expressing β-APP695, display early Alzheimer's disease-like histopathology. Ann N Y Acad Sci 695:224–227, 1993

Higgins LS, Holtzman DM, Rabin J, et al: Transgenic mouse brain histopathology resembles early Alzheimer's disease. Ann Neurol 35:598–607, 1994

Higgins LS, Rodems JM, Catalano R, et al: Early Alzheimer's disease-like histopathology increase with age in mice transgenic for β-APP751. Proc Natl Acad Sci U S A 92:4402–4406, 1995

Johnson SA, McNeil T, Cordell B, et al: Relation of neuronal APP-751/APP-695 mRNA ratio and neuritic plaque density in Alzheimer's disease. Science 248:854–857, 1990

Kang J, Lemaire H-G, Unterbeck A, et al: The precursor protein of Alzheimer's disease amyloid A4 protein resembles a cell-surface receptor. Nature 325:733–736, 1987

Kitaguchi N, Takahashi Y, Tokushima Y, et al: Novel precursor of Alzheimer's disease amyloid protein shows protease inhibitory activity. Nature 331:530–532, 1988

Mann DMA, Esiri MM: The pattern of acquisition of plaques and tangles in the brains of patients under 50 years of age with Down's syndrome. J Neurol Sci 89:169–179, 1989

Moran PM, Higgins LS, Cordell B, et al: β-APP751 mice exhibit impaired learning (abstract). Neurobiol Aging 15:48, 1994

Mullan M, Crawford F, Axelman K, et al: A pathogenic mutation for probable Alzheimer's disease in the APP gene at the N-terminus of β-amyloid. Nat Genet 1:345–347, 1992

Neve RL, Finch EA, Dawes LP: Expression of the Alzheimer amyloid protein gene transcript in the human brain. Neuron 1:669–677, 1988

Ponte P, Gonzalez-DeWhitt P, Schilling J, et al: A new A4 amyloid precursor contains a domain homologous to serine protease inhibitors. Nature 331: 525–527, 1988

Quon D, Wang Y, Catalano R, et al: Formation of β-amyloid protein deposits in brains of transgenic mice. Nature 352:239–241, 1991

Rumble B, Retallack R, Hilbich C, et al: Amyloid A4 protein and its precursor in Down's syndrome and Alzheimer's disease. N Engl J Med 320:1446–1452, 1989

Shoji M, Golde TE, Ghiso J, et al: Production of the Alzheimer β protein by normal protolytic processing. Science 258:126–129, 1992

Tanzi RE, Guezella JF, Watkins PC, et al: Amyloid β-protein gene: cDNA, mRNA distribution and genetic linkage near the Alzheimer locus. Science 235: 880–884, 1987

Tanzi RE, McCleachey AI, Lamperti ED, et al: Protease inhibitor domain encoded by an amyloid protein precursor mRNA associated with Alzheimer's disease. Nature 331:528–530, 1988

Wisniewski KE, Wisniewski HM, Wen GY: Occurrence of neuropathological changes and dementia of Alzheimer's diseases in Down's syndrome. Ann Neurol 17:278–281, 1985

Wolozin BL, Pruchnicke A, Dickson DW, et al: A neuronal antigen in the brains of Alzheimer's patients. Science 232:647–650, 1986

Zhong Z, Quon D, Higgins LS, et al: Increased amyloid production from aberrant β-amyloid precursor proteins. J Biol Chem 16:12179–12184, 1994

Chapter 14

Alzheimer's Disease and the Cholinergic System

An Introduction to Clinical Pharmacological Research

Paul A. Newhouse, M.D.

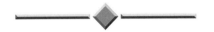

P atients with Alzheimer's disease exhibit a wide range of cognitive deficits. These deficits may be characterized broadly as problems with attention; acquisition, retention, and retrieval of knowledge; access to previously acquired knowledge; decisional processes; and processing capacity. The cellular derangements that underlie the development of this disease have been the subject of intense investigation over the past decade. These research efforts have focused on the role of β-amyloid—particularly its encoding, expression, and processing (Cordell 1994).

Although investigators have made great strides, the full nature of the disease process still eludes them. Furthermore, even if researchers fully understood the cellular events that led to disease expression, they still would need to study how these derangements lead to cognitive impairment. The brain is a complex set of neurochemical and cognitive systems that interact exquisitely to produce higher-order cognitive and behavioral functioning. Intelligently designed therapeutic strategies for patients with Alzheimer's disease will require an understanding of such interactions and how they relate to neurochemical/cognitive system deficits in the disorder. Although treatments aimed at basic cellular deficits in Alzheimer's disease may be helpful, such therapy is unlikely to eliminate the need for direct treatment of cognitive failings in Alzheimer's disease, which probably will require agents that directly interact with specific neurotransmitter systems.

Researchers have characterized the memory problems of early Alzheimer's disease as difficulties in the storage of new information. These memory problems occur along a gradient: memory deficits become more prominent as task difficulty increases—that is, as increasing organization and rehearsal of information are needed for efficient storage and retrieval. This conceptualization has led to the hypothesis that as Alzheimer's disease progresses, internal representations of information become increasingly degraded or "noisy"—and locating, storing, and retrieving information become harder (Nebes et al. 1986).

Patients with Alzheimer's disease also develop a liberal response bias on yes/no recognition and identification tasks (Brandt et al. 1992; Corwin 1992; Snodgrass and Corwin 1988). This defect appears to be characteristic of Alzheimer's disease; it may be related to the well-known tendency of Alzheimer's disease patients to make high numbers of intrusion errors (Fuld et al. 1982).

Overall, early deficits in Alzheimer's disease might be most simply described as difficulties with new learning caused by problems in organization and consolidation of information, coupled with a "noisy" semantic memory system. The degree to which these deficits can be ascribed to particular neurochemical defects is unclear. Such deficits in cognitive operations may be secondary to loss of central cholinergic innervation (Sunderland et al. 1989); they also may be influenced by nicotinic receptor modulation (Newhouse et al. 1994).

Although researchers have described a variety of neurochemical deficits in Alzheimer's disease, explanation of the nature of cognitive disturbances in the disorder has focused on the "cholinergic hypothesis." This theory implicates disturbances in central muscarinic cholinergic mechanisms in normal cognitive functioning and disorders of memory function (Bartus et al. 1982; Drachman 1977; Drachman and Leavitt 1974). Evidence supporting this hypothesis includes significant reductions in choline acetyltransferase (Corkin 1981) and cholinergic cell number (Whitehouse et al. 1982) in autopsy-confirmed Alzheimer's disease.

Antimuscarinic drugs such as scopolamine disrupt some cognitive functions in healthy individuals (Ghoneim and Mewaldt 1977; Peterson 1977); investigators have proposed such processes as a model of cognitive deficits in Alzheimer's disease (Caine et al. 1981; Sitaram et al. 1978).

Cholinergic probes using agents such as scopolamine (Sunderland et al. 1989) and atropine (Higgins et al. 1989) have been useful in evaluating the role of muscarinic systems in cognition. In particular, antagonists that have a high degree of specificity allow researchers to identify cognitive operations affected by the interruption of agonist neurotransmission. Furthermore, investigators can compare cognitive deficits that follow drug administration of antagonists with those of specific cognitive disorders such as Alzheimer's disease to evaluate the clinical significance of certain neurochemical defects. Although any attempt to model the whole range of cognitive pathology of a complex neurodegenerative disorder with a single antagonist would be overly simplistic, the effects may indicate which cognitive domains are influenced by lesions to the affected system (Weingartner et al. 1987).

In this chapter, I review research that has focused on attempts to systematically evaluate the role of the cholinergic system in Alzheimer's disease. These studies have relied on the pharmacological challenge as their basic paradigm. The pharmacological challenge takes advantage of the relatively short half-life of cholinergic agents to examine the effects of repeated administrations of a range of doses of agonists and antagonists in patients with the disease being studied, in healthy volunteers, and in patients with related or comparison disorders. This approach enables investigators to study the acute effects of these agents and evaluate in vivo models of intact and disordered cholinergic functioning regarding how closely they mimic important cognitive and behavioral symptoms of the disease of interest. This strategy also allows researchers to assess whether there is evidence, based on dose-response shifts, for increased sensitivity to cholinergic agents (particularly antagonists)—which would suggest that cholinergic lesions observed on autopsy may have functional significance. The studies that I review in this chapter were designed to evaluate the functional relevance of the cholinergic hypothesis for the treatment of Alzheimer's disease and to guide researchers about what they might realistically expect from treatment with cholinergic agents.

Muscarinic Cholinergic Investigations

Evidence for cholinergic functional deficits in the brains of patients with Alzheimer's disease provides a rationale for studying cholinergic drugs in the disease. The nucleus basalis of Meynert in the basal forebrain, which sends cholinergic projects to the cerebral cortex, degenerates extensively in Alzheimer's disease and shows a loss of acetylcholine-containing cells (Coyle et al. 1983). Patients with Alzheimer's disease exhibit loss of cholinergic cell bodies in the nucleus basalis, with accompanying loss of cortical markers of acetylcholine—including a decrease in choline acetyl transferase (the synthetic enzyme) and decreases in acetylcholinesterase, the enzyme responsible for breaking down acetylcholine (Bartus et al. 1982; Coyle et al. 1983). Researchers also have found important correlations between decreases in cholinergic markers and the presence of pathological hallmarks of Alzheimer's disease, such as plaques and tangles (Blessed et al. 1968).

Investigators have found evidence associating acute muscarinic cholinergic blockade with deficits in several areas of cognitive functioning (Drachman 1977; Drachman and Leavitt 1974):

- Acquisition: Studies suggest that muscarinic blockade decreases the ability of organisms to store new information into memory and apparently increases the time required to learn new material.
- Retrieval: Although recall of previously learned material appears to be unimpaired, recall of newly learned material appears to be affected during exposure to the drug.
- Attention: Attention to stimuli appears to decrease, and vigilance is impaired.
- Psychomotor: The speed of performance declines.

Drachman and Leavitt (Drachman 1977; Drachman and Leavitt 1974) studied the effects of small doses of subcutaneous scopolamine in healthy young individuals, compared with healthy elderly control subjects. They showed that a small dose of subcutaneous scopolamine administered to young subjects produced a degree of cognitive impairment that was similar to the performance of elderly control subjects at baseline. This result suggested an age-related decline in cholinergic function.

My colleagues and I hypothesized that we could extend this paradigm by using scopolamine as a pharmacological probe to evaluate the functional relevance of pathological findings of cholinergic system dysfunction in healthy elderly individuals and Alzheimer's disease patients. Our initial study to assess the importance of cholinergic lesions in

Alzheimer's disease focused on muscarinic receptors (Sunderland et al. 1989). This study involved 10 Alzheimer's disease patients (mean age 58.8 ± 4 years) and 10 healthy elderly control subjects (mean age 61.3 ± 11.2 years); the patients with Alzheimer's disease had average severity scores on the Global Deterioration Scale (Reisberg et al. 1982) of 4.0 ± 0.7, indicating a moderate degree of dementia. The study involved a 3-dose, double-blind trial, with 0.1 mg, 0.25 mg, or 0.5 mg scopolamine administered intravenously.

We conducted cognitive testing 90 minutes after drug administration; the cognitive measures consisted of assessments of new learning (Buschke Selective Reminding Task; Buschke 1973), vigilance tasks (recognition of repeated words), knowledge memory (category retrieval), sustained motor effort (dynamometer), and a computer-generated continuous performance task (see Sunderland et al. 1987). Behavioral measures at 1 and 2 hours post-drug administration included the Profile of Mood States (McNair et al. 1971), the NIMH Self-Rating Scale (Van Kammen and Murphy 1975), a physical side-effect rating scale, the Beck Depression Inventory (Beck 1978), and a mood visual analogue scale. A "blind" observer also completed the Brief Psychiatric Rating Scale (Overall and Gorham 1962), as well as visual analogue scales.

The healthy control subjects showed sensitivity to the muscarinic blocking effects of scopolamine only at the 0.5-mg dose; compared with the 100% placebo-day baseline, they showed a significant decrease in category retrieval and selective reminding performance and a decline in vigilance attention performance. The healthy control subjects displayed no significant change from baseline at the 0.25-mg and 0.1-mg doses, however. These results contrasted sharply with those in the Alzheimer's disease patients: these patients showed significant declines in cognitive functioning at the 0.25-mg dose, as well as at the 0.5-mg dose, on all three cognitive tasks. In fact, the degree of change in the patients with Alzheimer's disease at the 0.25-mg dose was similar to that in the healthy control subjects at the 0.5-mg dose. These results extended to behavioral measures as well.

My colleagues and I also were interested in whether elderly depressed patients, like Alzheimer's disease patients, would show increased sensitivity to muscarinic cholinergic blockade. Depression—particularly in elderly persons—produces cognitive changes that, at sufficient severity, may resemble dementia; researchers have referred to this condition as pseudodementia (Wells 1979). Newhouse et al. (1988b) examined the effects of cholinergic blockade in elderly patients with depression. We used the same scopolamine paradigm, with nine elderly patients—six men and three women (mean age 69.7 ± 6.1 years)—with a mean severity rating on the Hamilton Depression Rating Scale (Hamilton 1960) of 29.3 ± 7.

The results of a cognitive battery across five different measures—recognition, free recall, category retrieval, selective reminding, and continuous performance—showed that these patients did not exhibit sensitivity to scopolamine except at the 0.5-mg dose. Behavioral assessment presented a similar picture. These results suggest that the cognitive pathology in elderly patients with depression does not appear to be based on muscarinic cholinergic mechanisms; thus, although severe depression in elderly patients occasionally may resemble dementia, the mechanisms underlying such depression differentiate it from Alzheimer's disease.

The results of these muscarinic cholinergic blockade studies confirm in functional terms the relevance of cholinergic pathology in the brains of patients with Alzheimer's disease. Alzheimer's disease patients exhibited much steeper dose-response curves and increased sensitivity to muscarinic cholinergic blockade, compared with healthy elderly control subjects and elderly patients with depression. Furthermore, small doses of scopolamine in healthy elderly control subjects produced a cognitive picture similar to that of dementia patients at baseline. Thus, cholinergic functioning displayed not only age-related but also disease-related deterioration. These findings, which paralleled and extended the results of Drachman and others, suggest that further cholinergic studies are justified in the hope of finding ways to improve the functioning of this system.

Muscarinic Agonist Study

A second step in understanding the cholinergic pathology of Alzheimer's disease involves examination of the postsynaptic responsivity of patients with dementia to cholinergic agonists. Tariot et al. (1988), for example, studied 12 patients with Alzheimer's disease. Rather than nonspecifically challenging a system with known cholinergic abnormalities using indirect agents, however, the investigators chose the postsynaptic muscarinic cholinergic agonist arecoline based on the assumption that many cholinergic receptors in the brain are muscarinic.

The patients in this study received infusions of placebo or arecoline hydrobromide at a dose of 1 mg/hour, 2 mg/hour, or 4 mg/hour of base on 4 test days—separated by 48 hours—in a randomized, double-blind experiment. A formal cognitive battery at 0, 10, and 90 minutes included tests similar to those used in the scopolamine paradigm. The researchers also assessed speech characteristics, grammatical form, articulation, and phrase length in 9 of the patients at 0, 30, and 90 minutes. Based on a report that Alzheimer's disease patients showed improved picture recognition after administration of arecoline (Christie et al. 1981), the patients also performed a picture recognition task.

The patients did not improve in category retrieval or free recall at any of the arecoline doses; in fact, they exhibited a significant decrease in category retrieval after the 2- and 4-mg/hour doses. Inappropriate responses on category retrieval and selective reminding tasks did not vary across drug conditions. Ratings of verbal expressiveness and word finding did increase significantly 30 minutes after the 1-mg/hour infusion. There was no significant change on the test of picture recognition; when the 4 patients who scored perfectly on this test at baseline were excluded from the analysis, however, a one-tailed t test comparing the 2-mg/hour arecoline results with placebo showed significant improvement in the 8 remaining patients.

The results of this muscarinic cholinergic agonist study suggest that acute cholinergic postsynaptic stimulation does not necessarily reverse the effects of cholinergic lesions in Alzheimer's disease. These findings contrast with a study in which Sitaram et al. (1978) found enhanced performance on serial learning in young healthy individuals receiving subcutaneous arecoline doses of 6 mg but no difference with lower doses. These results and those of Christie et al. (1981) suggest that arecoline has beneficial effects only at low doses; these findings are consistent with the possibility that the threshold for cognitive changes is reduced in Alzheimer's disease or that the dose-response curve is shifted to the left. Studies of other muscarinic agonists (e.g., pilocarpine, bethanechol, oxo-tremorine, RS-86) have been similarly disappointing.

More recent developments have suggested that muscarinic receptors may be divided into five subtypes (M_1-M_5). Certain subtypes (e.g., M_2) may act as negative presynaptic autoreceptors. Arecoline and other previously examined muscarinic agonists appear to be nonselective; they may stimulate presynaptic and postsynaptic receptors. Direct stimulation with a postsynaptic-selective muscarinic agonist may produce different results; efforts to develop such an agent continue.

Nicotinic Cholinergic Studies

Researchers' understanding of the neurobiology of the central nervous system (CNS) nicotinic receptor has advanced considerably in the past decade. Analysis of the structure of this receptor has led to recognition of multiple molecular subtypes within the mammalian brain (Heinemann et al. 1991; Luetje et al. 1990). Although researchers have not fully worked out the pharmacology of these subtypes, the development of nicotinic ligands has enabled investigators to study the distribution of these receptors in brain tissue (Schwartz 1986), as well as the effects of aging and disease on their density (Aubert et al. 1992; Giacobini 1990).

Researchers' interest in the role of nicotinic systems in the cognitive deficits of Alzheimer's disease increased after the development of techniques to image and map CNS nicotinic receptors (Schwartz 1986). Whitehouse et al. (1986) and others (e.g., Aubert et al. 1992) showed that the brains of patients with Alzheimer's disease exhibited a marked reduction in nicotinic receptor density, compared with age-matched control subjects. These results contrasted with binding studies of muscarinic receptors—which generally show little change, unless subtypes are considered (Giacobini 1990).

Decreases in receptor number do not by themselves establish that these changes are responsible for the cognitive symptomatology of the disorder, however. Researchers must demonstrate functional or cognitive consequences from the loss of these receptors or their associated cell processes in vivo.

Until recently, attempts to assess this role have focused primarily on the effects of nicotine administration. In animals, nicotine facilitates task acquisition and memory consolidation (Nelson and Goldstein 1972; Nordberg and Bergh 1985); it also improves delayed match-to-sample performance in monkeys (Elrod et al. 1988) and reverses the effects of nucleus basalis lesions in rats (Ksir and Benson 1983). In humans, researchers have reported that nicotine increases arousal and attention, decreases reaction time, prevents decline in efficiency over time, and improves the ability to withhold inappropriate responses (Wesnes and Warburton 1983).

Researchers may take a number of approaches to verify that nicotinic receptor changes produce significant effects on cognitive abilities during the course of Alzheimer's disease. In the following sections, I review a series of studies on the effects of nicotinic agonists and antagonists on cognitive functioning in younger and older healthy individuals, as well as patients with Alzheimer's disease and Parkinson's disease.

Nicotine Agonist Studies

My colleagues and I have examined the effects of intravenous nicotine on cognitive, behavioral, and physiological functioning in healthy nonsmokers and patients with Alzheimer's disease (Newhouse et al. 1988a, 1990). We initially studied 12 Alzheimer's disease patients (7 women and 5 men) with moderate dementia and 11 young healthy nonsmokers (7 women and 4 men). We administered single-blind infusions of saline placebo or nicotine bitartrate for 60 minutes at doses of 0.125 µg/kg/minute, 0.25 µg/kg/minute, and 0.5 µg/kg/minute in a within-subjects design in which the subjects provided their own controls in a test of increasing doses. We performed cognitive testing at 0, 30, and 60 minutes and at 4, 8, and 24 hours after the start of the infusion. We also assessed patients and control subjects on behavioral and physiological measures at regular intervals. We used blood sampling to measure nicotine levels and to assess the effects on certain plasma hormones.

Cognitive assessment of the Alzheimer's disease patients showed that nicotine had no significant effect on immediate correct recall of a word list. Yet there was a significant dose-related decrease in intrusion errors on this task, with a "U"-shaped dose-response curve—in other words, the middle dose (0.25 µg/kg/minute) produced the biggest decrease in errors. The decline in errors was apparent for words presented 30 and 60 minutes after the beginning of the infusion. Furthermore, this decrease in intrusions was not caused simply by response suppression; total word production was no different across doses. In addition, analysis of long-term recall showed that words that were immediately recalled under the 0.25-µg dose were significantly more likely to be recalled 8 hours later than words immediately recalled under other doses or placebo, suggesting that nicotine had an effect on memory consolidation.

Behavioral measures also showed significant dose-related changes. Both groups exhibited significant increases in depressive affect and anxiety self-ratings, particularly after the 0.5-µg/kg/minute dose. The Alzheimer's disease patients seemed to be more sensitive to adverse behavioral effects, however. Moreover, they showed significant increases in anxiety and depression at the 0.25-µg/kg/minute dose as well. These behavioral effects were closely linked to the drug infusion period; they disappeared rapidly after the infusion was terminated.

Neuroendocrine measures confirmed that the doses were active at CNS nicotinic receptors. Adrenocorticotropic hormone (ACTH) and cortisol showed significant dose- and time-related increases in both groups. The ACTH increase was evident by 30 minutes postinfusion, whereas the cortisol increase was delayed until 60 minutes postinfusion, suggesting that nicotine had no direct effect on adrenal cortical cells. Prolactin exhibited a more inconsistent response, with large elevations in some individuals and negligible increases in others; these results suggested the absence of a uniform "stress response." Reports of physical side effects generally were minimal, although some individuals complained of mild headache. Neither group reported consistent nausea. Remote telemetry showed no cardiac rhythmic disturbances.

These studies demonstrated that acute treatment with nicotine—sufficient to stimulate CNS nicotinic receptors—could produce measurable changes in short-term recall errors and long-term recall consistency. Studies by Jones et al. (1992)—using subcutaneous administration of nicotine in patients with Alzheimer's disease—found that nicotine improved reaction time, sustained visual attention, and improved visual perception, but had no significant effects on memory. Investigators generally agree that nicotine improves attention and may improve short-term memory by facilitating attention to stimuli (Warburton et al. 1986). Moreover, nicotine may have a consolidative effect on memory as well, as demonstrated by the increase in long-term recall consistency in our study and studies by others that show that information learned before exposure to nicotine is better recalled at a later time (Colrain et al. 1992; Warburton et al. 1986).

Nicotinic Antagonist Studies

My colleagues and I also examined the effects of a temporary blockade of central nicotinic receptors by the drug mecamylamine on aspects of cognition. Mecamylamine is a centrally active noncompetitive antagonist of nicotine (and presumably acetylcholine) at C6 (ganglionic)-type nicotinic receptors (Martin et al. 1989). We previously showed that mecamylamine administered acutely to young and elderly healthy volunteers produced dose- and age-related impairment of several cognitive processes (Newhouse et al. 1992, 1994). Newhouse et al. (1994) provides a detailed description of our experimental methodology. In this section, I review data from studies in young and elderly healthy individuals and patients with Alzheimer's disease.

We administered 5-, 10-, and 20-mg doses of oral mecamylamine and placebo, in a double-blind procedure. We then conducted cognitive testing at 60 and 120 minutes postadministration. This cognitive testing consisted of a computer battery, one oral memory test, and behavioral ratings. Assessment instruments included the Repeated Acquisition Test (RAT), which tests a subject's ability to retrieve previously acquired information, as well as the ability to learn new information (Thompson 1973); the High-Low Imagery Test, a recognition memory test with high- and low-imagery words (Corwin et al. 1987); a choice reaction-time (CRT) test and a manikin spatial rotation test, both from the Walter Reed Performance Assessment Battery (Thorne et al. 1985); and the Selective Reminding Test.

Mecamylamine produced dose-related impairment of acquisition of new information, with group differences in sensitivity. These results were demonstrated most clearly on the RAT task (in which subjects learn a button-pushing sequence). The young healthy individuals showed a significant increase in errors only after the 20-mg dose. By contrast, the elderly healthy individuals exhibited significant impairment after the 10- and 20-mg doses, and the patients with Alzheimer's disease showed impairment after all three active doses. There were no significant dose-related impairments in retrieval condition (old learning) in any group.

The selective reminding task (which involves verbal learning) demonstrated a similar pattern. The young healthy individuals showed a small dose-related decline in total recall but no change in recall failure. The elderly healthy individuals showed a significant and substantial increase in recall failure after the 20-mg dose, and the patients with Alzheimer's disease had increased recall failure after the 10- and 20-mg doses. On the High-Low Imagery task (a test of recognition memory), both healthy groups showed dose-related decreases in discrimination; the elderly group showed a greater effect than the young group. More interestingly, mecamylamine produced a dose-related change in response bias in the elderly healthy individuals, with a significant liberal shift after the 20-mg dose.

With regard to psychomotor speed, mecamylamine produced dose-related slowing in a number of tasks that measured reaction time, including increases in mean reaction time for the CRT and manikin tasks; although there were no significant dose by group interactions for the speed measures, older individuals tended to show proportionately greater increases in reaction time than younger individuals. Physiological effects were consistent with peripheral ganglionic blockade.

In contrast to the results with the muscarinic antagonist scopolamine, mecamylamine produced minimal behavioral effects. Although there were small changes in the scores of some observer rating scales, these changes were clinically insignificant. There were no changes in ratings of subject mood or physical side effects.

Thus, exposure to a nicotinic antagonist produced cognitive impairment on several tasks. These effects included impairment of acquisition on the RAT task, impaired recall on the selective reminding task, slowing of reaction time, and impairment of discrimination and liberalization of response bias on the High-Low Imagery task. Young healthy individuals were proportionately less sensitive to the effects of mecamylamine than elderly healthy individuals, who in turn were less responsive than patients with Alzheimer's disease. This pattern suggests a continuum of increasing sensitivity with increasing receptor loss. The lack of clinically significant behavioral changes and physical side effects implies that cognitive effects were secondary to specific blockade of nicotinic receptors, not to nonspecific effects on arousal or overall well-being.

These results suggest that the loss of central nicotinic receptors in normal aging (Court et al. 1992) and in Alzheimer's disease and Parkinson's disease (Aubert et al. 1992) have functional consequences. The deficits produced by mecamylamine resemble in several respects those in Alzheimer's disease and, to a lesser extent, Parkinson's disease. Deficits in short- and long-term memory, impaired attention, liberal response bias, and decreases in reaction time are hallmarks of the dementia in these disorders. The age-related nature of some of these effects suggests that the decline in nicotinic receptors with age produces increased vulnerability to the effects of nicotinic blockade. This model of experimental nicotinic deficits may explain the derivation of some of the deficits in Alzheimer's disease and Parkinson's disease; given the fact that these experimental cognitive deficits are not contaminated by gross behavioral or physical effects, this paradigm may have particular explanatory power.

Discussion

The foregoing studies attempted to take a systematic approach to the evaluation of the functional significance of observed cholinergic system lesions in Alzheimer's disease by using a variety of pharmacological probes to test the function, responsiveness, and sensitivity of central cholinergic neurons in Alzheimer's disease. The results of these studies and others support the role of the cholinergic system in the cognitive pathology of Alzheimer's disease. Although these findings do not imply that degeneration of the cholinergic system is the sole explanation for cognitive deterioration in Alzheimer's disease, they do support further development of drugs designed to interact with this system.

Studies with acetylcholinesterase inhibitors such as tacrine suggest modest but measurable benefits (Gracon and Knapp 1994). These agents have nonselective effects; that is, they augment all cholinergic transmission. As a result, there may be a ceiling on their clinical effectiveness—either because peripheral side effects preclude sufficient dosage to positively influence appropriate CNS transmission or because promoting all cholinergic transmission augments negative feedback as effectively as positive feed-forward mechanisms. Nevertheless, researchers continue their attempts to develop CNS-selective anticholinesterases (e.g., eptastigmine, huperzine, CI-1002, MDL 73,745, metrifonate).

Researchers have not determined whether direct-acting selective muscarinic agonists can be more effective than nonselective agents. Development efforts continue, focusing particularly on M_1-selective agents. Agents currently under development include xanomeline, PD142505, CI-979, and others.

Researchers have identified other classes of drugs that increase stimulated or evoked release of acetylcholine. These drugs act through other neurotransmitters or directly through unknown mechanisms. One example is ondansetron, which releases acetylcholine by blocking $5\text{-}HT_3$ receptors. Investigators have evaluated ondansetron in Alzheimer's disease, but preliminary results have not been promising. Linopiridine (DUP996) enhances stimulated but not basal release of acetylcholine in vitro (Zaczek et al. 1994), perhaps through mechanisms related to potassium channels. Researchers currently are evaluating linopiridine for clinical efficacy.

The possibility that clinicians might use nicotine or other nicotinic agonists as chronic therapeutic agents for cognitive enhancement in Alzheimer's disease or Parkinson's disease clearly is worth further exploration. However, nicotine presents several potential problems. First, nicotine is a complex agent with a panoply of effects—some desirable, many undesirable. For example, nicotine provokes upregulation of its own receptor after chronic administration, perhaps through desensitization (Marks et al. 1983); whether these upregulated receptors remain in a low-affinity active state is unclear (Takayama et al. 1989). Researchers also do not know whether chronic nicotine will reproduce the positive effects observed after acute administration—especially in light of the known neurochemical effects of chronic administration. For instance, whereas nicotine acutely increases the release of dopamine and acetylcholine, on chronic administration it appears to decrease dopamine turnover, at least in striatum (Kirch et al. 1987), and increase dopamine binding in the nucleus accumbens (Reilly et al. 1987).

If nicotinic receptors are involved primarily in modulating the release of other neurotransmitters, chronic agonist-induced desensitization may not have the net effect of increasing signal traffic. However, if chronic agonist exposure increases stimulated release of neurotransmitters, the overall gain of such a system may increase. This effect may be beneficial to a patient with a deteriorating neurotransmitter system; it may explain, in part, improvement on attentional tasks after administration of nicotine.

Additional limitations with nicotine include its narrow therapeutic index, its relatively high acute toxicity, and its effects on mood and anxiety. Researchers have not determined, for example, whether nonsmoking patients can tolerate, on a chronic basis, doses of nicotine sufficient to produce sustained cognitive enhancement. Moreover, nicotine's gastrointestinal and cardiovascular toxicity may be significant; such toxicity might be particularly problematic for elderly patients with other complicating conditions.

Thus, although nicotinic modulation may alleviate or improve cognitive impairments in various dementing disorders that entail a loss of nicotinic receptors, nicotine is unlikely to be an ideal candidate for this task. Development of compounds that are more selective than nicotine may prove fruitful.

ABT-418, for example, is a novel, highly selective nicotinic agonist that appears to preferentially activate the $\alpha4\beta2$ nicotinic receptor subtype in the CNS (Arneric et al. 1994). Preclinical testing suggests that ABT-418 has cognition-enhancing and anxiolytic properties, as well as a large therapeutic index; that is, unlike nicotine, its effective dose range is well below its toxic dose. Studies in humans are under way. Researchers also have developed a series of anabasine derivatives that appear to be selective nicotinic agonists (Meyer 1994). Some of these compounds appear to have cognition-enhancing, as well as cytoprotective, properties.

The Future

Pharmacological challenge studies will continue to have their place in drug development and research in dementing disorders for several reasons. First, they offer a mechanism for initial evaluation of potential effects of putative cognition-enhancing agents. Perhaps more importantly, continued investigation of the cognitive effects of selective agonists and antagonists may help researchers to understand more clearly which neurotransmitter systems modulate specific cognitive operations or domains.

This understanding, in turn, may foster more realistic and focused expectations about the cognitive changes that investigators can expect from a particular therapeutic agent. For example, considerable evidence indicates that nicotine's salutary effects on cognition may be mediated through effects on attentional functioning (Warburton and Rusted 1993). More precise evaluation of the attentional effects of cholinergic agents in patients with Alzheimer's disease is needed; such research is under way.

Ultimately, treatment of Alzheimer's disease is unlikely to be based on a single therapeutic strategy such as neurotransmitter replacement or augmentation. Future treatment of Alzheimer's disease may come to resemble treatment of other chronic diseases, such as coronary artery disease, that are not curable in the traditional sense. Diagnosed patients or at-risk individuals (identified with genetic markers) may have a variety of therapeutic approaches to consider. These treatments may involve compounds that decrease the production or increase the breakdown of β-amyloid, anti-inflammatory compounds that slow the maturation of benign plaques, and neurotransmitter augmentation therapy to improve degraded cognitive functioning. For the foreseeable future, the latter therapeutic strategy is likely to be cholinergically based.

References

Arneric SP, Sullivan JP, Decker MW, et al: Cholinergic channel activators (ChCAs) as therapeutics for CNS disorders: ABT 418 as a prototype ChCA to treat Alzheimer's disease (abstract). Neuropsychopharmacology 10(3S):395S, 1994

Aubert I, Araujo DM, Cécyre D, et al: Comparative alterations of nicotinic and muscarinic binding sites in Alzheimer's and Parkinson's diseases. J Neurochem 58:529–541, 1992

Bartus R, Dean R, Beer B, et al: The cholinergic hypothesis of geriatric memory dysfunction. Science 217:408–417, 1982

Beck AT: Depression Inventory. Philadelphia, PA, Philadelphia Center for Cognitive Therapy, 1978

Blessed G, Tomlison BE, Roth M: The association between quantitative measures of dementia and of senile changes on the cerebral grey matter of elderly subjects. Br J Psychiatry 114:797–811, 1968

Brandt J, Corwin C, Krafft L: Is verbal recognition memory really different in Huntington's and Alzheimer's disease? J Clin Exp Neuropsychol 14:773–784, 1992

Buschke H: Selective reminding for analysis of memory and learning. Journal of Verbal Learning and Behavior 12:543–550, 1973

Caine E, Weingartner H, Ludlow DL, et al: Qualitative analysis of scopolamine-induced amnesia. Psychopharmacology 74:74–80, 1981

Christie JE, Shering A, Ferguson J, et al: Physostigmine and arecoline: effects of intravenous infusions in Alzheimer presenile dementia. Br J Psychiatry 138: 46–50, 1981

Colrain IM, Mangan GL, Pellet OL, et al: Effects of post-learning smoking on memory consolidation. Psychopharmacology 108:448–451, 1992

Cordell B: β-amyloid formation as a potential therapeutic target for Alzheimer's disease. Annu Rev Pharmacol Toxicol 34:69–89, 1994

Corkin S: Acetylcholine, aging, and Alzheimer's disease: implications of treatment. Trends in Neuroscience 4:287–290, 1981

Corwin J: Assessing olfaction: cognitive and measurement issues, in Science of Olfaction. Edited by Serby M, Chobor K. New York, Springer-Verlag, 1992, pp 335–354

Corwin J, Peselow E, Fieve R, et al: Memory in untreated depression: severity and task requirement effects. Paper presented at American College of Neuropharmacology Annual Meeting, San Juan, Puerto Rico, December 1987

Court JA, Piggott MA, Perry EK, et al: Age associated decline in high-affinity nicotine binding in human brain frontal-cortex does not correlate with the changes in choline-acetyltransferase activity. Neuroscience Research Communications 10:125–133, 1992

Coyle JT, Price DL, DeLong MR: Alzheimer's disease: a disorder of cholinergic innervation. Science 219:1184–1190, 1983

Drachman D: Memory and cognitive function in man: does the cholinergic system have a specific role? Neurology 27:783–790, 1977

Drachman D, Leavitt J: Human memory and the cholinergic system. Arch Neurol 30:113–121, 1974

Elrod K, Buccafusco J, Jackson W: Nicotine enhances delayed match-to-sample performance by primates. Life Sci 43:277–281, 1988

Fuld P, Katzman R, Davies P, et al: Intrusions as a sign of Alzheimer dementia: chemical and pathological verification. Ann Neurol 11:155–159, 1982

Ghoneim M, Mewaldt S: Studies on human memory: the interactions of diazepam, scopolamine, and physostigmine. Psychopharmacology 52:1–6, 1977

Giacobini E: Cholinergic receptors in human brain: effects of aging and Alzheimer's disease. J Neurosci Res 27:548–560, 1990

Gracon SI, Knapp MJ: Tacrine: an overview of efficacy in two parallel group studies, in Alzheimer Disease: Therapeutic Strategies. Edited by Giacobini E, Becker R. Boston, MA, Birkhäuser, 1994, pp 145–149

Hamilton MA: A rating scale for depression. J Neurol Neurosurg Psychiatry 23: 56–62, 1960

Heinemann S, Boulter J, Connolly J, et al: The nicotinic receptor genes. Clin Neuropharmacol 14:S45–S61, 1991

Higgins ST, Woodward BM, Henningfield JE: Effects of atropine on the repeated acquisition and performance of response sequences in humans. J Exp Anal Behav 51:5–15, 1989

Jones GMM, Sahakian BJ, Levy R, et al: Effects of acute subcutaneous nicotine on attention, information processing and short-term memory in Alzheimer's disease. Psychopharmacology 108:485–494, 1992

Kirch DG, Gerhardt GA, Shelton RC, et al: Effects of chronic nicotine administration on monoamine and monoamine metabolite concentrations in rat brain. Clin Neuropharmacol 10:376–383, 1987

Ksir C, Benson D: Enhanced behavioral response to nicotine in an animal model of Alzheimer's disease. Psychopharmacology 81:272–273, 1983

Luetje CW, Patrick J, Seguela P: Nicotine receptors in the mammalian brain. FASEB J 4:2753–2760, 1990

Marks MJ, Burch JB, Collins AC: Effects of chronic nicotine infusion on tolerance development and nicotine receptors. J Pharmacol Exp Ther 226:817–825, 1983

Martin BR, Onaivi ES, Martin TJ: What is the nature of mecamylamine's antagonism of the central effects of nicotine? Biochem Pharmacol 38:3391–3397, 1989

McNair DM, Loor M, Droppleman LF: Profile of Mood States. San Diego, CA, Educational and Industrial Testing Service, 1971

Meyer EM: A nicotinic approach for neuroprotection and memory enhancement: studies with anabasine derivatives. Neuropsychopharmacology 10(3S):393S, 1994

Nebes RD, Boller F, Holland A: Use of semantic context by patients with Alzheimer's disease. Psychol Aging 1:261–269, 1986

Nelson JM, Goldstein L: Improvement of performance on an attention task with chronic nicotine treatment in rats. Psychopharmacologia 26:347–360, 1972

Newhouse PA, Sunderland T, Tariot P, et al: Intravenous nicotine in Alzheimer's disease: a pilot study. Psychopharmacology 95:171–175, 1988a

Newhouse PA, Sunderland T, Tariot P, et al: The effects of acute scopolamine in geriatric depression. Arch Gen Psychiatry 45:906–912, 1988b

Newhouse PA, Sunderland T, Narang P, et al: Neuroendocrine, physiologic, and behavioral responses following intravenous nicotine in nonsmoking healthy volunteers and patients with Alzheimer's disease. Psychoneuroendocrinology 15:471–484, 1990

Newhouse PA, Potter A, Corwin J, et al: Acute nicotinic blockade produces cognitive impairment in normal humans. Psychopharmacology 108:480–484, 1992

Newhouse PA, Potter A, Corwin J, et al: Age-related effects of the nicotinic antagonist mecamylamine on cognition and behavior. Neuropsychopharmacology 10:93–107, 1994

Nordberg A, Bergh C: Effect of nicotine on passive-avoidance behavior and motoric activity in mice. Acta Pharmacol Toxicol 56:337–341, 1985

Overall JE, Gorham DR: The Brief Psychiatric Rating Scale. Psychol Rep 10: 799–812, 1962

Peterson R: Scopolamine-induced learning failures in man. Psychopharmacology 52:283–289, 1977

Reilly MA, Lapin EP, Maker HS, et al: Chronic nicotine administration increases binding of [^{3}H] domperidone in rat nucleus accumbens. J Neurosci Res 18: 621–625, 1987

Reisberg B, Ferris SH, DeLean MJ, et al: The global deterioration scale for assessment of primary degenerative dementia. Am J Psychiatry 139:1136–1139, 1982

Schwartz R: Autoradiographic distribution of high affinity muscarinic and nicotinic cholinergic receptors labeled with [^{3}H]acetylcholine in rat brain. Life Sci 38:2111–2119, 1986

Sitaram N, Weingartner H, Gillin J: Human serial learning: enhancement with arecoline and choline and impairment with scopolamine. Science 201: 274–276, 1978

Snodgrass J, Corwin J: Pragmatics of recognition memory: application to dementia and amnesia. J Exp Psychol Gen 117:34–50, 1988

Sunderland T, Tariot PN, Cohen RM, et al: Anticholinergic sensitivity in patients with dementia of the Alzheimer type and age matched controls: a dose-response study. Arch Gen Psychiatry 44:418–426, 1987

Sunderland T, Tariot PN, Newhouse PA: Differential responsivity of mood, behavior, and cognition to cholinergic agents in elderly neuropsychiatric populations. Brain Res 13:371–389, 1989

Takayama H, Majewska D, London ED: Interactions of noncompetitive inhibitors with nicotinic receptors in rat brain. J Pharmacol Exp Ther 253:1083–1089, 1989

Tariot PN, Cohen RM, Welkowitz JA, et al: Multiple dose arecoline infusion in Alzheimer's disease. Arch Gen Psychiatry 95:901–905, 1988

Thompson D: Repeated acquisition as a behavioral base line for studying drug effects. J Pharmacol Exp Ther 184:506–514, 1973

Thorne D, Genser S, Sing H, et al: The Walter Reed performance assessment battery. Neurobehav Toxicol Teratol 7:415–418, 1985

Van Kammen DP, Murphy DL: Attenuation of the euphoriant and activating effects of D- and L-amphetamine by lithium carbonate treatment. Psychopharmacologia 44:215–224, 1975

Warburton DM, Rusted JM: Cholinergic control of cognitive resources. Neuropsychobiology 28:43–46, 1993

Warburton DM, Wesnes K, Shergold JM: Facilitation of learning and state dependency with nicotine. Psychopharmacology 89:55–59, 1986

Weingartner H, Cohen R, Sunderland T, et al: Diagnosis and assessment of cognitive dysfunctions in the elderly, in Psychopharmacology: The Third Generation of Progress. Edited by Melzer H. New York, Raven, 1987, pp 909–919

Wells CE: Pseudodementia. Am J Psychiatry 136:895–900, 1979

Wesnes K, Warburton D: Smoking, nicotine, and human performance. Pharmacol Ther 21:189–208, 1983

Whitehouse P, Martino A, Antuono P, et al: Nicotinic acetylcholine binding sites in Alzheimer's disease. Brain Res 371:146–151, 1986

Whitehouse PJ, Price DL, Struble RG, et al: Alzheimer's disease and senile dementia—loss of neurons in the basal forebrain. Science 215:1237–1239, 1982

Zaczek R, Chorvat RJ, Earl RA, et al: Neurotransmitter release as a possible therapy for neurodegenerative diseases: an update on linopiridine (DUP996), in Alzheimer Disease: Therapeutic Strategies. Edited by Giocobini E, Becker R. Boston, MA, Birkhäuser, 1994, pp 252–258

Chapter 15

The Spokane Elder Care Program

Community Outreach Methods and Results

Ray Raschko, M.S.W.

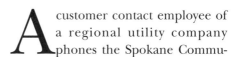

A customer contact employee of a regional utility company phones the Spokane Community Mental Health Center's Elder Services program. The utility employee is concerned about a 79-year-old woman who has been a faithful customer of the company for more than 40 years. The woman has not paid her utility bill for 2 months; when the customer service representative contacted her, she sounded "very confused" and was unable to comprehend the nature of the problem.

A bank manager calls Elder Services about a 74-year-old widowed man who comes to the bank demanding to withdraw funds from an account he had closed 2 days earlier. He refuses to believe the evidence the bank produces and accuses the bank of stealing his money.

An apartment building manager phones Elder Services concerning an 81-year-old single male tenant. The building manager describes the tenant as increasingly isolated and forgetful; the previous evening, he had a small grease fire in his apartment when he left a pan on the stove.

In each of these cases, Elder Services had trained the referral source employees as gatekeepers. Elder Services designed this structured case-finding component to identify isolated, at-risk, community-dwelling elderly individuals who do not self-refer and/or do not have a support system able and willing to refer them and provide them with access to appropriate resources.

Theory and Philosophy

Professionals in the field of aging have long argued that low utilization of mental health and other community services by at-risk elderly persons relates primarily to problems of access. In response, service providers have committed resources such as telephone information and referral, public education, transportation, and even most forms of case management in the aging system to overcoming problems of access. The underlying assumption has been that older adults—including those with dementia—know that they have serious problems, and want assistance for those problems, but do not know how or where to get assistance.

High-risk, home-dwelling, elderly persons with depression, dementia, substance abuse disorders, and/or other serious disturbances generally do not self-refer for community services, however. Almost always, they use such services only because someone else—spouses, children, other relatives, physicians, or hospitals—identifies them as being in need and assists them in overcoming problems of access (Flaherty and Raia 1994).

One-third of all elderly persons live alone (Aging America 1991), and most severe mental health problems—including dementia—have late-life onset; thus, pervasive lack of self-identification and resulting low utilization of services are understandable. Elder Services has collected referral data regarding its interdisciplinary clinical case management component for 12 years. Approximately 1% of all elderly persons referred and admitted to this program were self-referred (Table 15–1).

Community mental health providers share responsibility for low utilization, in part, because the system is passive; by waiting for elderly persons to contact them, these providers screen out individuals most at risk, especially those with no support system (Raschko 1990a). A report to the U.S. Congress by the Office of Technology Assessment (OTA 1990) recommended creation of an active case-finding system for persons with dementia to help address this situation.

When the Spokane Community Mental Health Center created and organized the Elder Services program, our major premise was that the system must first identify target populations—such as individuals with

Table 15–1. Admissions in 1993 to interdisciplinary in-home clinical case management program

Referral source	Number	%
Gatekeepers	335	37
Physicians and hospitals	275	30
Area agency on aging and funded programs	119	13
Relatives, friends, and neighbors	112	12
Other community agencies	63	7
Self	10	1

dementia who live alone and/or have an inadequate support system (or none at all)—before addressing issues of access and service delivery. Traditional case-finding efforts have succeeded in locating higher-functioning elderly persons who can seek help on their own or at-risk individuals with positive family supports. However, in almost all areas of the United States, persons with dementia who do not have positive support systems become progressively worse—until their lack of self-care, inability to care for their living environment, and/or resulting behavioral states make them visible enough to warrant their removal from the community. We therefore concluded that we could overcome service delivery problems more effectively by initiating active as well as passive referral/intake procedures to identify community-dwelling elderly individuals most at risk.

The Gatekeeper Case-Finding Component

In addition to access problems inherent in the system of care, at-risk elderly individuals are subject to conditions that may help to account for their resistance to intervention. For example, resistance often is a cover for pervasive feelings of shame, suspicion, and fear. Moreover, denial and lack of insight often reduce elderly individuals' capacity to acknowledge problems. The very nature of disorders that elderly persons often exhibit—such as memory loss, depression, anxiety, or paranoia—can render these individuals incapable of understanding and action (Raschko 1991).

The American school system—public and private—plays a gatekeeping role in identifying at-risk children, especially when parents or parental surrogates are unable or unwilling to do so. Furthermore, in the past several decades, the number of employee assistance programs in the workplace has increased considerably. One function of these programs is to identify troubled individuals who do not self-identify, whose families are unable to convince them to seek help, and whose work performance is seriously affected. The gatekeeper component created by Elder Services is an attempt to organize an identification system that functions for isolated, at-risk, community-dwelling elderly individuals as school and workplace programs function for younger persons.

Since 1979 Elder Services has trained gatekeepers on an annual basis to assist in identifying and referring isolated elderly persons. These gatekeepers are staff members and employees of Spokane businesses and organizations typically considered to be nontraditional referral sources; these businesses and organizations, however, are convinced of their importance in a community-based, long-term care system. Elder Services has developed manuals, videos, and a curriculum to provide training concerning cognitive, emotional, behavioral, and other signs and symptoms indicating that an elderly person is at risk and may not be able to remain at home.

As of 1995 the gatekeeper component of Elder Services consisted of a variety of businesses, agencies, and organizations:

- Customer contact and meter-reader employees of major electrical and natural gas utilities, as well as employees of companies that sell other forms of energy (such as furnace oil)
- Installers and other employees of the local cable television company
- Tellers and other personnel from several banks
- Letter carriers from the U.S. Postal Service
- Resident apartment managers in housing authorities, as well as in private housing
- Police and sheriff department personnel
- Code enforcement and other staff members of city and county government
- Emergency medical response teams of various fire departments
- Ambulance companies
- Residential property appraisers from the county assessor's office
- Telephone company employees

The gatekeeper component must be "owned" and operated by the system of care, not by any one member organization or business.

Research supports the underlying philosophy for establishing a gatekeeper component to identify isolated elderly individuals. Investigators have shown that an active case-finding component can overcome the shortcomings of passive case-finding systems in locating isolated, severely impaired elderly persons (Atkinson and Stuck 1991; Buckwalter et al. 1991; Gerson et al. 1992; Knight et al. 1982; Raschko 1985, 1990b, 1991; Roca et al. 1990; Toseland et al. 1979).

Establishing a gatekeeper component as part of a service delivery system requires a systematic, ongoing community organization effort. We have found that most corporations and organizations are willing to allow access to their employees. Periodic scheduled training, communication after referral, and the system's ability to work appropriately with highly resistant elderly individuals are essential in maintaining the gatekeeper component.

Interdisciplinary Clinical Case Management

Elder Services' interdisciplinary clinical case management program includes several elements:

- Active identification of the target population (gatekeeper) in addition to accepting referrals from traditional sources
- Crisis intervention available 24 hours a day, 7 days a week
- Interdisciplinary in-home evaluation and care planning
- Family and support system conferences
- Supportive therapy
- Coordination and brokering of services
- Advocacy
- Continuity of care

Elder Services provides 24-hours-a-day, 7-days-a-week crisis intervention in emergency situations for all elderly persons, regardless of whether they are active or enrolled in Elder Services. This intervention is available to all referral sources.

In nonemergency referrals, a clinical case manager and a nurse team leader conduct an initial home visit within 2 days. Their first task is to gain acceptance, engage the individual, and begin an in-home evaluation. In some cases, several visits are required simply to gain admission to the home; perseverance is a key intervention technique. We expect resistance; most often, we see it as a cover for anxiety, fear, suspicion, depression, and so forth. The case managers and team leaders have become highly skilled, however, in engaging at-risk individuals and establishing positive relationships. Whenever clinically possible—in some elderly persons with dementia, this ability has been lost—this relationship provides a conduit for evaluation, care planning, and continuity of care.

Based on the initial evaluation, the clinical case management team generates a service/treatment or care plan. This plan may include medical, psychiatric, socioeconomic, or environmental manipulation and medication modalities. When support systems exist, the team holds family conferences.

Elder Services has six clinical case management teams, each comprising three clinical case managers and one team leader. A full-time psychiatrist also is available; this psychiatrist rotates through the six teams. The psychiatrist makes home visits with team members and provides additional evaluation and treatment. The psychiatrist also provides a great deal of consultation to primary care physicians. In addition, resident physicians from Family Medicine, a residency program of the University of Washington, spend 10 hours a month making home visits with clinical case managers and providing additional evaluation and treatment.

The six team leaders do not carry separate caseloads; instead, they field-train the case managers, accompany them at initial intake and subsequent home visits, and provide daily backup. Above all, however, they add an important interdisciplinary element to the service delivery system. In our experience, clinical case management is a more effective service when the case manager is a skilled relationship builder and counselor as well as a service broker, linker, advocate, and coordinator.

The Area Agency on Aging provides half of the funding for Elder Services, which is the lead or focal agency in a system of community-based, long-term care. Elder Services integrates aging and mental health services: we can deliver a network of preventive, supportive, and rehabilitative in-home services.

We have negotiated 16 written coordination and referral agreements with other agencies, most of which are funded by the Area Agency on Aging. These agreements detail each agency's role, referral mechanisms, methods of resolving problems, and how training and other resources are shared. Clinical case managers most often use personal care/homemaker services, home health services, in-home nutrition services, day health/day care, support groups, respite care, and physician services, in addition to core services provided directly by Elder Services.

Research on the Gatekeeper Case-Finding System

The gatekeeper model's success and low cost of implementation has attracted a great deal of attention across the United States. Several replication projects are under way, and literature in the field of aging has called for additional research on the gatekeeper concept (Colenda and Van Dooten 1993).

Unfortunately, however, until recently we were unable to provide interested agencies and communities with data on the characteristics of individuals identified by gatekeepers and whether those persons differed from individuals identified by traditional sources such as relatives, hospitals, or physicians. In 1993, however, the Washington Institute for Mental Illness Research and Training submitted a grant proposal to the Retirement Research Foundation to supply this important information. Under this grant, *Clinical Characteristics and Service Needs of Elderly Referred to a Community Mental Health Center: An Evaluation of the Gatekeeper Casefinding Technique,* we collected data during 1994 on 568 persons referred to Elder Services (Dyck et al. 1995).

Gatekeepers made 34% of the referrals to Elder Services during the first 11 months of 1994. Of the remaining referrals, 32% were made by medical sources such as hospitals, physicians, and home health agencies; 35% were made by other sources, including social service agencies, relatives, friends, and neighbors. Three attributes characterized the demographic profile: age, sex, and marital status.

One of the areas in which gatekeepers had a significant influence was finding the "oldest old"—that is, persons older than 85 years. As Table 15–2 shows, the mean age at the time of referral was the same among the three referral groups. Focusing only on the oldest old, however, 38% of individuals older than 85 years were referred by gatekeepers, compared with 28% by medical sources and 33% by other referral sources.

There was no appreciable difference between the referral sources with regard to the sex of individuals referred. Of individuals referred by medical sources, 37% were men; 32% of those referred by gatekeepers and 35% of those referred by other sources were men.

With regard to marital status, we expected that gatekeepers would identify elderly individuals without spouses more frequently than other, more traditional, sources would identify such persons. In fact, marital status differed significantly across referral sources: 28% of the individuals

Table 15–2.   Referral of 102 elderly individuals by mean age, and "oldest old"

Referral source	Mean age (years)	% Older than 85 years
Gatekeepers	77	38
Medical	77	28
Other	77	33

referred by gatekeepers were married at the time of referral, compared with 39% for medical and other referral sources. Interestingly, 13% of the gatekeeper-referred individuals were persons who had never been married—compared with 2% of those referred by medical sources and 6% of those from other referral sources.

We assessed psychological isolation by asking clinical case managers to rate the emotional disturbance and cognitive impairment of each elderly person on a five-point scale (with 0 indicating no problem and 5 indicating either a major disturbance or complete impairment). As Table 15–3 shows, there were no significant differences between referral sources.

Two measures of economic status indicated that gatekeeper-referred individuals were more economically disadvantaged than those referred by traditional sources. Gatekeepers identified more elderly persons with incomes below the poverty line than did other referral sources: 45% of gatekeeper-referred individuals had incomes below the poverty line, compared with 29% of those referred by medical sources and 35% of those from other referral sources. We also asked clinical case managers to assess whether economic problems had a significant impact on the elderly person's life; 25% of gatekeeper-referred individuals had significant economic problems, whereas only 13% of those referred by medical sources and 15% of those referred by other sources were significantly affected by economic problems.

In the area of medical care, we wanted to determine whether there were any differences regarding access to a primary care physician; on these measures too, individuals differed by referral source. Thus, elderly persons identified by gatekeepers were less likely to have a family physician: 22% of these individuals lacked a primary care physician, compared with 5% of those referred by medical sources and 11% of those referred by other sources. Furthermore, gatekeeper-referred individuals were less

Table 15–3. Emotional disturbance and cognitive impairment in referred elderly individuals

Referral source	Emotional disturbance		Cognitive impairment	
	n	Mean	*n*	Mean
Gatekeeper	153	2.2	154	1.7
Medical	142	2.2	142	1.7
Other	160	2.3	161	1.9
Total	455	2.2	457	1.8

likely to have seen a physician in the month before referral; 33% had not seen a physician during that period, compared with 10% of those referred by medical sources and 20% of those referred by other sources.

A major assumption underlying creation of the gatekeeper component was that gatekeepers would locate at-risk elderly individuals who would not self-refer and who did not have someone who would seek help for them. Thus, we expected gatekeepers to find socially isolated elderly persons. Indeed, social isolation was higher among gatekeeper referrals than medical referrals but lower than "other" (Table 15–4). Other measures of social isolation supported this finding. Table 15–5, for example, shows that gatekeeper-identified individuals were more likely to live alone and more likely to have no significant other providing them with emotional support. Furthermore, when clinical case managers indicated areas that had a significant impact on the person's life, 54% of the gatekeeper-referred individuals were assessed as socially isolated, compared with 36% of those referred by medical sources and 34% of those from other referral sources.

Thus, gatekeeper-referred individuals were more socially isolated than persons referred through traditional channels. These findings lend strong support to the claim that gatekeeper-referred persons are different from others: they represent a population that traditional sources are unlikely to find and treat.

Table 15–4. Social isolation of elderly individuals by referral source

Referral source	*n*	Mean
Gatekeepers	151	2.3
Medical	141	1.3
Other	161	1.3
Total	453	1.6

Table 15–5. Elderly individuals who live alone and have no emotional support

Referral source	Live alone (*n*)	No emotional support (*n*)
Gatekeepers	64	22
Medical	48	8
Other	48	7

Elderly persons living alone constituted 52% of all referrals. As Table 15–6 shows, when all diagnoses were included, gatekeepers referred 39% of all individuals who lived alone; medical sources referred 28%, and other sources referred 32%. By comparison, Table 15–7 reflects, by diagnosis, individuals who did not live alone. Gatekeepers referred 26% of these persons, whereas medical sources referred 35% and other referral sources identified 39%.

Conclusion

At-risk, community-dwelling elderly individuals require a proactive system of care that uses an organized gatekeeper component. An integrated and comprehensive continuum of aging and mental health services can effectively maintain such persons in the community. The rapidly growing

Table 15–6.   Axis I diagnosis for individuals living alone, by referral source

Diagnosis	Gatekeeper		Medical		Other	
	n	%	n	%	n	%
Dementia	32	31.7	30	41.1	36	43.9
Depression	18	17.8	14	19.2	12	14.6
Adjustment disorder	4	4.0	3	4.1	6	7.3
Anxiety	3	3.0	7	9.6	4	4.9
Schizophrenia	4	4.0	0	0.0	2	2.4
Other	40	39.6	19	26.0	22	26.8
Total	101	39.5	73	28.5	82	32.0

Table 15–7.   Axis I diagnosis for individuals not living alone, by referral source

Diagnosis	Gatekeeper		Medical		Other	
	n	%	n	%	n	%
Dementia	18	30.5	42	52.5	43	48.3
Depression	10	16.9	15	18.8	12	13.5
Adjustment disorder	7	11.9	7	8.8	7	7.9
Anxiety	1	1.7	6	7.5	5	5.6
Schizophrenia	2	3.4	0	0.0	2	2.2
Other	21	35.6	10	12.5	20	22.5
Total	59	25.9	80	35.1	89	39.0

population of elderly individuals who live alone or have inadequate support systems will "blindside" our care systems if we do not assertively seek them out for assistance and treatment.

References

Aging America: Trends and Projections. Washington, DC, U.S. Senate Special Committee on Aging, American Association of Retired Persons, Federal Council on Aging and U.S. Administration on Aging, 1991

Atkinson V, Stuck B: Mental health services for the rural elderly: the SAGE experience. Gerontologist 31:548–550, 1991

Buckwalter K, Smith M, Zevenbergen P, et al: Mental health services of the rural elderly outreach program. Gerontologist 31:408–412, 1991

Colenda C, Van Dooten H: Opportunities for improving community mental health services for elderly persons. Hosp Community Psychiatry 44:531–533, 1993

Dyck D, Florio E, Rockwood T, et al: Clinical characteristics and service needs of elderly referred to a community mental health center: an evaluation of the gatekeeper casefinding technique. Final report to Retirement Research Foundation, January 1995

Flaherty G, Raia P: Beyond risk: protection and Alzheimer's disease. Journal of Elder Abuse and Neglect 6:75–93, 1994

Gerson L, Schelble E, Wilson J: Using paramedics to identify at-risk elderly. Ann Emerg Med 21:688–692, 1992

Knight B, Reinhart R, Field P: Senior outreach services: a treatment-oriented team in community mental health. Gerontologist 22:544–547, 1982

Office of Technology Assessment (OTA): Confused minds, burdened families: finding help for people with Alzheimer's disease and other dementias. Washington, DC, U.S. Government Printing Office, July 1990

Raschko R: System integration at the program level: aging and mental health. Gerontologist 25:460–463, 1985

Raschko R: Gatekeepers do the casefinding in Spokane. Aging 361:38–40, 1990a

Raschko R: The gatekeeper model for the isolated at-risk elderly, in Psychiatry Takes to the Streets. Edited by Cohen N. New York, Guilford, 1990b, pp 195–209

Raschko R: Spokane community mental health center elderly services, in The Elderly with Chronic Mental Illness. Edited by Light E, Lebowitz B. New York, Springer, 1991, pp 232–244

Roca R, Stoven D, Robbins B, et al: Psychogeriatric assessment and treatment in urban public housing. Hosp Community Psychiatry 41:916–920, 1990

Toseland R, Decker J, Blissner J: A community outreach program for socially isolated older persons. Journal of Gerontological Social Work 1:211–224, 1979

Chapter 16

Neurotransmitter Abnormalities and the Psychopharmacology of Alzheimer's Disease

Murray A. Raskind, M.D., and Elaine R. Peskind, M.D.

———◆———

During the past two decades, researchers have devoted substantial attention to the status of classic central nervous system (CNS) neurotransmitter systems in Alzheimer's disease. These efforts have been based on investigators' belief that delineating specific neurochemical abnormalities underlying cognitive and noncognitive behavioral manifestations of Alzheimer's disease may suggest effective approaches to pharmacotherapy.

This approach seems reasonable because of its successful application to Parkinson's disease, another common neurodegenerative disorder of later life. In Parkinson's disease, the discovery of a CNS dopaminergic deficit led to successful development of dopaminergic enhancement therapies, which effectively ameliorated motor signs and symptoms of Parkinson's disease.

Could a similar approach be equally successful in the treatment of Alzheimer's disease? In this chapter, we address this seemingly straightforward yet quite complex question by reviewing the status of several major brain neurotransmitter systems in Alzheimer's disease and the implications of abnormalities in these systems for the development and application of pharmacotherapeutic strategies.

Brain Cholinergic Systems

Research has clearly established that acetylcholine is involved in the modulation of cognitive function in the mammalian brain (Drachman et al. 1974). Investigators documented a deficiency of brain cholinergic systems in Alzheimer's disease by demonstrating decreased concentrations of the acetylcholine synthetic enzyme choline acetyltransferase, as well as nucleus basalis atrophy, in postmortem analysis of brain tissue from patients with Alzheimer's disease (Davies and Maloney 1976; Whitehouse et al. 1982). Subsequent studies confirmed a presynaptic cholinergic deficiency in Alzheimer's disease (see Davis and Haroutunian 1993).

The status of postsynaptic cholinergic receptors in Alzheimer's disease is more controversial. Although most earlier studies found unchanged muscarinic receptor binding status in Alzheimer's disease, researchers have reported increased and decreased muscarinic ligand binding (see Quirion et al. 1986). Subsequent reports suggested that high-affinity agonist binding to cortical M_1 muscarinic receptors and muscarinic receptor–G protein coupling were diminished in Alzheimer's disease (Flynn et al. 1991; Warpman et al. 1993).

Clinical studies that demonstrated increased behavioral sensitivity to centrally active muscarinic antagonist challenge protocols supported the presence of postsynaptic muscarinic cholinergic abnormalities in Alzheimer's disease (Sunderland et al. 1988). Postsynaptic nicotinic cholinergic receptors also appear to be decreased and/or dysfunctional in Alzheimer's disease (see Chapter 14).

Research findings documenting cholinergic deficits in Alzheimer's disease have stimulated numerous attempts to improve cognitive function in patients with the disorder by enhancing central cholinergic activity. Although precursor-loading strategies using choline and lecithin—in a manner analogous to L-dopa therapy in Parkinson's disease—have not been successful, investigators now generally acknowledge that muscarinic and nicotinic cholinergic agonists, as well as cholinesterase inhibitors, improve cognitive function in at least some Alzheimer's disease patients (Asthana et al. 1995; Christie et al. 1981; Farlow et al. 1992; Knapp et al. 1994; Sunderland et al. 1988). However, cholinergic enhancement strategies generally provide only modest improvement, and only a minority of patients show a clinically meaningful response to such therapy.

Other neurotransmitter and neuromodulator abnormalities in Alzheimer's disease (see "Brain Serotonergic Systems" and "Brain Noradrenergic Systems") probably contribute to disappointing therapeutic responses to cholinergic enhancement strategies. Pharmacokinetic factors also may frustrate these efforts. Soncrant et al. (1993), for example, demonstrated that a carefully titrated intravenous administration protocol could increase the percentage of patients with Alzheimer's disease responding reliably to cholinergic muscarinic agonist therapy. These investigators gave continuously escalating intravenous infusions of the mixed M_1 and M_2 muscarinic agonist arecoline to nine patients with Alzheimer's disease; five had replicable and significant memory increments, at doses that varied fourfold across patients. Cognitive response exhibited an inverted U-shaped relationship to dose: maximal improvement occurred at infusion rates of 0.17–0.67 mg/hour, whereas dosing rates of less than 0.05 mg/hour or greater than 1 mg/hour were ineffective.

Individual titration of cholinesterase inhibitor therapy to the degree of cholinesterase inhibition achieved also may improve therapeutic response to cholinergic enhancement strategies. Asthana et al. (1995) demonstrated that memory enhancement by the cholinesterase inhibitor physostigmine in Alzheimer's disease correlated directly with the magnitude of plasma cholinesterase inhibition.

Large-scale clinical trials of cholinesterase therapy (e.g., Knapp et al. 1994) did not take individual differences in tacrine or other cholinesterase inhibitor pharmacokinetics or the degree of cholinesterase inhibition into consideration in dosing decisions. Theoretically, undesirable agonist activity at presynaptic M_2 autoinhibitor receptors also may have compromised the efficacy of nonselective muscarinic cholinergic agonists. Cholinergic agonists that are more selective for the postsynaptic M_1 receptor are undergoing large-scale clinical trials.

Cholinergic Enhancement for Noncognitive Behavioral Problems in Alzheimer's Disease

Acute blockade of brain cholinergic systems can produce agitation and psychotic symptoms (Longo 1966). Two studies explored the potential efficacy of cholinesterase inhibitor therapy in Alzheimer's disease patients with disruptive agitated behaviors. Cummings et al. (1993) reported that two Alzheimer's disease patients with delusions and agitation responded as well to treatment with physostigmine as with the standard antipsychotic drug, haloperidol. In a more extensive study, Gorman et al. (1993) administered physostigmine to 13 Alzheimer's disease patients who exhibited disruptive agitation. Physostigmine and haloperidol were equally effective in reducing target symptoms, and physostigmine was better tolerated than haloperidol. Although neither of these studies included a placebo control group, they highlight the importance of exploring the possible involvement of cholinergic systems in noncognitive behaviors of patients with Alzheimer's disease.

Researchers have suggested that increased brain cholinergic activity may precipitate depressive signs and symptoms (Janowsky et al. 1972). A study of the effects of the cholinesterase inhibitor tacrine combined with lecithin on mood in patients with Alzheimer's disease (Vida et al. 1989), however, may allay this concern. These investigators used the Geriatric Depression Scale (Yesavage and Brink 1983) to evaluate the effects of tacrine combined with lecithin in 18 patients with Alzheimer's disease; they found that this approach to CNS cholinergic enhancement had no adverse effect on patients' moods.

Cholinesterase inhibitors also may affect behavior in Alzheimer's disease indirectly by modulating behaviorally relevant noncholinergic systems that are cholinergically regulated. Peskind et al. (1995) studied the effect of long-term (6 weeks) oral physostigmine treatment in patients with Alzheimer's disease; concentrations of norepinephrine in cerebrospinal fluid (CSF) were significantly lower during the period of treatment with physostigmine than during a placebo comparison period. Pomara et al. (1992) demonstrated that arecoline increased CSF concentrations of the dopamine metabolite homovanillic acid (HVA) in Alzheimer's disease, and Davis et al. (1981) found a similar increase in HVA following infusion of physostigmine.

Brain Serotonergic Systems

Serotonin appears to be involved in the mediation of cognitive function (Altman and Normile 1988), and brain serotonergic systems appear to be damaged in Alzheimer's disease: researchers have consistently reported atrophy of brain-stem raphe serotonergic nuclei in patients with the disorder (Mann and Yates 1983; Yamamoto and Hirano 1985; Zweig et al. 1988). Concentrations of serotonin and its primary metabolite, 5-hydroxyindoleacetic acid (5-HIAA), are decreased in postmortem brain tissue from patients with Alzheimer's disease (Arai et al. 1984; D'Amato et al. 1987), as is ligand binding to serotonergic receptors (Reynolds et al. 1984). CSF 5-HIAA concentrations also are reduced in Alzheimer's disease (Blennow et al. 1991; Volicer et al. 1985).

Although the data supporting serotonergic deficiencies in Alzheimer's disease probably are as compelling as data supporting cholinergic deficiencies, only a few studies have evaluated serotonin enhancement as a cognitive treatment strategy in Alzheimer's disease. For example, Olafsson et al. (1988)—a small, open, pilot study—reported significant improvement on neuropsychological tests in four of eight elderly patients with dementia who were treated with the serotonin reuptake inhibitor fluvoxamine.

In a larger double-blind, placebo-controlled study, however, Olafsson et al. (1992) found no significant improvement on neuropsychological tests—including picture recall and recognition, trail making, and finger-tapping—in elderly patients with Alzheimer's disease or vascular dementia. Furthermore, Nyth and Gottfries (1990) were unable to confirm cognitive enhancement in patients with Alzheimer's disease and vascular dementia who were treated with the serotonin reuptake inhibitor citalopram.

The patients in the two foregoing studies were diagnostically heterogeneous, however. Selection for "pure" Alzheimer's disease patients in mild to moderate stages of the disease—as is typical for Phase III studies in the United States (e.g., Knapp et al. 1994)—might improve investigators' ability to detect cognition-enhancing effects of serotonin reuptake inhibitor therapy.

However, serotonin reuptake inhibitor therapy may be effective in ameliorating noncognitive behavioral disturbances in patients with Alzheimer's disease. Deficient serotonergic activity appears to be involved in the pathophysiology of depression, at least in persons without dementia (Meltzer and Lowy 1987), and researchers have documented decreased brain serotonergic activity in persons without dementia who exhibit impulsive aggressive behavior (Eichelman et al. 1981; Greenwald et al. 1976).

In the Nyth and Gottfries (1990) study of patients with Alzheimer's disease and vascular dementia, for example, citalopram was more effective than placebo in the treatment of irritability, anxiety, fear, depressed mood, and restlessness. In a subsequent study of elderly persons with and without concomitant dementing disorders, Nyth et al. (1992) demonstrated that citalopram was more effective than placebo in the treatment of depressive signs and symptoms. Olafsson et al. (1992) found that fluvoxamine tended to be more effective than placebo for irritability, anxiety, fearfulness, depressed mood, and restlessness. In addition, several case-report studies (e.g., Pinner and Rich 1988; Simpson and Foster 1986) suggested that the serotonergic-enhancing drug trazodone may be useful in the management of disruptive agitation in Alzheimer's disease.

Brain Noradrenergic Systems

Abnormalities of brain noradrenergic systems clearly are present in Alzheimer's disease. Nevertheless, postmortem neurohistological and neurochemical studies are difficult to reconcile with studies of CNS noradrenergic activity in premortem patients.

Consistent reports of substantial loss of pigmented neurons in the noradrenergic locus coeruleus in postmortem Alzheimer's disease brain tissue (Bondareff et al. 1982; Mann et al. 1980; Tomlinson et al. 1981) support CNS noradrenergic deficiency. Neurochemical studies in postmortem Alzheimer's disease brain tissue are more difficult to interpret, however. Several studies have found decreased concentrations of norepinephrine but normal or increased concentrations of the norepinephrine metabolite 3-methoxy-4-hydroxyphenylglycol (MHPG) (Francis et al. 1985; Winblad et al. 1982). In one study of carefully obtained and preserved brain tissue from Alzheimer's disease patients who were free of antipsychotic drug treatment (D'Amato et al. 1987), norepinephrine concentrations actually tended to be increased in the frontal cortex (130% of central norepinephrine concentrations). These postmortem neurochemical studies are compatible with increased norepinephrine release into brain tissue; they suggest that reparative mechanisms compensate for the loss of locus coeruleus neurons (Bondareff 1987).

In vivo studies of CNS noradrenergic activity comparing resting concentrations of norepinephrine and/or MHPG in CSF among Alzheimer's disease patients, healthy elderly persons, and healthy young individuals produced even more unexpected results. Raskind et al. (1988), for example, found increased CSF norepinephrine in healthy elderly persons; this age-associated increase in resting CSF norepinephrine and MHPG was retained in Alzheimer's disease outpatients with mild or moderate dementia and further increased in Alzheimer's disease patients with severe dementia (Raskind et al. 1984; Tohgi et al. 1992). Thus, resting CSF norepinephrine and MHPG concentrations fail to decline—and actually may increase as the patient loses locus coeruleus noradrenergic neurons through the stages of Alzheimer's disease.

Resolution of these paradoxical findings could have important implications for efforts to understand and treat Alzheimer's disease. If locus coeruleus neuronal loss found in postmortem tissue accurately reflects a CNS noradrenergic deficiency, pharmacological enhancement of CNS noradrenergic activity might improve cognitive function (Arnsten and Cai 1993; Bierer et al. 1993). Alternatively, if in vivo CSF norepinephrine and MHPG findings accurately reflect increased central noradrenergic responsiveness in normal aging and Alzheimer's disease, this phenomenon could contribute to the disruptive hyperactive behavioral problems that frequently complicate Alzheimer's disease (Raskind 1995).

Functional studies measuring CSF norepinephrine responses to pharmacological challenges would enhance researchers' understanding of the status of CNS noradrenergic activity in Alzheimer's disease and aging. Peskind et al. (1995) recently reported the results of one such study. We compared the effects of Alzheimer's disease and advanced age on CSF norepinephrine responses with the α_2-adrenergic antagonist yohimbine, the α_2-agonist clonidine, and placebo among patients with Alzheimer's disease, healthy elderly persons, and healthy young individuals. Yohimbine-induced increases in CSF norepinephrine were greater in Alzheimer's disease patients and healthy elderly persons than in young individuals (see Figure 16–1). Ratings of tension, excitement, and anxiety following administration of yohimbine were significantly greater in Alzheimer's disease patients than in the other two groups.

The results of this study suggest that CNS noradrenergic changes in Alzheimer's disease are complex. Despite locus coeruleus neuron loss, remaining noradrenergic neurons appear capable of robust response to removal of α_2-adrenergic inhibition. The fact that this robust noradrenergic response in Alzheimer's disease patients was associated with behavioral hyperarousal suggests that abnormal sensitivity to CNS noradrenergic activation plays a role in some of the problematic agitation that occurs in the middle and late stages of Alzheimer's disease. Anecdotal reports of therapeutic reduction of agitated behaviors in Alzheimer's disease following treatment with the centrally active β-adrenergic antagonist propranolol lend some support to this possibility (Nielson et al. 1993; Weiler et al. 1988; Yudofsky et al. 1981; Zubenko 1992).

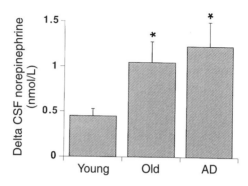

Figure 16–1. Delta cerebrospinal fluid (CSF) norepinephrine (difference between placebo and yohimbine conditions) in 18 young and 10 old healthy individuals and 10 patients with Alzheimer's disease (AD). * = greater than in young healthy individuals; $P < .05$; one-way analysis of variance followed by Newman-Keuls post hoc tests.

Effects of Estrogen on Behavior in Alzheimer's Disease

Interest in the potential use of estrogen as a pharmacotherapeutic agent in Alzheimer's disease has been stimulated by preliminary data from epidemiological and open treatment trials. Paganini-Hill and Henderson (1994), for example, estimated that the risk of Alzheimer's disease in elderly women was lower among estrogen users than among nonusers (odds ratio = 0.69) and that the apparent protective effect of estrogen increased with dosage and duration of therapy. Furthermore, Henderson et al. (1994) demonstrated that community-dwelling, postmenopausal women with Alzheimer's disease were significantly less likely to have been maintained on estrogen replacement therapy than 92 older women without dementia.

In an open trial of estradiol therapy, Fillit et al. (1986) reported memory improvement in patients with Alzheimer's disease; Honjo et al. (1989) reported improvement in cognitive function in an open trial of estrone sulfate in patients with Alzheimer's disease. The results of these pilot clinical studies, combined with evidence for the effects of estrogen on CNS systems that are affected in Alzheimer's disease and involved in cognitive function (Gibbs et al. 1994; Sherwin 1988; Toran-Allerand et al. 1992), provide a rationale for clinical outcome trials assessing the effects of estrogen on cognitive function and disease progression in Alzheimer's disease. Such clinical trials currently are under way.

Conclusion

The search for effective neuropharmacological therapies for Alzheimer's disease has enriched the medical profession's knowledge of the pathophysiology of this most common of late-life dementing disorders. Attempts to find "magic bullets" to compensate for neurochemical deficits in Alzheimer's disease have been disconcertingly complex; some of the frustration with the slow rate of progress may relate to unrealistically high expectations. Nevertheless, such efforts are beginning to result in clinically useful pharmacological agents (Knapp et al. 1994). Innovative approaches involving pharmacological enhancement strategies are likely soon to improve the management of cognitive and noncognitive manifestations of Alzheimer's disease.

References

Altman HJ, Normile HJ: What is the nature of the role of the serotonergic nervous system in learning and memory: prospects for development of an effective treatment strategy for senile dementia. Neurobiol Aging 9:627–639, 1988

Arai H, Kosaka K, Iizuka R: Changes in biogenic amines and their metabolites in postmortem brains from patients with Alzheimer-type dementia. J Neurochem 43:388–393, 1984

Arnsten AFT, Cai JX: Postsynaptic alpha-2 receptor stimulation improves memory in aged monkeys: indirect effects of yohimbine versus direct effects of clonidine. Neurobiol Aging 14:597–603, 1993

Asthana S, Greig NH, Hegedus L, et al: Clinical pharmacokinetics of physostigmine in patients with Alzheimer's disease. Clin Pharmacol Ther 58:299–309, 1995

Bierer LM, Aisen PS, Davidson M, et al: A pilot study of oral physostigmine plus yohimbine in patients with Alzheimer disease. Alzheimer Dis Assoc Disord 7:98–104, 1993

Blennow K, Wallin A, Gottfries CG, et al: Significance of decreased lumbar CSF levels of HVA and 5-HIAA in Alzheimer's disease. Neurobiol Aging 13: 107–113, 1991

Bondareff W: Changes in the brain in aging and Alzheimer's disease assessed by neuronal counts. Neurobiol Aging 8:562–563, 1987

Bondareff W, Mountjoy CQ, Roth M: Loss of neurons of origin of the adrenergic projection to cerebral cortex (nucleus locus coeruleus) in senile dementia. Neurology 32:164–168, 1982

Christie JE, Shering A, Ferguson J, et al: Physostigmine and arecoline: effects of intravenous infusions in Alzheimer's presenile dementia. Br J Psychiatry 138: 46–50, 1981

Cummings JL, Gorman DG, Shapira J: Physostigmine ameliorates the delusions of Alzheimer's disease. Biol Psychiatry 33:536–541, 1993

D'Amato RJ, Zweig RM, Whitehouse PJ, et al: Aminergic systems in Alzheimer's disease and Parkinson's disease. Ann Neurol 22:229–246, 1987

Davies P, Maloney AJF: Selectiveness of central cholinergic neurons in Alzheimer's senile dementia. Nature 288:279–280, 1976

Davis K, Haroutunian V: Strategies for the treatment of Alzheimer's disease. Neurology 43(suppl 4):S52–S55, 1993

Davis KL, Faull KF, Hollister LE, et al: Alterations in cerebrospinal fluid dopamine metabolites following physostigmine infusion. Psychopharmacology 72:155–160, 1981

Drachman DA, Leavitt J, Chicago MA: Human memory and the cholinergic system. Arch Neurol 30:113–121, 1974

Eichelman B, Elliot GR, Barchas JD: Biochemical, pharmaceutical and genetic aspects of aggression, in Biochemical Aspects of Aggression. Edited by Hamburg D, Trudeau MB. New York, Alan R. Liss, 1981, pp 51–84

Farlow M, Gracon SI, Hershey LA, et al: A controlled trial of tacrine in Alzheimer's disease. JAMA 268:2527–2529, 1992

Fillit H, Weiner H, Cholst I, et al: Observations in a preliminary open trial of estradiol therapy for senile dementia–Alzheimer's type. Psychoneuroendocrinology 11:337–345, 1986

Flynn DD, Weinstein DA, Mash DC: Loss of high affinity agonist binding to muscarinic receptors in Alzheimer's disease: implications for failure of cholinergic replacement therapies. Ann Neurol 29:256–262, 1991

Francis PT, Palmer AM, Sims NR, et al: Neurochemical studies of early-onset Alzheimer's and Parkinson's disease. Arch Neurol 313:7–11, 1985

Gibbs R, Wu D, Hersh LB, et al: Effects of estrogen replacement on the relative levels of choline acetyltransferase, trkA, and nerve growth factor messenger RNAs in the basal forebrain and hippocampal formation of adult rats. Exp Neurology 129:70–80, 1994

Gorman G, Read S, Cummings JL: Cholinergic therapy of behavioral disturbances in Alzheimer's disease. Neuropsychiatry, Neuropsychology and Behavioral Neurology 6:229–234, 1993

Greenwald BS, Marin DB, Silverman SM: Depressed 5-hydroxyindole levels associated with hyperactive and aggressive behavior: relationship to drug response. Arch Gen Psychiatry 33:331–336, 1976

Henderson V, Paganini-Hill A, Emanuel C, et al: Estrogen replacement therapy in older women: comparisons between Alzheimer's disease cases and nondemented control subjects. Arch Neurol 51:896–900, 1994

Honjo H, Ogino Y, Naitoh K, et al: In vivo effects by estrone sulfate on the central nervous system—senile dementia (Alzheimer's type). J Steroid Biochem 34: 521–525, 1989

Janowsky DS, El-Yousef MK, Davis JM, et al: A cholinergic-adrenergic hypothesis of mania and depression. Lancet 1:632–635, 1972

Knapp MJ, Knopman DS, Solomon PR, et al: A 30-week randomized controlled trial of high dose tacrine in patients with Alzheimer's disease. JAMA 271: 985–991, 1994

Longo VG: Behavioral and electroencephalographic effects of atropine and related compounds. Pharmacol Rev 18:965–996, 1966

Mann DMA, Yates PO: Serotonin nerve cells in Alzheimer's disease. J Neurol Neurosurg Psychiatry 46:96–98, 1983

Mann DMA, Lincoln J, Yates PO, et al: Changes in the monoamine containing neurones of the human CNS in senile dementia. Br J Psychiatry 136:533–541, 1980

Meltzer HY, Lowy MT: The serotonin hypothesis of depression, in Psychopharmacology: The Third Generation of Progress. Edited by Meltzer HY. New York, Raven, 1987, pp 513–526

Nielson KA, Shankle WR, Cotman CW: Neurobiological correlates of aggression and agitation in dementia provide bases for effective treatment: a study of propranolol. Society for Neurosciences Abstracts 19:400, 1993

Nyth AL, Gottfries CG: The clinical efficacy of citalopram in treatment of emotional disturbances in dementia disorders (a Nordic multicenter study). Br J Psychiatry 157:894–901, 1990

Nyth AL, Gottfries CG, Lyby K, et al: A controlled multicenter clinical study of citalopram and placebo in elderly depressed patients with and without concomitant dementia. Acta Psychiatr Scand 86:138–145, 1992

Olafsson K, Bille A, Palsby A, et al: Serotonin reuptake-inhibitor in the treatment of dementia. Nord Psykiatr Tidsskr 42:533–535, 1988

Olafsson K, Jorgensen S, Jensen HV, et al: Fluvoxamine in the treatment of demented elderly patients: a double-blind, placebo-controlled study. Acta Psychiatr Scand 85:453–456, 1992

Paganini-Hill A, Henderson V: Estrogen deficiency and risk of Alzheimer's disease in women. Am J Epidemiol 140:256–261, 1994

Peskind ER, Wingerson D, Pascualy M, et al: Oral physostigmine in Alzheimer's disease: effects on norepinephrine and vasopressin in cerebrospinal fluid and plasma. Biol Psychiatry 38:532–538, 1995

Pinner E, Rich CL: Effects of trazodone on aggressive behavior in seven patients with organic mental disorders. Am J Psychiatry 145:1295–1296, 1988

Pomara N, Stanley M, LeWitt PA, et al: Increased CSF HVA response to arecoline challenge in Alzheimer's disease. J Neural Transm 90:53–65, 1992

Quirion R, Martel JC, Robitaille Y, et al: Neurotransmitters and receptor deficits in senile dementia of the Alzheimer's type. Can J Neurol Sci 13:503–510, 1986

Raskind MA: Alzheimer's disease: treatment of noncognitive abnormalities, in Psychopharmacology: The Fourth Generation of Progress. Edited by Kupfer D, Bloom F. New York, Raven, 1995, pp 1427–1435

Raskind MA, Peskind ER, Halter JB, et al: Norepinephrine and MHPG levels in CSF and plasma in Alzheimer's disease. Arch Gen Psychiatry 4:343–346, 1984

Raskind MA, Peskind ER, Veith RC, et al: Increased plasma and cerebrospinal fluid norepinephrine in older men: differential suppression by clonidine. J Clin Endocrinol Metab 66:438–443, 1988

Reynolds P, Arnold L, Rossor MN, et al: Reduced binding of (3H)ketanserin to cortical 5-HT2 receptors in senile dementia of the Alzheimer type. Neurosci Lett 44:47–51, 1984

Sherwin B: Estrogen and/or androgen replacement therapy and cognitive functioning in surgically menopausal women. Psychoneuroendocrinology 13: 345–357, 1988

Simpson DM, Foster D: Improvement in organically disturbed behavior with trazodone treatment. J Clin Psychiatry 47:191–193, 1986

Soncrant TT, Raffaele KC, Asthana S, et al: Memory improvement without toxicity during chronic low-dose intravenous arecoline in Alzheimer's disease. Psychopharmacology 112:421–427, 1993

Sunderland T, Tariot PN, Newhouse PA: Differential responsivity of mood, behavior, and cognition to cholinergic agents in elderly neuropsychiatric populations. Brain Res 13:371–389, 1988

Tohgi H, Ueno T, Takahashi S, et al: Concentrations of monoamines and their metabolites in the cerebrospinal fluid from patients with senile dementia of the Alzheimer type and vascular dementia of the Binswanger's type. J Neural Transm Park Dis Dement Sect 4:69–77, 1992

Tomlinson BE, Irving D, Blessed G: Cell loss in the locus coeruleus in senile dementia of the Alzheimer type. J Neurol Sci 49:419–428, 1981

Toran-Allerand C, Miranda R, MacLusky N, et al: Estrogen receptors colocalize with low-affinity nerve growth factor receptors in cholinergic neurons of the basal forebrain. Proc Natl Acad Sci U S A 89:4668–4672, 1992

Vida S, Gauthier L, Gauthier S: Canadian collaborative study of tetrahydroaminoacridine (THA) and lecithin treatment of Alzheimer's disease: effect on mood. Can J Psychiatry 34:165–170, 1989

Volicer L, Direnfeld LK, Freedman M, et al: Serotonin and 5-hydroxyindoleacetic acid in CSF: differences in Parkinson's disease and dementia of the Alzheimer's type. Arch Neurol 42:127–129, 1985

Warpman U, Alafuzoff I, Nordberg A: Coupling of muscarinic receptors to GTP proteins in postmortem human brain—alterations in Alzheimer's disease. Neurosci Lett 150:39–43, 1993

Weiler PG, Mungas D, Bernick C: Propranolol for the control of disruptive behavior in senile dementia. J Geriatr Psychiatry Neurol 1:226–230, 1988

Whitehouse PJ, Price DL, Struble RG, et al: Alzheimer's disease and senile dementia: loss of neurons in the basal forebrain. Science 215:1237–1239, 1982

Winblad B, Adolfsson R, Carlsson A, et al: Biogenic amines in brains of patients with Alzheimer's disease, in Alzheimer's Disease: A Report of Progress. Edited by Corder S. New York, Raven, 1982, pp 25–33

Yamamoto T, Hirano A: Nucleus raphe dorsalis in Alzheimer's disease: neurofibrillary tangles and loss of large neurons. Ann Neurol 17:573–577, 1985

Yesavage JA, Brink TL: Development and validation of a geriatric depression screening scale: a preliminary report. J Psychiatr Res 17:37–49, 1983

Yudofsky S, Williams D, Gorman J: Propranolol in the treatment of rage and violent behavior in patients with chronic brain syndromes. Am J Psychiatry 138:218–220, 1981

Zubenko GS: Biological correlates of clinical heterogeneity in primary dementia. Neuropsychopharmacology 6:77–93, 1992

Zweig RM, Ross CA, Hedreen JC, et al: The neuropathology of aminergic nuclei in Alzheimer's disease. Ann Neurol 24:233–242, 1988

Chapter 17

Effects of a Multicomponent Support Program on Spouse-Caregivers of Alzheimer's Disease Patients

Results of a Treatment/Control Study

Mary S. Mittelman, Dr.P.H.,
Steven H. Ferris, Ph.D., Emma Shulman, M.S.,
Gertrude Steinberg, M.A.,
Abby Ambinder, Ed.D., and Joan Mackell, Ph.D.

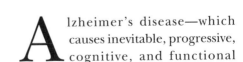

Alzheimer's disease—which causes inevitable, progressive, cognitive, and functional deterioration—poses unique problems for family caregivers. Caregivers who are married to patients with Alzheimer's disease almost invariably want to keep their husband or wife at home rather than put their

This work was supported by a grant from the National Institute of Mental Health (1R01 MH42216).

spouse in a nursing home. We set out to find out if we could help these caregivers.

For many years, counselors at the New York University Aging and Dementia Research Center (NYU-ADRC) had formed and led support groups and provided informal counseling to caregivers of NYU-ADRC patients (Ferris et al. 1985). These experiences induced us to develop a multicomponent intervention for caregivers of Alzheimer's disease patients. The goals of this intervention were to help the caregivers survive the illness and to postpone nursing home placement of the patient; the treatment program we designed successfully achieved both of these goals.

With support from the National Institute of Mental Health, we have conducted a longitudinal study to evaluate the potential benefits of this program since 1987. We restricted the study to spouse-caregivers—both because spouses are the primary caregivers for approximately two-thirds of Alzheimer's disease patients and because we felt that the impact of the illness would be different for husbands and wives of Alzheimer's disease patients than for other family members. Spouse-caregivers generally are elderly themselves, and they may no longer be in optimal physical health. Many elderly people rely largely on their spouses for companionship and become socially isolated when their spouses exhibit dementia. Unlike other family caregivers, most spouse-caregivers are living with the patient rather than in separate households.

Issues in Designing an Alzheimer's Disease Caregiver Treatment Study

The design of a caregiver treatment program must consider the nature of the illness. In particular, we had to consider the fact that Alzheimer's disease is a chronic illness that frequently lasts for many years. Previous studies of interventions for caregivers entailed treatment for a relatively short time. Haley et al. (1987), for example, compared education in groups, education and stress management in groups, and no treatment. The groups were time-limited (10 sessions), however, and after 4 months of follow-up, there was no evidence for the effectiveness of either treatment. This intervention might have been successful if it had not been terminated after such a short time.

Furthermore, with Alzheimer's disease the nature of the illness changes over time. Caregivers often report that the methods they use initially to cope with patient symptoms become useless after a short time, as these symptoms disappear and new symptoms replace them. Thus, caregivers need access to someone who can help them develop new techniques for patient management and provide them with information about appropriate resources.

Moreover, each individual caregiver has different specific problems and needs; to be effective, treatment must address these individual circumstances. An intervention that depends entirely on treatment in group settings cannot adequately address these individualized needs.

Many spouse-caregivers become homebound themselves either because of reluctance or inability to leave the patient alone or because of illness of their own. A study that requires caregivers to travel to a clinic for assessments as well as treatment probably would experience difficulty in recruiting and retaining caregivers in the study.

Although some form of control group is essential in assessing the effectiveness of treatment, psychosocial interventions generally are provided by members of caring professions such as social workers, family counselors, and psychologists. As a result, ethical considerations preclude the possibility of denying treatment entirely to anyone. In addition, preventing counselors from providing at least some assistance to every caregiver would be demoralizing. Moreover, caregivers who feel they are receiving valuable services have an incentive to remain in the study.

We incorporated several strategies to overcome the challenges we faced in designing and implementing a successful intervention study. Counselors were available on evenings and weekends so we could accommodate the schedules of caregivers and their families rather than requiring them to accommodate the schedule imposed by the typical working day. In addition, counselors went to the caregivers' homes, if necessary, for intake and follow-up assessments, as well as for individualized components of the intervention. We also designed the study to provide some basic support services to all study subjects.

The study design incorporated longitudinal follow-up to determine long-term outcome. Caregivers remained in the study throughout the course of the disease, whether the patient was at home or in a nursing home. We also interviewed caregivers 1 and 2 years after the death of each patient.

Components of the Treatment

All aspects of the treatment had a common aim: to provide support for the caregiver. Published studies, as well as our own clinical experience and research findings, indicated that the amount of support and assistance the caregiver receives from family members and others is one of the most important factors in caregiver well-being (Cantor 1983; Ferris et al. 1987; Glosser and Wexler 1985; Gwyther and Blazer 1984; Gwyther and Matteson 1983; Kahan et al. 1985; Scott et al. 1986; Simons and West 1985; Teusink and Mahler 1984; Toseland et al. 1990; Wasow 1986; Zarit and Zarit 1983; Zarit et al. 1987). Furthermore, diversity and variability in caregiver problems emphasized the need for a multicomponent caregiver treatment package, including elements designed to improve family support and provide group support, with the objective of alleviating the burden of caring for patients with Alzheimer's disease (Zarit et al. 1985a).

Increasing family and social support for caregivers was a major focus of our intervention strategy. According to Cobb (1976), social support is a mediator of stress in all phases of life from birth to death, and there is "strong and often hard evidence, repeated over a variety of transitions in the life cycle from birth to death, that social support is protective" against mental and physical disorder and improves an individual's ability to recover from illness.

Most families want to keep their impaired relatives out of institutions as long as possible. The well-being of the caregiver plays an important role in the decision to institutionalize the patient (Colerick and George 1986). Although our intervention focused on caregivers, we hypothesized that support for these caregivers also would enable them to maintain their spouse-patients at home for a longer time.

Our treatment program had three components. The first component consisted of individual and family counseling sessions. Before we designed this study, Simons and West (1985) reported that family support is an important buffer against poor health caused by stress. Zarit and Zarit (1983) proposed individual and family counseling as a clinical intervention to address problems that a group setting would not address effectively, including a caregiver's reluctance to ask for help and the involvement of potential supporters who have different ideas about what should be done.

Investigators also have suggested that individual and family counseling might improve understanding and communication between the caregiver and the family (Glosser and Wexler 1985; Teusink and Mahler 1984), resolve conflicts resulting from the impact of Alzheimer's disease on the patient's family (Gwyther and Blazer 1984; Wasow 1986), and convince family members of the need for caregiver respite (Scott et al. 1986). Prior research suggested that the extent of the burden on family members depends on their ability to cope with specific problems, their resources, and their responses to the patient's disabilities (Zarit et al. 1980). Individualized interventions address these problems most effectively.

All individual and family counseling sessions were task-oriented. These sessions had several major aims:

- Education to promote understanding of the nature of the disease and how it affects each person in the family.
- Promotion of communication, including listening, understanding, noncritical advice, feedback, encouragement, and praise where deserved, enabling family members to express and understand one another's needs.
- Problem solving: Because Alzheimer's disease is so overwhelming, we emphasized breaking problems into manageable pieces and informing the caregiver about available options. The counselor could help the caregiver choose among options and put them into practice to solve a particular piece of the problem. The counselor also would make the family and caregiver aware of all of the formal and informal services that were available and provide information about auxiliary resources at affordable prices, as well as where to obtain legal and financial advice.
- Patient behavior management: Counseling sessions incorporated role-play exercises to illustrate techniques for possible prevention or handling of difficult situations.
- Concrete planning to enhance caregiver support: This element included having family members other than the designated primary caregiver agree to an explicit plan to take over specific tasks to relieve the caregiver and getting the family to provide emotional support to the caregiver by scheduling activities with the primary caregiver but without the patient.
- Making families aware of the availability of psychopharmacological treatment to manage treatable dementia symptoms (e.g., depression, agitation, night-time wandering).

The second component of the intervention entailed ongoing support-group participation by the primary caregiver. These caregiver support groups were led by individuals experienced in working with caregivers and Alzheimer's disease patients, the family counselors conducting this study, counselors at the Alzheimer's Association, or counselors trained by or known to them.

A major focus of these group sessions was to provide a place for caregivers to express their feelings. Caregivers discussed how the illness affected their relationships with patients and other family members. The process of learning how to cope with Alzheimer's disease and deal with changes in patients who were becoming dependent on them helped caregivers develop techniques for managing problems provoked by the illness. The caregiver support-group leaders provided education about Alzheimer's disease and suggested appropriate resources for information and referral. These sessions also included discussion about financing long-term care, obtaining health care proxies, powers of attorney, and other issues. Group members learned techniques from each other for how to manage the competing demands on their time from their own needs, the needs of other family members, and the need to provide care to the patient; how to hire and manage paid help for the caregiver; and how to cope with problem patient behaviors.

The third component of the treatment consisted of unlimited ad hoc consultation. We did not originally formulate this element as a separate component of the treatment; as the study progressed, however, we became aware of the importance of the availability of the counselor to the caregiver and the family for help as they themselves determined the need for it. Coming to terms with the fact that the Alzheimer's disease patient, though physically unchanged, is no longer the person the caregiver once knew is difficult—and takes time. Ad hoc consultation was a vital component of the intervention; it acknowledged and addressed the constantly changing nature of the disease and its demands on the family, as well as the necessity for ongoing crisis intervention.

Counselors were available for telephone consultation at any time, including evenings and weekends in the event of a crisis. The need for ad hoc consulting varied; it depended, in part, on whether the patient's dementia symptoms were stable or changing and whether the caregiver was having conflicts with other demands or other family members. Counselors provided informal consultation for a variety of reasons, including changes in symptoms of dementia in the patient; physical problems of the patient and/or the caregiver; requests for and complaints about physicians, attorneys, aides, social services, nursing homes, and other individuals or services; miscellaneous family problems; the need for additional resource information; and changes in family composition and location.

The treatment schedule provided for individual and family counseling in the first 4 months after intake into the study. Treatment began with an individual counseling session; during that session, the counselor asked the caregiver to list family members he or she wanted to participate in subsequent family sessions. Four family counseling sessions followed, at times and places that were convenient for the caregiver and family members. These sessions could be held at NYU-ADRC, in the home of the caregiver or another family member, or at some other location specified by the caregiver. Treatment also included an additional individual counseling session with the spouse-caregiver.

The intervention protocol mandated that caregivers join a support group meeting weekly. Caregivers also were informed at intake into the study that consultation with the counselor was available to them and their families at any time. In addition, counselors provided resource information and referrals for auxiliary help, financial planning, and management of patient behavior problems.

Study Design

To be eligible for the study, subjects had to be married to a patient with Alzheimer's disease who had received a diagnosis from NYU-ADRC or another qualified medical facility. Caregivers had to be living with the patient at the time of intake into the study and to have at least one family member in the New York City metropolitan area.

The study was modeled after standard drug trial protocols. Caregivers were randomly assigned to a treatment group or a control group. All caregivers who agreed to participate completed an extensive structured intake interview. After the interview, the counselor opened a sealed envelope containing the caregiver's group assignment.

Each caregiver in the treatment group underwent all of the interventions, and each was provided with support for an unlimited time. Regular follow-up interviews of all caregivers contained all measures used in the intake interview. These follow-up interviews were conducted every 4 months for the first year and every 6 months thereafter.

This schedule was maintained when a patient entered a nursing home. The schedule was modified, however, when a patient died: in that case, the caregiver participated in two short, unstructured interviews—for the purpose of maintaining contact only—6 and 18 months after the death of the patient, and two structured interviews (eliminating the elements that dealt with patient care) 1 and 2 years after the patient's death.

Although the intake and follow-up interviews included structured instruments, counselors conducted these interviews informally, listening carefully to the caregivers' problems. Caregivers have told the counselors that they considered these sessions helpful.

The study design mandated that caregivers in the control group receive resource information and help on request only; these caregivers received no formal treatment. In reality, however, we provided some services to all caregivers. In fact, we received many letters of appreciation from caregivers in the control group, thanking counselors for their help. Caregivers in both groups reported that one of the most important things we provided was someone to listen to their problems. Moreover, we did not differentiate between treatment and control group caregivers if they asked for help in emergencies.

We provided resource information to any caregiver on request. In addition, NYU-ADRC publishes regular newsletters, which include tips about patient care, as well as other information about the latest advances in Alzheimer's disease research; we sent these newsletters to all caregivers in the study. We also sent birthday cards to all caregivers. These birthday cards were a symbol of the caring attitude we wanted to convey to our patients and caregivers, and caregivers frequently called us to thank us for remembering them.

One major difference between the support we provided to caregivers in the treatment and control groups involved counselors' responses to caregivers' telephone inquiries: treatment group caregivers received active help, whereas control group caregivers received only the information they requested. For example, if a caregiver in the control group telephoned to ask a counselor about hiring an aide, the counselor would provide the caregiver with the names and phone numbers of several agencies or aides they felt comfortable recommending. If a caregiver in the treatment group called with the same request, however, he or she would receive information on how to hire and train an aide; in some cases, counselors visited the homes of treatment group caregivers and trained the aides themselves.

Another important difference between the two groups was that the treatment group caregivers and their families took part in six formal, scheduled counseling sessions; no one in the control group received formal counseling. As a result, the counselors knew and interacted with the families of patients and caregivers, as well as caregivers themselves, in the treatment group; in the control group, however, they knew only the caregivers. Family members of treatment group caregivers frequently called counselors for advice or help with problems they were having with the primary caregivers or with the patients, whereas family members of control group caregivers never had contact with the counselors. Thus, the level of support provided to caregivers and their families was far greater in the treatment group than in the control group.

The emphasis placed on participation in a support group also was quite different between the two groups. Such participation was required of treatment caregivers, who agreed in writing to join a support group at the time of intake into the study. Of course, control group caregivers could initiate support group participation on their own, but the counselors did not urge them to do so.

Caregivers in both groups completed a large, comprehensive battery of structured questionnaires at intake and at each follow-up interview. All primary caregivers of NYU-ADRC research subjects complete the caregiver questionnaire as part of the standard patient evaluation protocol; caregivers recruited from elsewhere completed this questionnaire on entry into the study. All caregivers completed the entire caregiver assessment battery. This battery evaluates several dimensions of caregiver well-being including psychological, physical, financial, and environmental problems and social support. It also includes an evaluation of patient and family problems, with particular emphasis on issues and problems relevant to caregiver well-being and the precipitation of institutionalization.

The caregiver assessment battery included several elements:

- Caregiver questionnaire (developed at NYU-ADRC); readministered if more than 1 month had elapsed between entry into the study and previous administration
- Caregiver physical health questionnaire, adapted from the physical health questionnaire in Older American Resources and Services (OARS) (Duke University 1978)
- Patient physical health questionnaire, adapted from physical health questionnaire in OARS (Duke University 1978)
- Social network list, including satisfaction scale (Stokes 1983)
- Family cohesion, from Family Adaptability and Cohesion Evaluation Scale (Faces III) (Olson et al. 1987)
- Short Psychiatric Evaluation Scale (SPES) (Pfeiffer 1979)
- Affective Rating Scale (Yesavage et al. 1983)
- Burden interview (Zarit et al. 1985a)
- Memory and Behavior Problems Checklist (Zarit et al. 1985b)
- Caregiver home evaluation (safety checklist developed at NYU-ADRC)
- NEO Personality Inventory (Costa and McCrae 1985)

Results

Recruitment into the original study (Mittelman et al. 1995) ended in February 1991 with the enrollment of 206 caregivers. (We currently are enrolling a second group of 200 caregivers.) Table 17–1 presents some characteristics of the study subjects. Of the caregivers, 58% were women, and 42% were men. At intake into the study, 32% of the patients had mild dementia (Global Deterioration Scale [GDS] 4), 40% had moderate dementia (GDS 5), and 28% had moderately severe dementia (GDS 6) (Reisberg et al. 1982). We have continued the intervention with the original group of caregivers, evaluating all subjects at regular intervals to assess the long-term consequences of the intervention and caregiving in general.

The results of our study indicate that caregivers in the treatment group benefited greatly from the intervention. Most spouse-caregivers were reluctant to place their husbands or wives in institutions; a primary benefit of the program was that it enabled caregivers in the treatment group to maintain their spouses at home.

Effect of Intervention on Nursing Home Placement and Death of Patients

As of August 1, 1995, 25.2% of treatment group patients were still at home, compared with 12.6% of control group patients. Moreover, caregivers in the treatment group postponed placement of patients into nursing homes considerably longer than caregivers in the control group. Since the beginning of the study, 52 treatment group caregivers and 65 control caregivers had placed patients in nursing homes (see Table 17–2). Furthermore, caregivers in the treatment group kept patients who eventually were placed in nursing homes at home for an average of 194 days

Table 17–1.   Study variables at baseline

Variable	
Caregiver gender	Female = 58%
	Male = 42%
Severity of patient dementia (GDS)	Mild = 32%
	Moderate = 40%
	Moderately severe = 28%

(approximately 4.6 months) longer than caregivers in the control group. Many more patients in the control group died (67) than patients in the treatment group (45), and virtually all of the excess deaths occurred among patients who had been placed in nursing homes: 25 patients in each group died while living at home, whereas 42 patients in the control group died after nursing home placement versus 20 patients in the treatment group.

Because caregivers were randomly assigned to the treatment and control groups, and there was no significant difference in GDS or physical health status at intake in the two groups, the higher number of deaths among control group patients cannot be attributed to the fact that one group had more severe dementia than the other at intake. The fact that the time from nursing home placement to death was less among control group patients than among treatment group patients may indicate that patients in the control group were more physically ill at the time of nursing home placement than those in the treatment group. Although our intervention strategy was not designed specifically to maintain the physical health of patients, the extra education and counseling that the treatment group caregivers and their families received may have provided an unintended benefit in this regard.

The effect of our intervention strategy on nursing home placements was particularly striking in the first 12 months after intake into the study (see Table 17–3). During this period, 35 patients were placed in nursing homes. Fewer than half as many treatment group patients (11) were placed in nursing homes as control group patients (24), however (χ^2 = 5.8, P < .05) (Mittelman et al. 1993).

Table 17–2.   Effects of intervention: average number of days from intake to outcome

| Outcome | Treatment group | | Control group | | Difference |
	Days	N	Days	N	(days)
Patient placed in nursing home	810.2	52	640.5	65	169.7
Patient died	1,032.8	45	1,025.4	67	7.4
After nursing home placement	1,366.8	20	1,053.8	42	313.0
While living at home	765.7	25	977.8	25	–212.1
Caregiver died	1,479.9	12	807.6	11	672.5
Total time patients have remained at home	1,087.4	103	893.5	103	193.9

We also used hierarchical logistic regression to assess the effects of treatment and other predictors on nursing home placement. We entered caregiver gender, caregiver age, patient age, patient income, and caregiver difficulties with patient behavior into the multiple predictor model, one at a time, as covariates. We then estimated the effect of treatment group membership over and above the effects of these covariates. Being in the treatment group rather than in the control group had a statistically significant effect ($\chi^2 = 4.4$, $P < .05$). Controlling for caregiver sex and age, patient age, income, and need for assistance with activities of daily living, the odds of nursing home placement for treatment group patients were less than half those for control group patients (odds ratio = 0.40).

Effect of Intervention on Depression in Caregivers

Researchers have frequently documented the negative effects that living with and caring for a family member with Alzheimer's disease have on the mental health of caregivers. Previous systematic studies of interventions for caregivers of patients with dementia (e.g., Haley et al. 1987; Kahan et al. 1985; Lawton et al. 1989) have demonstrated little or no effect on depression.

We examined the effect of our intervention strategy on depression reported by caregivers ($N = 206$) in the first year after intake into the study (Mittelman et al. 1995). We hypothesized that caregivers in the treatment group would become less depressed or remain stable, whereas caregivers in the control group would become more depressed.

Table 17–3.   Outcome 12 months after baseline

Status	Treatment group (N = 103)		Control group (N = 103)		Total (N = 206)	
	n	%	n	%	n	%
Patient at home	83	80.6	74	71.8	157	76.2
Patient placed in nursing home	11	10.7	24	23.3	35	17.0
Patient died before nursing home placement	9	8.7	5	4.9	14	6.8
Patient died after nursing home placement	0	0.0	4	3.9	4	1.9

We measured caregiver depression at intake and all follow-up evaluations with the Geriatric Depression Scale (Yesavage et al. 1983), a 30-item symptom checklist (α = .94). At intake, more than 40% of the caregivers (50% of the women and 30% of the men) had scores of 11 or higher, indicating possible clinical depression; this cutoff has a sensitivity of .84 and a specificity of .95 for clinical depression (Brink et al. 1982). The mean score at intake was 9.8 (SD = 6.5).

Overall, the intervention had a positive effect on depression among caregivers (Mittelman et al. 1995). Because a multivariate analysis of covariance found a significant positive interaction between time and treatment group membership, we conducted three hierarchical multiple regression analyses, corresponding to the change from baseline to the three follow-ups (4, 8, and 12 months) in the first year after intake (see Table 17–4). The difference in the amount of change in depression between the treatment and control groups increased from the 4-month (b = –.71, F = 1.25, not significant) to the 8-month (b = –1.35, F = 5.02, P < .05) to the 12-month follow-up (b = –2.91, F = 15.94, P < .001); the control group became more depressed, while the treatment group remained stable. By the 12-month follow-up, the average difference between the treatment and control groups was almost three points.

Not surprisingly, depression at baseline was a significant predictor of depression at follow-up, although the effect of baseline depression on follow-up depression decreased with time. Although analysis of baseline data suggested that female caregivers entered the study with significantly more depressive symptoms than male caregivers (b = 3.13, t = 3.5, P < .001), the caregiver's sex was not a significant predictor of change in depression from baseline to follow-up. Increase in severity

Table 17–4.   Predictors of depression at follow-up

		Months from baseline		
Step	Predictor	4 (n = 192)	8 (n = 181)	12 (n = 173)
1	Depression at baseline	.83[a]	.80[a]	.67[b]
2	Caregiver female	.75	–.37	.61
3	Increase in severity of dementia in patient	2.26[a]	.60	.54
4	Treatment group	–.71	–1.35[c]	–2.91[a]

Note.   Figures are unstandardized regression coefficients.
[a]P < .001; [b]P < .01; [c]P < .05

of patient dementia was a significant predictor of increase in symptoms of depression in the caregiver only from baseline to the 4-month follow-up (b = 2.26, F = 9.17, P < .001); this factor was less predictive and not statistically significant at later follow-ups. Further exploratory analyses showed that differential improvement in satisfaction with social networks in the treatment and control groups accounted for about half of the difference in change in depression between the two groups.

Changes in depression were small for most caregivers, but 21% of caregivers (n = 44) changed more than one standard deviation (7 points or more) between baseline and 12-month follow-up. Moreover, 71% of treatment group caregivers who changed substantially became less depressed, compared with 30% of control group caregivers. These findings suggest that the NYU-ADRC intervention has the potential to alleviate some of the deleterious effects of caregiving on mental health.

Effect of Intervention on Social Support for Caregivers

Which aspects of the intervention contributed to the effectiveness of the treatment? Many researchers have theorized that social support mediates the stress of caring for a patient with Alzheimer's disease (Pearlin et al. 1990).

We examined the effect of our intervention strategy on caregivers' social systems to help explicate the effects of the treatment on depression in caregivers. We conducted two sets of hierarchical regression analyses. The results showed that caregivers in the treatment group experienced greater family cohesion (as measured by scores on FACES III) than those in the control group. The intervention also had a marked effect on caregivers' satisfaction with their social networks, which increased from baseline to the 4-month follow-up and still further from baseline to the 8-month follow-up.

We inferred that family counseling, which occurred in the first 4 months, and participation in a support group, which began after the 4-month follow-up, each added to the satisfaction of caregivers with their social support. Caregivers frequently included family counselors in their lists of members of social networks with whom they felt close. Thus, by directly providing caregivers with social support in their relationships with family counselors, the intervention increased caregivers' satisfaction with their social networks. The difference between the treatment and control groups did not diminish with time—predictably, because the availability of family counselors and support groups also remained constant.

The intervention enhanced social support for caregivers within 4 months of intake into the study (see Table 17–5), whereas its effect on caregiver depression became substantial only at later follow-up points. Social support was a significant predictor of depression cross-sectionally at baseline. This finding provides evidence to substantiate the theory that social support mediates between the primary stress of caregiving, as well as outcomes such as depression.

Conclusion

The results of the NYU-ADRC caregiver study indicate that the intervention achieved both of its goals. It significantly improved the ability of spouse-caregivers to cope with Alzheimer's disease and thereby significantly postponed nursing home placement.

The results of this study demonstrate that a multicomponent intervention can be effective in improving social support for the primary caregiver, largely by increasing the involvement of other family members in addition to the spouse. At follow-up interviews, caregivers in the treatment group reported increased family cohesion and greater satisfaction with the informal support provided by family and friends. This increase in social support appears to have a substantial effect on depression among some caregivers.

The intervention also was instrumental in enabling caregivers to postpone or avoid placing patients in nursing homes. This finding is especially

Table 17–5. Predictors of caregiver satisfaction with social network at follow-up

		Months from baseline		
Step	Predictor	4 ($n = 192$)	8 ($n = 181$)	12 ($n = 173$)
1	Satisfaction with social network at baseline	.73[a]	.59[b]	.58[a]
2	Caregiver female	−.22	.02	.05
3	Increase in severity of dementia in patient	−.23	−.09	.24
4	Increase in family cohesion	.02[c]	.03[c]	.04[b]
5	Treatment group	.48[a]	.66[a]	.68[a]

Note. Figures are unstandardized regression coefficients.
[a]$P < .001$; [b]$P < .01$; [c]$P < .05$

notable: if a pharmacological treatment produced equivalent effects on time to institutionalization, it would be hailed as a major breakthrough.

Clearly, the broad application of strategies similar to those embodied in the NYU-ADRC intervention would be likely to have a major impact on the social and economic cost of Alzheimer's disease. We are currently conducting research at NYU-ADRC to determine the economic cost of caregiving and the economic benefit of the intervention.

References

Brink TL, Yesavage JA, Owen L, et al: Screening tests for geriatric depression. Clin Gerontol 1:37–43, 1982

Cantor M: Strain among caregivers: a study of experience in the United States. Gerontologist 23:597–604, 1983

Cobb S: Social support as a moderator of life stress. Psychosom Med 38:300–314, 1976

Colerick EJ, George LK: Predictors of institutionalization among caregivers of patients with Alzheimer's disease. J Am Geriatr Soc 34:493–498, 1986

Costa PT, McCrae RR: The NEO Personality Inventory Manual. Odessa, FL, Psychological Assessment Resources, 1985, pp 1–43

Duke University, Center for the Study of Aging & Human Development: Multidimensional Functional Assessment: The OARS Methodology, 2nd Edition. Durham, NC, Duke University Press, 1978

Ferris SH, Steinberg G, Shulman E, et al: Institutionalization of Alzheimer's disease patients: reducing precipitating factors through family counseling. Home Health Care Serv Q 8:23–51, 1987

Glosser G, Wexler D: Participants' evaluation of educational/support groups for families of patients with Alzheimer's disease and other dementias. Gerontologist 25:232–238, 1985

Gwyther LP, Blazer DG: Family therapy and the dementia patient. Am Fam Physician 29:149–156, 1984

Gwyther LP, Matteson MA: Care for caregivers. J Gerontol Nurs 9:93–116, 1983

Haley WE, Brown SL, Levine EG: Family caregiver appraisals of patient behavioral disturbance in senile dementia. Clin Gerontol 6:25–34, 1987

Kahan J, Kemp B, Staples FR, et al: Decreasing the burden in families caring for a relative with a dementing illness. J Am Geriatr Soc 33:664–670, 1985

Lawton MP, Brody EM, Superstein AR: A controlled study of respite service for caregivers of Alzheimer's patients. Gerontologist 29:8–16, 1989

Mittelman M, Ferris S, Steinberg G, et al: An intervention that delays institutionalization of Alzheimer's disease patients: treatment of spouse-caregivers. Gerontologist 33:730–740, 1993

Mittelman M, Ferris S, Shulman E, et al: A comprehensive support program: effect on depression in spouse-caregivers of AD patients. Gerontologist 35: 792–802, 1995

Olson DH, Portner J, Lavee Y: Family Adaptability and Cohesion Evaluation Scales III, in Handbook of Measurements for Marriage and Family Therapy. Edited by Fredman N, Sherman R. New York, Brunner/Mazel, 1987, pp 181–184

Pearlin LI, Mullin JT, Semple SJ, et al: Caregiving and the stress process: an overview of concepts and their measures. Gerontologist 30:583–594, 1990

Pfeiffer E: A short psychiatric evaluation schedule: a new 15-item monotonic scale indicative of functional disorder, in Brain Function in Old Age: Proceedings of Bayer Symposium VII. New York, Springer-Verlag, 1979, pp 228–236

Reisberg B, Ferris SH, deLeon MJ, et al: The global deterioration scale for assessment of primary degenerative dementia. Am J Psychiatry 139:1136–1139, 1982

Scott JP, Roberto KA, Hutton JT: Families of Alzheimer's victims: family support to the caregivers. J Am Geriatr Soc 34:348–354, 1986

Simons RL, West GE: Life changes, coping resources, and health among the elderly. Int J Aging Hum Dev 20:173–189, 1985

Stokes JP: Predicting satisfaction with social support from social network structure. Am J Community Psychol 11:141–152, 1983

Teusink JP, Mahler S: Helping families cope with Alzheimer's disease. Hosp Community Psychiatry 35:152–156, 1984

Toseland RW, Rossiter CM, Peak T, et al: Comparative effectiveness of individual and group interventions to support family caregivers. Social Work 35:209–217, 1990

Wasow M: Support groups for family caregivers of patients with Alzheimer's disease. Soc Work 31:93–97, 1986

Yesavage JA, Brink TL, Rose TL, et al: The geriatric depression rating scale: comparison with other self-report and psychiatric rating scales, in Assessment in Geriatric Psychopharmacology. Edited by Crook T, Ferris SH, Bartus R. New Canaan, CT, Mark Powley Associates, 1983, pp 153–165

Zarit SH, Anthony CR, Boutselis SM: Interventions with caregivers of dementia patients: comparison of two approaches. Psychol Aging 2:225–232, 1987

Zarit SH, Zarit JM: Families under stress: interventions for caregivers of senile dementia patients. Psychotherapy 19:461–471, 1983

Zarit S, Reever K, Bach-Peterson J: Correlates of feelings of burden. Gerontologist 20:649–655, 1980

Zarit SH, Orr NK, Zarit JM: The burden interview, in Families Under Stress: Caring for the Patient With Alzheimer's Disease and Related Disorders. New York, New York University Press, 1985a

Zarit SH, Orr NK, Zarit JM: The memory and behavior problems checklist, in Families Under Stress: Caring for the Patient With Alzheimer's Disease and Related Disorders. New York, New York University Press, 1985b

Chapter 18

Caring for Persons With Dementing Illnesses
A Current Perspective

Peter V. Rabins, M.D., M.P.H.

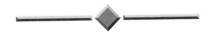

Throughout this century, most people with dementia have been cared for by family members in their homes. There are currently approximately 3 million persons in the United States with dementia; 2 million of these individuals reside at home. There are many misconceptions about the care that patients with dementia receive. For example, although people widely believe that Americans simply "dump" frail elderly persons into nursing homes, numerous studies demonstrate that nursing home residents with dementia are more severely ill, older, and less likely to have children or relatives available to care for them than those living at home (Colerick and George 1986). Moreover, clinical experience suggests that many families delay placement as long as possible—sometimes to the detriment of the patient and the family.

Nevertheless, institutions have played an important role in the care of the most severely ill persons. In 1920 approximately 18% of patients admitted to New York State mental facilities had organic mental disorders (Grob 1983). Although some of these individuals undoubtedly had neurosyphilis, many had the dementing illnesses that we now refer to as vascular dementia and Alzheimer's disease. Indeed, Alois Alzheimer himself was the superintendent of a psychiatric hospital; his early descriptions of both vascular dementia (Alzheimer 1896) and Alzheimer's disease (Alzheimer 1987) remain classics.

Although state psychiatric hospitals still provide care for a small number of severely ill persons with dementia, nursing homes have become the locus of care for most persons with dementia who require institutional care (Rovner et al. 1986). Approximately one-third of all persons with dementia reside in such institutions. Researchers know little about professional caregivers, however; clearly, more study of this important group is needed. In this chapter, therefore, I focus on persons who provide caregiving to family members at home; investigators have studied this group most extensively.

Caregiving and Caregiver Morbidity

Recognition that caring for persons with dementia can have significant adverse effects on family members dates to studies in Great Britain during the mid-1960s (Grad and Sainsbury 1963, 1968). In the late 1970s, pioneering work by Lezak (1978), Zarit et al. (1980), and others in the United States led to an explosion of research on the effects of caregiving on the family care provider.

Many studies have shown that some family members experience adverse emotional and physical outcomes that relate to their roles as caregivers (e.g., Baumgarten et al. 1994; Cohen and Eisdorfer 1988; George and Gwyther 1986; Gilleard et al. 1984; Grafstrom et al. 1992; Haley et al. 1987a; Rabins et al. 1982). Although the study methodologies and rates of reported morbidity varied widely, the median rate of negative impact in most studies was approximately 40%—two to three times higher than base rates of emotional distress in general population surveys.

Several caveats apply to these findings, however. Most studies, for example, examined care providers of persons attending memory assessment clinics, research programs, or social service agencies. Individuals who do not use these services probably are different in many ways from those who do (O'Connor et al. 1990). The results of a community-based study from England (Eagles et al. 1987) support this conjecture; the study found that the rates of emotional morbidity in elderly caregivers were no higher than those in noncaregivers.

The measures these investigators used to detect distress also varied widely in their psychometric properties. Some were developed to measure emotional or physical disorders in a variety of settings; others were specific to the caregiving setting. For example, Zarit introduced the term *burden* and developed an instrument to measure the concept in the late 1970s (Zarit et al. 1980). Yet although researchers have used this scale widely, they have not firmly established its validity. Moreover, burden probably is a multidimensional concept (Deimling and Bass 1986) that is influenced more by the caregiver's perception of the disease than by objective measures of disease severity (see Wright et al. 1993).

Nevertheless, recognition that dementia can have significant adverse effects on the physical and psychological well-being of family care providers (Kiecolt-Glaser et al. 1990; O'Connor et al. 1990) and demonstration of the extensive efforts that many caregivers undertake in attempting to keep the person with dementia at home as long as possible (Hinrichsen and Niederehe 1994) have been important advances in researchers' understanding of the social context of chronic care. Continued development of valid outcomes measures is needed (e.g., Gerritsen and van der Ende 1994).

The positive aspects of caregiving often are lost in such studies. Many caregivers report that providing care has emotional and spiritual rewards (Gilhooly 1984; Lawton et al. 1991). For example, one-third of the caregivers in a small convenience sample study reported a positive overall mood (Rabins et al. 1990a). Investigators' tendency to focus on the negative outcomes of caregiving may arise from their desire to bring the problem to public attention and increase the availability of services to persons in need. Nevertheless, this perspective can "pathologize" caregiving, even though it is a normative event for many people (Brody 1985). Researchers should guard against this attitude.

Yet the emphasis on the impact of dementia in the family has had one beneficial result: researchers now recognize that impairments in noncognitive symptoms—such as function (e.g., dressing, bathing, eating) and behavior (e.g., aggression)—are closely linked to caregiving difficulties (Deimling and Bass 1986; Pruchno and Resch 1989). Because treatment can relieve or improve some of these behavioral and functional impairments (Hinrichsen and Niederehe 1994; see also Table 18–1), these difficulties provide a focus for active approaches in a disease that currently offers no primary prevention and minimal benefits from cognitive enhancement therapies.

Research on the impact of dementia on caregivers also has suggested that a variety of services can relieve the caregiver of some of the difficulties associated with care and benefit the patient by active stimulation (Collins et al. 1994). Resources such as family support groups, activity

Table 18–1. Published studies of caregiver intervention with appropriate control/comparison groups

| | Outcome studies: Caregiver treatment | | |
Study	Treatment	Outcomes	Magnitude
Kahan et al. (1985) (N = 40)	Education/support versus no treatment	Decreased burden Decreased depression Increased knowledge	P < .001
Farran (in press) (cited in Collins et al. 1994) (N = 139)	Education versus support versus no treatment	Education and support increased distress (adverse outcome)	P < .02
Lovett and Gallagher (1988) (N = 111)	Life satisfaction versus problem solving versus wait list	Decreased depression Improved morale	P < .01 P < .05
Chiverton and Caine (1989) (N = 40)	Education versus control	Increased competence Increased knowledge	P < .01 P < .001
Zarit et al. (1987) (N = 184)	Counseling versus support versus wait list	Decreased burden Counseling better than support	Not significant
Perkins and Poynton (1990) (N = 12)	Counseling versus wait list	Improved morale	P < .001

Sutcliffe and Larner (1988) ($N = 15$)	Information versus support versus no treatment	Emotion-focused: decreased Beck Score Information-focused: increased knowledge	$P < .05$
Mohide et al. (1990) ($N = 30$)	Education/support versus control	Increased quality of life Increased satisfaction Mood/anxiety unchanged	20% difference; not significant
Brodaty and Peters (1991) ($N = 96$)	Support group versus memory retraining techniques versus wait list	Decreased placement Decreased caregiver distress Memory training: increased caregiver distress	$P < .01$
Mittelman et al. (1993) ($N = 206$)	Group versus available treatment	Decreased nursing home placement	$P < .05$

centers, day care (Sands and Suzuki 1983), and brief overnight respite care have sprung up as options to nursing home care. Although some studies have found that such programs fail to prevent nursing home placement (Lawton et al. 1989), others suggest that day care may decrease emotional distress (Lokk 1990) and delay nursing home placement (Brodaty and Peters 1991).

Most notably, however, 7 of 10 studies with appropriate control/comparison groups found that family-member-focused support groups were beneficial (Table 18–1). One of these studies (Mittelman et al. 1993) showed that patients randomized to a family-member-focused support group entered nursing homes later than those receiving typical care. This development may be one of the better-documented areas of the effectiveness of mental health intervention. Stevens and Baldwin (1994) found that emotion-focused groups were more effective than education-focused groups; this intriguing finding bears replication.

Another area of caregiver intervention that deserves further study is whether such interventions should focus on all caregivers or only those at high risk. For example, a reanalysis (Whitlatch et al. 1991) of one of the aforementioned studies (Zarit et al. 1987)—in which intervention was not effective—demonstrated that such intervention was effective for the subset of distressed caregivers. The question of whether whole populations or high-risk groups only should be the target of prevention efforts has been a matter of significant contention (Rose 1992); the answer might be different for different populations, different situations, and different disorders.

A Proposed Model

The study of caregivers also has provided opportunities for investigators to study how individuals respond to specific chronic stressors and identify factors that modify these responses (Schulz and Williamson 1991; Vitaliano et al. 1991). Research on caregiving has demonstrated that the severity of dementia—at least as measured by degree of cognitive decline—is a minor correlate of caregiver outcome. However, caregiver *perception* of the situation is a significant correlate of outcome. That is, caregivers who identify a specific set of symptoms as problematic are more likely to have an adverse outcome than caregivers who rate the same symptoms as not problematic (Fopma-Loy and Austin 1993).

Likewise, the perceived adequacy of social supports appears to be more important than the size of the network (Haley et al. 1987b).

Intrinsic caregiver characteristics such as personality (Hooker et al. 1992; Rabins et al. 1990b) and coping style (Harvis and Rabins 1989; Stephens et al. 1988) also are strong correlates of outcome. Other variables that correlate with caregiver outcome include the availability of family resources, financial status (Moritz et al. 1989), ethnic background (Dilworth-Anderson and Anderson 1994), and prior relationship between patient and caregivers (Cantor 1983; Williamson and Schulz 1990). Wright et al. (1993) provide an excellent overview of many of these issues. Although research demonstrates that family support services can moderate caregiver morbidity (see Table 18–1), use of such services by persons residing in the community is determined more by caregiver characteristics than by availability.

The fact that lifelong personality characteristics, the severity of behavioral symptoms, and the availability of social, financial, and environmental supports independently predict emotional state in caregivers suggests a paradigm that researchers have called the *person/ provocation or predisposition/provocation* model (Kenrick and Funder 1988; Mischel 1979). As Figure 18–1 illustrates, this model postulates that intrapersonal resources such as personality and intellect predispose individuals to respond to a stressor or provocation in a predictable fashion. Variables that modify this response include interpersonal resources, financial resources, and family resources (Baillie et al. 1988). One implication of this model is that some individuals are at higher risk for adverse outcome given a specific stress (Shore et al. 1986). This effect suggests potential preventive interventions for high-risk individuals.

To date, however, investigators have generated few data with which to estimate the weight or degree of influence of individual factors in this model. Moreover, the nonrepresentative nature of most study populations dictates caution in generalizing their findings. Nevertheless, such research has important potential because health care workers do not know whether identifying high-risk individuals and focusing intervention efforts on their inclusion in treatment trials or general population-focused intervention would produce the highest cost/benefit ratio and have the greatest impact (Rose 1992).

Furthermore, some factors that the model identifies as "modifiers" might be predispositions. For example, perceived adequacy of the social network and perceived severity of the stressor have conceptual and measurement overlap with "coping style" and "personality" (i.e., characteristics that vary dimensionally among individuals).

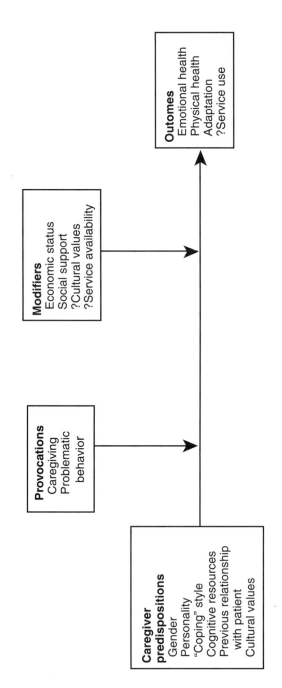

Figure 18–1.   Person/provocation model of stress response; variables associated with caregiving listed as predispositions, provocations, or modifiers.

One interesting issue that this model raises is whether caregiving for a person with Alzheimer's disease is a unique stressor. That is, does caregiving in the context of Alzheimer's disease differ from other difficult situations, and does the type of disease the ill person has affect caregiver outcome (Yeatman et al. 1993)? One difficulty in answering these questions has been the challenge of matching for severity of stressor. Although the findings are somewhat variable (Rabins et al. 1990a), several studies suggest that caring for a person with Alzheimer's disease may lead to poorer caregiver outcome than caring for a person after a stroke (Tompkins et al. 1988), caring for a person with cancer (Clipp and George 1993), or caring for a person with Parkinson's disease (Dura et al. 1990).

Conclusion

What have we learned over the past two decades about caregivers for persons with dementia? Several issues are clear:

- Most care is provided by family and friends.
- Institutional care is a necessity in some circumstances; it should be an integral part of the care system for Alzheimer's disease.
- Caring for persons with chronic illness brings with it both burdens and blessings. People respond to this stressor in a variety of ways, based on variations in the disease and the person who has it.
- The most humane care system recognizes the variability of the disease and the variability in caregiver resources. Providing a variety of services is most likely to meet the needs of most people.
- The reformulation of senility as a disease has opened many important avenues. It has not only provided the impetus for research into the pathogenesis and biological treatment of Alzheimer's disease but also empowered patients and family members to pursue treatment for what is currently treatable, seek whatever knowledge currently is available, and force health care professionals to consider the types of care such individuals need.
- The financial impact of dementia is clear. Nursing home costs are a significant proportion of this expense—and are likely to remain so.

References

Alzheimer A: Die arteriosklerotische Atrophie des Gehirns. Alig Zschr Psychiatr u psychisch-gerichtl Med 52:533–594, 1896

Alzheimer A: A characteristic disease of the cerebral cortex, in The Early Story of Alzheimer's Disease. Translated and edited by Bick K, Armaducci L, Pepeu G. New York, Raven, 1987, pp 1–3

Baillie V, Norbeck JS, Barnes LEA: Stress, social support, and psychological distress of family caregivers of the elderly. Nurs Res 37:217–222, 1988

Baumgarten M, Hanley JA, Infante-Rivard C, et al: Health of family members caring for elderly persons with dementia. Ann Intern Med 120:126–132, 1994

Brodaty H, Peters K: Cost effectiveness of a training program for dementia carers. Int Psychogeriatr 3:11–22, 1991

Brody EM: Parent care as a normative family stress. Gerontologist 25:19–29, 1985

Cantor MH: Strain among caregivers: a study of experience in the United States. Gerontologist 23:597–604, 1983

Chiverton P, Caine ED: Education to assist spouses in coping with Alzheimer's disease: a controlled trial. J Am Geriatr Soc 37:593–598, 1989

Clipp EC, George LK: Dementia and cancer: a comparison of spouse caregivers. Gerontologist 33:534–541, 1993

Cohen D, Eisdorfer C: Depression in family members caring for a relative with Alzheimer's disease. J Am Geriatr Soc 36:885–889, 1988

Colerick EJ, George LK: Predictors of institutionalization among caregivers of patients with Alzheimer's disease. J Am Geriatr Soc 34:493–498, 1986

Collins CE, Given BA, Given CW: Interventions with family caregivers of persons with Alzheimer's disease. Nurs Clin North Am 29:195–207, 1994

Deimling GT, Bass DM: Symptoms of mental impairment among elderly adults and their effects on family caregivers. J Gerontol 41:778–784, 1986

Dilworth-Anderson, Anderson NB: Dementia caregiving in blacks: a contextual approach to research, in Stress Effects on Family Caregivers of Alzheimer's Patients. Edited by Ught E, Niederehe G, Lebowitz BD. New York, Springer, 1994, pp 385–409

Dura JR, Haywood-Niler E, Kiecolt-Glaser JK: Spousal caregivers of persons with Alzheimer's and Parkinson's disease dementia: a preliminary comparison. Gerontologist 30:332–336, 1990

Eagles JM, Rawlinson ACF, Restall DB, et al: The psychological well-being of supporters of the demented elderly. Brit J Psychiatry 150:293–298, 1987

Fopma-Loy J, Austin JK: An attributional analysis of formal caregivers' perception of agitated behavior of a resident with Alzheimer's disease. Arch Psychiatr Nurs 7:217–225, 1993

George LK, Gwyther LP: Caregiver well-being: a multidimensional examination of family caregivers of demented adults. Gerontologist 26:253–259, 1986

Gerritsen JC, van der Ende PC: The development of a care-giving burden scale. Age Ageing 23:483–491, 1994

Gilhooly MLM: The impact of care-giving on care-givers: factors associated with the psychological well-being of people supporting a dementing relative in the community. Br J Med Psychol 57:35–44, 1984

Gilleard CJ, Belford H, Gilleard E, et al: Emotional distress amongst the supporters of the elderly mentally infirm. Br J Psychiatry 145:172–177, 1984

Grad J, Sainsbury P: Mental illness and the family. Lancet 9:544–547, 1963

Grad J, Sainsbury P: The effects that patients have on their families in a community care and a control psychiatric service—a two-year follow-up. Br J Psychiatry 114:265–278, 1968

Grafstrom N, Fratiglioni L, Sandman PO, et al: Health and social consequences for relatives of demented and non-demented elderly: a population-based study. J Clin Epidemiol 45:861–870, 1992

Grob G: Mental Illness and American Society, 1875–1940. Princeton, NJ, Princeton University Press, 1983

Haley WE, Levine EG, Brown SL: Stress, appraisal, coping, and social support as predictors of adaptational outcome among dementia caregivers. Psychol Aging 2:323–330, 1987a

Haley WE, Levine EG, Brown SL, et al: Psychological, social, and health consequences of caring for a relative with senile dementia. J Am Geriatr Soc 35: 405–411, 1987b

Harvis K, Rabins PV: Dementia: helping family caregivers cope. J Psychosoc Nurs Ment Health Serv 27:7–12, 1989

Hinrichsen GA, Niederehe G: Dementia management strategies and adjustment of family members of older patients. Gerontologist 34:95–102, 1994

Hooker K, Monahan D, Shrifren K, et al: Mental and physical health of spouse caregivers: the role of personality. Psychol Aging 7:367–375, 1992

Kahan J, Kemp B, Staples FR, et al: Decreasing the burden in families caring for a relative with a dementing illness: a controlled study. J Am Geriatr Soc 33:664–670, 1985

Kenrick ST, Funder DC: Profiting from controversy: lessons from the person-situation debate. Am Psychol 43:23–34, 1988

Kiecolt-Glaser KJ, Dura JR, Speicher CE, et al: Spousal caregivers of dementia victims: longitudinal changes in immunity and health. Psychosom Med 53: 345–362, 1990

Lawton MP, Brody EM, Saperstein AR: A controlled study of respite service for caregivers of Alzheimer's patients. Gerontologist 29:8–16, 1989

Lawton MP, Moss M, Kleban MH, et al: A two-factor model of caregiving, appraisal and psychological well-being. J Gerontol 46:P181–P189, 1991

Lezak MD: Living with the characterologically altered brain injured patient. J Clin Psychiatry 39:592–598, 1978

Lokk J: Emotional and social effects of a controlled intervention study in a day-care unit for elderly patients. Scand J Prim Health Care 8:165–172, 1990

Lovett S, Gallagher D: Psychoeducational interventions for family caregivers: preliminary efficacy data. Behavior Therapy 19:321–330, 1988

Mischel W: On the interface of cognition and personality: beyond the person-situation debate. Am Psychol 34:740–754, 1979

Mittelman M, Ferris S, Steinberg G, et al: An intervention that delays institutionalization of Alzheimer's disease patients: treatment of spouse-caregivers. Gerontologist 33:730–740, 1993

Mohide EA, Pringle DM, Streiner DL, et al: A randomized trial of family caregiver support in the home management of dementia. J Am Geriatr Soc 38:446–454, 1990

Moritz DJ, Kasl SV, Berkman LF: The health impact of living with a cognitively impaired elderly spouse: depressive symptoms and social functioning. G Gerontol 44:S17–S27, 1989

O'Connor DW, Pollit PA, Roth M, et al: Problems reported by relatives in a community study of dementia. Br J Psychiatry 156:835–841, 1990

Perkins RE, Poynton CF: Group counselling for relatives of hospitalized presenile dementia patients: a controlled study. Br J Clin Psychol 29:287–295, 1990

Pruchno RA, Resch NL: Aberrant behaviors and Alzheimer's disease: mental health effects on spouse caregivers. J Gerontol 44:177–182, 1989

Rabins PV, Mace NL, Lucas MJ: The impact of dementia on the family. JAMA 248:333–335, 1982

Rabins PV, Fitting MD, Eastham J, et al: Emotional adaptation over time in caregivers for the chronically ill elderly. Age Ageing 19:185–190, 1990a

Rabins PV, Fitting MD, Eastham J, et al: The emotional impact of caring for the chronically ill. Psychosomatics 31:331–336, 1990b

Rose GA: The Strategy of Preventive Medicine. New York, Oxford University Press, 1992

Rovner BW, Kafonek K, Filipp L, et al: Prevalence of mental illness in a community nursing home. Am J Psychiatry 143:1446–1449, 1986

Sands D, Suzuki T: Adult day care for Alzheimer's patients and their families. Gerontologist 23:21–23, 1983

Schulz R, Williamson GM: A 2-year longitudinal study of depression among Alzheimer's caregivers. Psychol Aging 6:569–578, 1991

Shore JH, Tatum EL, Vollmer WM: Psychiatric reactions to disaster: the Mount St. Helens experience. Am J Psychiatry 143:590–595, 1986

Stephens MAP, Norris VK, Kinney JM, et al: Stressful situations in caregiving: relations between caregiver coping and well-being. Psychol Aging 3:208–209, 1988

Stevens GL, Baldwin BA: Comparative efficacy of didactic versus psychotherapeutic modalities, in Stress Effects on Family Caregivers of Alzheimer's Patients. Edited by Light E, Niederehe G, Lebowitz B. New York, Springer, 1994

Sutcliffe C, Larner S: Counselling carers of the elderly at home: a preliminary study. Br J Clin Psychol 27:177–178, 1988

Tompkins CA, Schulz R, Rau MT: Post-stroke depression in primary support persons: predicting those at risk. Journal of Clinical and Consulting Psychology 50:2–8, 1988

Vitaliano PP, Russo J, Young HM, et al: Predictors of burden on spouse caregivers of individuals with Alzheimer's disease. Psychol Aging 6:392–402, 1991

Whitlatch CJ, Zarit SH, von Eye A: Efficacy of interventions with caregivers: a reanalysis. Gerontologist 31:9–14, 1991

Williamson GM, Schulz R: Relationship orientation, quality of prior relationship, and distress among caregivers of Alzheimer's patients. Psychol Aging 5:502–509, 1990

Wright LK, Clipp EC, George LK: Health consequences of caregiver stress. Med Exerc Nutr Health 2:181–195, 1993

Yeatman R, Bennetts K, Allen N, et al: Is caring for elderly relatives with depression as stressful as caring for those with dementia? A pilot study in Melbourne. International Journal of Geriatric Psychiatry 8:339–342, 1993

Zarit SH, Reever KE, Bach-Petersen J: Relatives of the impaired elderly: correlates of feelings of burden. Gerontologist 20:649–655, 1980

Zarit SH, Anthony CR, Boutselis M: Interventions with caregivers of dementia patients: comparison of two approaches. Psychol Aging 2:225–232, 1987

Index

Page numbers in **boldface** *type refer to figures and tables.*